COLONIZING MADNESS

COLONIZING MADNESS

Asylum and Community in Fiji

Jacqueline Leckie

University of Hawai'i Press
Honolulu

Printed in the United States of America

25 24 23 22 21 20   6 5 4 3 2 1

Library of Congress Cataloging-in-Publication Data

Names: Leckie, Jacqueline, author.
Title: Colonizing madness : asylum and community in Fiji / Jacqueline Leckie.
Description: Honolulu, Hawaii : University of Hawaiʻi Press, 2019. | Includes bibliographical references and index.
Identifiers: LCCN 2019021696 | ISBN 9780824878009 (cloth)
Subjects: LCSH: Mental illness—Social aspects—Fiji. | Mentally ill—Fiji—Suva. | Asylums—Fiji—Suva—History.
Classification: LCC RA790.7.F47 L43 2019 | DDC 362.196/890099611—dc23
LC record available at https://lccn.loc.gov/2019021696

ISBN 978-0-8248-8846-6 (pbk.)

University of Hawaiʻi Press books are printed on acid-free paper and meet the guidelines for permanence and durability of the Council on Library Resources.

MM	Methodist Mission Collection
MO	Medical officer
MP	Minute paper
MS	Medical superintendent
NAF	National Archives of Fiji
NC	Native commissioner
NMP	Native medical practitioner
PLA	Public Lunatic Asylum
PN	Patient number
PIMHnet	Pacific Islands Mental Health Network
PS	Permanent secretary
PSA	Psychiatric Survivors' Association
SG	St Giles Hospital, Suva, Fiji
STG	St Giles Hospital, files
SM	Stipendiary magistrate
SS	Secretary of State for the Colonies
WHO	World Health Organization

CHAPTER 1

Introducing the Colonization of Madness into Fiji

In 1884, Qaqa—a Fijian prisoner in Suva Gaol—attacked two European prisoners with a spade and fatally cleft the skull of John Murray.[1] Mr. Halkett, Fiji's superintendent of prisons, despaired that he could not manage prisoners like Qaqa, who "should be sent to an asylum as soon as it was built."[2] Two years earlier on the island of Ovalau, Qaqa had viciously assaulted newlywed Isabella Moore with an ax while she was sitting on her verandah at Waidu doing embroidery. When he attacked his fellow prisoners in 1884, Qaqa was found not guilty on grounds of insanity, a "victim of homicidal mania."[3] Qaqa had "acted like a maniac since his birth that the community to which he belongs have ever regarded him as a maniac."

> His wont is to challenge trees, the moon—the sea, or a mountain height—dancing round like a Sioux Indian and inviting Nature generally to "come on"—Hence his name "Qaqa"—The Brave, The Warrior.

Qaqa was admitted to Suva's Public Lunatic Asylum in 1884 and died there two years later, age thirty-five and emaciated with tuberculosis.[4]

More than a hundred years later, Apete Kaisau, another Fijian, was charged with the double murder of John Scott and his partner Gregory Scrivener.[5] The killer had forced his way into their home in Suva early on the morning of July 1, 2001, and almost decapitated the couple with a cane knife. The court found Kaisau not guilty by reason of insanity: "the accused killed both men whilst suffering from a mental illness called schizophrenia and that the killings were motivated by delusions that he was acting on the instructions of God."[6] On August 6, 2003, Kaisau was confined indefinitely to Fiji's only psychiatric facility—St Giles—the successor to the asylum in which Qaqa had been confined. Whereas Qaqa's maniacal violence had highlighted the inadequacy of prisons to control the mentally ill, Kaisau's admission to St Giles conversely evoked concern over whether it was an appropriate facility for incarcerating those who had committed forensic crimes. The horrific consequences of Qaqa's and Kaisau's insanity

highlight, in entirely different contexts, contentious debates over the protection of the community, the treatment and rights of the mentally ill, and the role of the asylum. Or, as Judge Salesi Temo stated in 2015, when Kaisau appealed to be permanently discharged from the hospital into the community, "law, fairness of the accused person and the protection of society" must be considered.[7] To the outside observer, it appeared that Kaisau had been sentenced to an institution little different in purpose or physical structure from the colonial asylum. Health professionals, however, could point out the substantial shifts in patient outcomes made during the colonial era. Mortality rates had fallen dramatically. Furthermore, the use of psychotropic medication enabled patients to participate in a greater range of activities than a hundred years earlier; by 2014, Kaisau's lawyers could thus argue for his discharge.

Temo's statement about mental illness and the community links back to the asylum's opening on August 26, 1884, only ten years after Fiji became a British colony.[8] His words raise questions about the meaning and impact of madness and mental disorder among Fiji's many ethnic communities.[9] How did the entanglement of community and the asylum delineate illness and normality, and how did this change within Fiji's colonial history? Initially it might appear that this dynamic was determined by Western biomedicine and British colonialism and resulted in racially defined madness. The following chapters, however, reveal how cultural, religious, gendered, economic, and political nuances within Fiji's communities also shaped the colonization of madness. I do not deny that colonization entailed the brutal imposition of power over indigenous peoples and induced the dislocation of migrants. But communities had their own boundaries of tolerable behavior and what constituted wellness within daily life. The colonization of madness brought new institutions, legislation, and medicine that filtered into communities and also more subtly inculcated concepts of civilization, modernity, and sanity, akin to

> power in the passive voice, the gradual Western saturation of medical knowledge and justice, the aesthetics of dress and the sociality of food, the conception of thinking and the representation of the body. Thus the everyday, the routines, the "givens" of everyday life.[10]

Colonizing madness was not simply about state hegemony or controlling minds through asylum building or lunacy legislation. It also reflected tensions and prejudices within homes, villages, workplaces, and churches, and—sadly for insane destitutes—also when those communities failed. Mental despair could also be an outcome of the destruction and displacement wrought by migration and

colonialism. Rather than place the incursion of colonial madness management against the extremes of either a humane civilizing mission or hegemonic social control, this book explores the way the practices and discourse of modern biomedicine and mental health were articulated in local communities as well as in the asylum.

Unlike Qaqa and Kaisau, most asylum patients never killed or attacked anyone. They were considered dangerous, however, to their families, their communities, or themselves. That threat might remain hidden in the screams and silences of the mad, but in some instances it exploded into unpredictable physical violence against people and property. Fear of the insane was also directed at a few prominent Fijians who were considered potentially dissident.

Those who were committed to Fiji's new asylum were representative of the colony's emergent ethnic complexity, the first patients being indigenous Fijians, Rotumans, Indians, Europeans, Polynesians, Kailoma (people of mixed ethnic ancestry), and other immigrants.[11] The behavior of the first six patients in 1884, like that of all patients, was deemed beyond reason. The first, Bhagal, could not sleep, singing for hours and bursting into idiotic laughter.[12] Janki talked all night about his imagined great riches, including sugar plantations.[13] Sukudaia, alternating between sullenness and mania, was obsessed with sexual matters.[14] An-

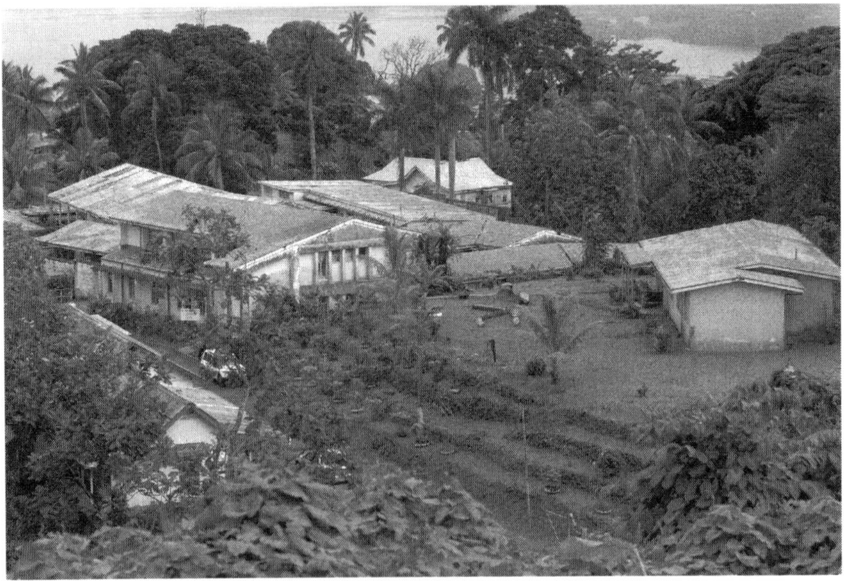

Figure 1.1. View of part of St Giles Hospital, 2014. Source: *Fiji Times*, February 6, 2014.

other woman, admitted with puerperal insanity, had tried to drown herself and attack her husband. Another was an extremely emaciated fifteen-year-old Polynesian who would not speak or move but had "a fixed stare in his countenance" and at other times continually masturbated and "had long fits of crying."[15] These descriptions seem typical of psychiatric patients worldwide. Most psychiatrists today accept common organic and biochemical foundations as well as the pivotal role of the community as explaining madness, although anthropologists and historians emphasize social, cultural, and environmental factors.[16] Historian Jonathan Sadowsky rejects binary extremes of madness as either universal or relative, suggesting instead that "madness appears to be a feature of all known human societies, but one that nevertheless has distinctive features in each."[17] So too was the profound suffering that glimpses of patient voice or others' observations revealed.

This book focuses on mental difference in colonial Fiji at its most extreme: among people legally certified as lunatics or as of unsound mind. That story is told here primarily through the remaining records of former patients at St Giles to explore the nebulous condition and label of madness and states of mental difference. These records were the result of opinions and observations made by family, friends, indigenous leaders, police, employers, magistrates, and medical personnel, and sometimes patient experience. The records are dominated by European voices because Europeans filled out the lunacy certificates, although indigenous voices and testimony were often included. It is not my intention to diagnose patients retrospectively to ascertain their madness or sanity. Instead, I am concerned with reading the lunacy archive to address how madness was constructed and managed and how it affected individuals and communities in colonial Fiji.

The asylum archive also offers a rich and new source about the historical and cultural complexities of a colonial society in the Pacific. That Qaqa was considered mad did not quash other social tensions from being raised to explain his violence. A medical officer suggested that Qaqa probably "would not have attacked Moore 'had she not been alone.'" That Moore lived on land dispossessed from a "leading" Fijian woman of Bureta was cited as another factor.[18] The *Fiji Times* rejected these rumors and asserted that Qaqa's madness was the reason for the attack.[19] Likewise, context and rumor are significant in understanding Kaisau's brutal slaying of Scott and Scrivener during a period of intense political upheaval, religious fundamentalism, and Fijian nationalism. Scott was from a prominent European family in Fiji, and as director general of the Fiji Red Cross was pivotal in visiting and in the release of parliamentary hostages during a coup in 2000; many people assumed that Scott had

been assassinated because he had knowledge that would incriminate the rebels.[20] Just as Moore had been blamed for Qaqa's attack, Scott and Scrivener were blamed for Kaisau's actions. Some people asserted that the victims' homosexuality, flamboyant and alleged depraved lifestyle triggered Kaisau's violence.[21]

Qaqa's voice is absent from the archive, as are those of so many sufferers of mental illness. The asylum records are fragmentary, often scribbled in shorthand by colonial officials and the doctors who sanctioned the confinement of these patients. Their caregivers—variously termed warders, attendants, orderlies, or mental health assistants—were also usually not part of the historical narrative. Histories of madness have tended to dismiss subject voices and the content of delusions and expression of these as raving.[22] Throughout this book, patients' delusions are disentangled to shed light on the communities in which patients lived. The patient's voice could mirror past and present external realities and be a way, however imperfect, of coping with that world. Delusions of grandeur could be, as Megan Vaughan has suggested, a way for colonized and oppressed peoples to invert the social order or to fling "back at the conquerors their own images of superiority in disturbingly distorted forms."[23] Fantastic delusions might also be symptoms of organic and neurological illness (for a discussion of general paralysis of the insane, see chapter 5).

Displaced Minds: Institutional Solutions

The colonization of madness in Fiji was forged by the entanglement of colonial institutions and cultures and cast within a wider world of colonial psychiatry, Western biomedicine, and asylum building. This book extends the emergent literature on the social history of medicine in the tropical Pacific,[24] in which little attention is paid to mental health with the exception of Michael Goddard's ethnography of madness and critique of psychiatry in Papua New Guinea and my own previous work.[25] Although I emphasize the timing, environment, multiethnic complexity, and Oceanic cultures within which colonial psychiatry became embedded in Fiji, the literature on madness, asylums, and psychiatry in nonsettler colonies outside Oceania informed this study.[26] My research also builds on substantial historiography from Australia and New Zealand that shows how colonial psychiatry and the construction of the insane patient diverged from metropolitan patterns.[27] Pioneering work by Barbara Brookes, Catharine Coleborne, Stephen Garton, and Bronwyn Labrum went past institutional and legalistic histories to explore gender, class, and race as markers of colonial difference in asylums.[28] Historians found that, in contrast to the colonial record for Fiji, in

New Zealand Māori patients were marginalized within European categories, and indigenous voices were virtually absent from asylums in Australia.[29] Two significant books in 2015 took the study of colonial asylums and madness in Australia and New Zealand into the wider context of migration and transnationalism.[30] Coleborne focused on the discourse of gender, class, and ethnicity in nineteenth-century asylums in Victoria (Australia) and Auckland (New Zealand) to shed light on colonial "identity making" (especially whiteness). McCarthy's exploration of ethnicity and madness in New Zealand uniquely traced the impact of the voyage out on immigrant mental health between 1860 to 1910. This work diverged from Coleborne's tracing how the colonial binary of whiteness and Other was constructed and replicated in the asylum. McCarthy instead disentangled the category European to investigate ethnicity and nationality among these patients.

Fiji's asylum was one of the first in the Pacific Islands outside New Zealand and Australia when many other parts of the Pacific Islands were still being colonized and where medical and legal infrastructure had barely emerged. Fiji was a key plantation-based colony in the southwest Pacific with a rapidly increasing migrant population. The asylum in Fiji was preceded by the Oahu Insane Asylum in Hawaiʻi, established in 1866, and was condemned by Dr. George Tucker: "It would not be humane to herd wild beasts in such a place."[31] It closed in 1930 when patients were relocated to a new hospital in Kaneohe. Since 1868, some mentally ill people in the French colony of New Caledonia were treated at l'hôpital du Marais, but a psychiatric hospital did not open until 1936—the Nouville Asylum, today known as the Centre Hospitalier Spécialisé Albert Bousquet.[32] Asylums were intermittently set up in the British colonies of the Gilbert and Ellice Islands (Kiribati and Tuvalu) and Solomon Islands during the first half of the twentieth century.[33]

When Fiji's was founded in the 1880s, asylums were well established in British settler colonies, but provision of care varied across its other colonies. Following revelations from 1858 to 1861 of appalling conditions and abuses in the Kingston Lunatic Asylum in Jamaica, the Colonial Office surveyed the state of hospitals and asylums across the British empire.[34] The ensuing report pushed the Colonial Office to become more centrist in the regulation and governance of asylums.[35] Locally, the origins of the Fiji asylum were embedded in the development of policing, prisons, and public health; legal and social control became linked to the management of the insane. As in other colonies, the imperative was to separate "insane" and "normal" prisoners.[36] Similar concerns were raised over hospital patients when mentally disturbed patients could not be accommodated separately.

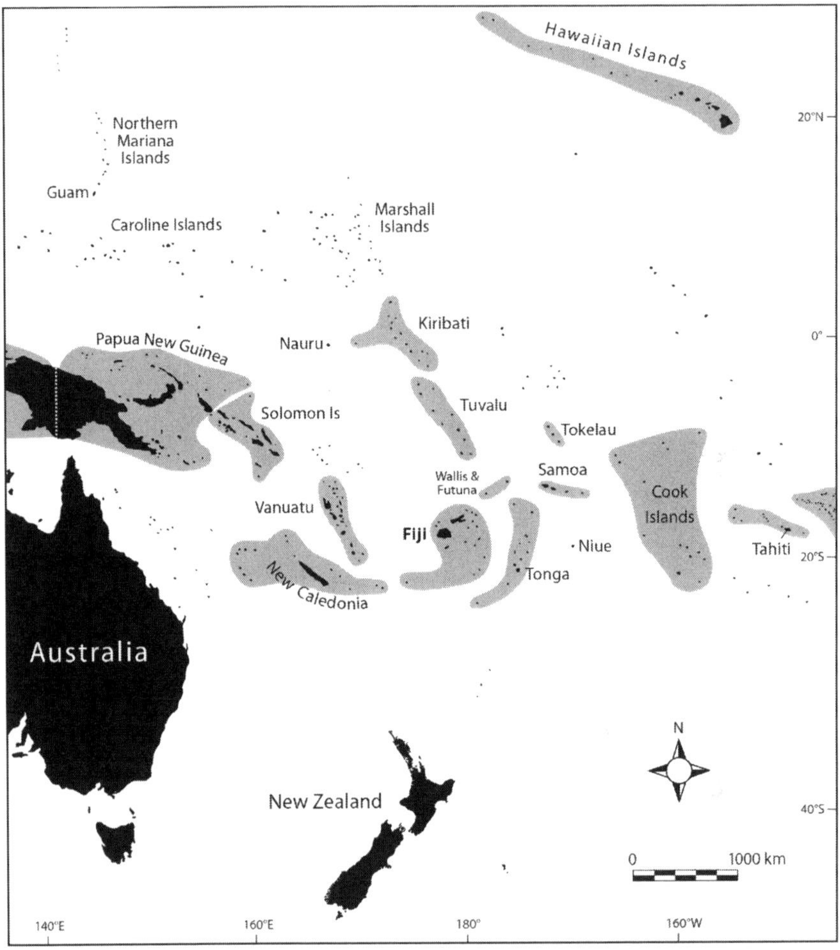

Map 1. South Pacific. Source: Les O'Neill.

In 1881, William Seed, the police superintendent, alerted Governor George William Des Voeux that lunatics in Fiji required special accommodation rather than confinement inside prisons.[37] Des Voeux passed this recommendation on to the Colonial Office.[38] Before lunacy legislation was introduced in Fiji, mentally disturbed people could only be confined if convicted as criminally insane. They came under prison jurisdiction, where medical authorities determined whether they could be released.[39]

Qaqa tested the limitations of care for mad and violent prisoners. Prison and medical authorities were divided over how to manage the extremes of his violent,

manic, and calm periods. At first, in Levuka Gaol, he was mechanically restrained because he knocked his head against the cell's walls. In Suva Gaol, he was quiet and allowed to work in the prison gang, but by January 1, 1883, "a change seemed to come over him and he became very troublesome." He was "attacked with another fit of insanity" and assaulted Sergeant Riley, after which he was confined to a solitary stone cell for two months but released for daily exercise, during which his hands were cuffed behind his back. Prison Superintendent Halkett denied that this was punishment, asserting that it was necessary to isolate Qaqa and "prevent annoyance to the other prisoners." Halkett despaired that he was "not conversant with the management of lunatics" and could not rely on the native warders to supervise Qaqa.[40] He also frequently informed the visiting surgeon that the jail was an unsuitable place to confine Qaqa. Halkett's frustration over controlling insane prisoners made establishment of an asylum urgent.

Part of the rationale for an asylum was that it could be a place of observation to determine whether a criminal was really insane. Qaqa's changeable mental state and behavior created such uncertainties that in 1883 it was recommended that he "be detained in the Asylum for observation if found eventually to be an

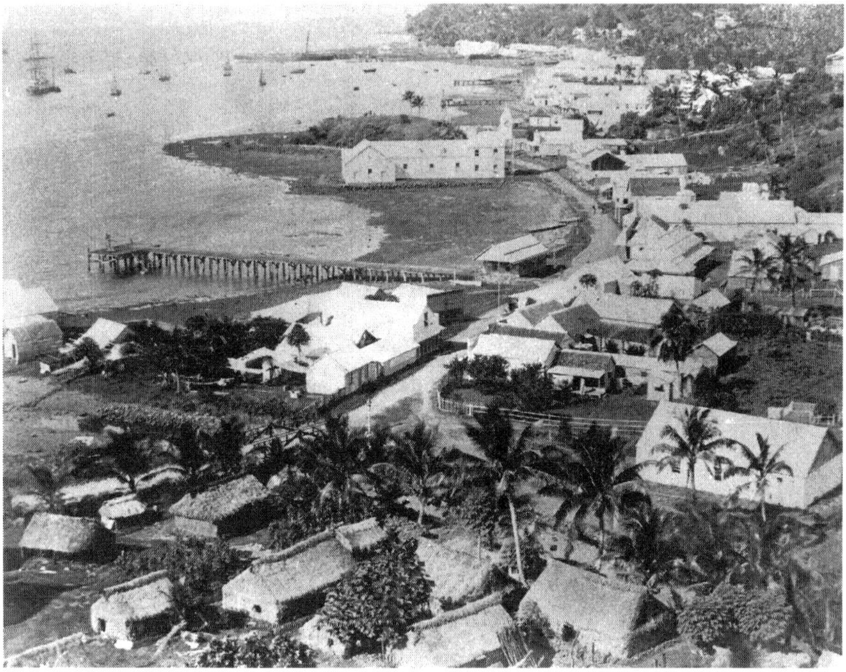

Figure 1.2. Levuka, 1880s. Source: M5561, NAF.

imposter let him be dealt with accordingly; if mad he will be soon be found out under continuous observation" (emphasis in the original).[41] But before the asylum was functioning, Qaqa killed the prisoner Murray. The state's ability to control mad prisoners evoked public outcry: "A very painful feeling has been stirred against the authorities for allowing a so well-known furious brute to go among other prisoners and to have access to iron implements."[42]

Prison and medical authorities also advocated for an asylum in Fiji because it would enable more humane management of insane prisoners. In 1884, Dr. David Blyth warned that the excessive use of mechanical devices was counterproductive to the treatment and cure of mentally ill prisoners. Blyth had great faith in the curative possibilities of moral management but believed this could only be possible if the insane were separated from other criminals.[43] Moral management stressed self-discipline and orderly routine rather than mechanical restraints. Blyth's study of Wilson, a prisoner in Levuka Gaol, vindicated this approach:

> the use of handcuffs is entirely uncalled for, and that their adoption would be highly injudicious. Restraint of this kind would greatly irritate the man, and arouse his temper, which, in the absence of restraint and unnecessary interference would not become violent, or uncontrollable. . . . in Wilson's care, the use of handcuffs would be productive of incalculable mischief, and impel him to actions which otherwise he would not commit. . . . The same remarks apply to Leg-irons as to handcuffs; they are unnecessary, and therefore could only be productive of evil results . . . To attempt to cure insanity in a common gaol, instead of in an Institution set apart for the reception of lunatics, would be futile, but at the same time I have all along endeavoured to carry out rational treatment in Wilson's case to the best of my ability, always recognizing the fact that a line of treatment adapted to one case of insanity may be wholly unfitted to another. Solitary confinement, handcuffs, strait-jacket etc may be occasionally necessary in treating maniacs, but in Wilson's case their adoption would be a mistake in my opinion. To restrain him, and surround him with Warders, to restrict his time out of doors to two hours daily, and to load him with chains, would certainly be the most likely means of developing in the man periodical outbursts of mania. . . . Let him be <u>strictly watched</u>; have all dangerous weapons out of his reach by night and by day. . . . .do not shut him up in his cell by day on any account; and do not adopt mechanical restraint in the shape of leg-irons etc. [emphasis in the original][44]

Blyth's suggestion of moral management and moral therapy for Wilson was not possible in Fiji's early prison system. Halkett's budget had no leeway to employ extra European staff to provide "incessant vigilance" over insane prisoners. Native staff were cheaper, but Halkett considered them "wholly unreliable in dealing with lunatics."

Uncontrollable, mentally disturbed patients also presented a problem in the operation of Fiji's early hospitals. By 1881, Des Voeux and again in 1883 John Bates Thurston advocated a separate ward for mentally ill patients distant from other hospital patients.[45] Thurston informed the Legislative Council that hospital attendants had "been greatly embarrassed by the violent behaviour of lunatics, and the excitement and disturbance caused to patients."[46]

Another pressure on early health services in Fiji was the introduction of indentured labor, or *girmitiyas,* from India beginning in 1879.[47] Colonial authorities in Fiji were responsible for confining and repatriating these "unfortunates" to India. By 1883, Des Voeux urged that an asylum be erected in Fiji because "the arrival lately of several lunatics among the Coolie Immigrants brought matters to a crisis."[48]

Sukudaia was one of these immigrants. Her sad fate as a twenty-six-year-old vagrant featured in the October 29 edition of the *Suva Times* in 1881:

> There is an insane Indian woman who wanders about, choosing the most populous parts of the town, in a state of sometimes more than semi-nudity. She has long been an eyesore to residents, and to our personal knowledge is a difficult subject to restrain. Usually her child accompanies her and the whole conduct of the two is most repulsive to anyone with the most remote sense of decency.

Sukudaia was variously depicted as "one poor, helpless, homeless creature . . . amongst us whom no one chooses to care for" and "a disgrace to our civilization."[49] The acting agent general of immigration ordered that Sukudaia and her daughter, Ramsomjh, be returned to India because Fiji had no lunatic asylum.[50] A temporary solution was offered, in which the state paid an Indian couple in rations to care for Sukudaia and her child.[51] Sukudaia would be the asylum's first female patient—a story we will return to later.

Colonial officials were also reluctant to support insane Europeans. Before the asylum opened, a prison doctor recommended that European lunatics be "kept in one of the neighbouring colonies possessing a temperate climate. The lunatic would benefit and probably the pecuniary cost to us would be less."[52] One such case was James Allen, who sailed to Fiji in 1883 from Dunedin, New Zealand. He apparently had been promised work in Fiji, but, after unsuccessfully searching

Abbreviations

AG	Attorney general
AMO	Assistant medical officer
AMP	Assistant medical practitioner
AR	Annual report
BB	*Blue Book of Fiji*
BOV	Board of Visitors
CB	Casebook
CMO	Chief medical officer
CO	Colonial Office
CP	Council Paper of the Fiji Legislative Council
CPN	Community psychiatric nursing
CS	Colonial Secretary
CSO	Colonial Secretary's Office Series, Suva
CW	Chief warder
CWM	Colonial War Memorial Hospital
DC	District commissioner
DMS	Director, medical services
DMO	District medical officer
DO	District officer
DSM	Diagnostic and Statistical Manual of Mental Disorders
ECT	Electroconvulsive therapy
GMH	Global Mental Health
GPI	General paralysis of the insane
ICD	International Classification of Diseases, Injuries, and Causes of Death
ICT	Insulin coma therapy
LC	Legislative Council

My second research space in Suva has long been the National Archives of Fiji. I cannot express how grateful I am for the superb assistance of staff there, going back to my dear friend the late Margaret Patel. I continue to be amazed at the fantastic service provided by archives under Director Opeta Alefaio. My thanks also to the staff at the Pacific Collection, University of the South Pacific, Fiji School of Medicine Library, University of Otago Library, Hocken Library, Public Records Office and Wellcome Library in London, and the *Fiji Times* (especially Reapi Mateinaniu). My research has also been provoked through feedback and advice—too many people to name—but I thank especially Sue Heydon, Odille Chang, Cathy Coleborne, Waltraud Ernst, Judy Bennett, Angela McCarthy, Brij Lal, Vicki Luker, and Yoram Mouchenik. Feedback from anonymous reviewers of my manuscript has hopefully made this a better book. Morgan Tuimaleali'ifano, Clive Moore, Alan Howard, Ranjana Narayan, Robert Macgregor, Jan Tent, and Dr. M. P. Deva have generously supplied photographs and information. Superb research assistance was provided by Sue Heydon, Karin Reid, Bonnie Scarth, Willow McKay, Louise Pearman-Beres, Tui Clery, Marsa Dodson, Kristin Clift, and Stephanie Dobson. Lisa Marr offered superb editing and indexing, Les O'Neill designed the maps, and Graham Boyle patiently compiled and presented much of the quantitative data.

The writing of this book has been an exercise in persistence, particularly when I was faced with a traumatic disruption to my working life. The research for this project did not start this way. I received research grants from the University of Otago, including a Prestigious Writing Grant. I also thank the Wellcome Trust for a Travel Grant. The completion of the book, though, would not have been possible without the warm support of colleagues, friends, and family, and in particular without the love, understanding, and wonderful conversations of Graham and Tara. I am most grateful for editor Masako Ikeda, who has steadfastly supported me in the completion of this publication, and the fantastic production team from University of Hawai‘i Press, including Helen Glenn Court, Debra Tang, and Grace Wen. Above all, I would like to thank my great colleagues at the Stout Research Centre for New Zealand Studies at Victoria University of Wellington for providing a most congenial writing environment during 2018, enabling me to complete this book.

Acknowledgments

Almost everyone is touched by the pain, unpredictability, boredom, frustration, and craziness of mental illness—whether themselves, a loved one, a colleague, or a stranger. I was acutely aware as a child of the profound suffering mental illness could bring to a family, but it was as an anthropology student that I began to take an intellectual interest in the cultural meaning of madness. Professor Peter Wilson's humanity and insights, and his book *Oscar: An Inquiry into the Nature of Sanity?* unearthed for me a fascination with understanding how different cultures perceived madness, and how social transgressions, marginality, and stigma could open a rich but disturbing window to understanding cultures, past and present. Much later in life through research with health workers in Fiji and *talanoa* with Matron Jane Erasito and Dr. Issac Karim, I learned that a lunatic asylum had been established early in Fiji's colonial history. I was enthusiastically welcomed by former medical superintendent Dr. Jude Ohaeri to pursue research at St Giles Psychiatric Hospital. This support was generously endorsed by later superintendents, especially Dr. Shish Narayan, Dr. Peni Biukoto, and Dr. Odille Chang. My research would not have been possible without the assistance and hospitality of the administrative and nursing staff at St Giles, who provided me and my research assistant Sue Heydon with working space, access to records, and cups of tea, answering endless questions and provoking much laughter. Although I did not interact directly with patients, my presence induced curiosity and I sincerely thank them for kindly sharing their space. My biggest thanks go to the patients and families I will never meet but whom I had the privilege to encounter through the archive. I hope that I have been respectful in how I have treated peoples' recorded pasts and written about their shattered lives. I argue that the silenced lives of people once deemed mad should be part of Pacific history and not hidden away in fear of shame. Equally, it is important to be mindful of different cultural understandings of insanity and illness. But these concepts have changed over time and in today's world the removal of stigma may help counteract the growing burden of mental illness within many Pacific societies.

CONTENTS

for his employer in the Rewa district, was remanded in Suva Gaol for vagrancy and lunacy. The acting superintendent of police warned that if Allen stayed in Fiji he was likely to remain in jail and probably die there. This case could create a precedent that "neighbouring colonies may take advantage of to rid themselves at the expense of this colony of inconvenient and troublesome burdens."[53]

Although Fiji had limited financial resources during the 1880s,[54] economic considerations justified the need for a separate space to manage insane prisoners and insane hospital patients. Meager funds were allocated to build an asylum—a portent of how the asylum would be underresourced and remain low among priorities for health provision in Fiji. The acquiescence of local legislature and the Colonial Office in approving the building during a period of financial stringency was probably due to concerns about prison management, immigration, and public health. In 1882, Dr. William MacGregor and the commissioner of works discussed the erection of a new public hospital, including an asylum, in the colony's capital, Suva. A draft was submitted to the Colonial Office in 1883.[55] The asylum started as an annex to Suva Hospital but was relocated to its present site above the Suva Gaol and the former Polynesian Depot for indentured laborers by April 15, 1885.[56]

MacGregor was the driving force behind establishing Fiji's colonial medical services. As well as being chief medical officer (CMO) between 1875 and 1888, he was treasurer and after 1883 became colonial secretary. He was appalled at the inadequate medical personnel and facilities in the colony; from 1883 he recruited medical students from his homeland, Scotland, and founded the Fiji Native Medical School in 1885 to train native medical practitioners (NMPs).[57] MacGregor had previous experience in treating the insane as a surgeon at the Royal Lunatic Asylum in Aberdeen and as superintendent of the lunatic asylum in Mauritius, where *girmitiyas* would have been numerous.[58] Like many colonial administrators, MacGregor traversed colonial networks from Aberdeen to the Seychelles, Mauritius, Fiji, British New Guinea, Lagos, Newfoundland, and Queensland before retiring to Scotland. Professional networks and personnel were essential to the circulation of ideologies between disparate colonial centers and to the establishment of colonial health systems and colonial psychiatry. New colonial relationships formed through these fragile "webs of empire" but were still defined by the metropolis, the center of the web.[59]

Lunacy Legislation

Legislation was a key web of empire. Lunacy legislation in Fiji came early in the history of the Pacific Islands with the Public Lunatic Asylum Ordinance of 1884.[60] This ordinance, which included only a few amendments, enshrined the legal definition and treatment of mental illness in Fiji until mental health legislation was overhauled in the twenty-first century. A public lunatic asylum could not be legally established until legislation was enacted to "care for the maintenance of lunatics and idiots." The ordinance equated admission to the asylum with the legal definition of mental illness: a lunatic being "every person of unsound mind and every person being an idiot." Two committal schedules were required, issued either by a doctor and a stipendiary magistrate, or by two registered medical practitioners with a relative's authority. A magistrate could order police to bring a lunatic "at large"—that is, not under proper care or control—or being cruelly treated or neglected for examination by the magistrate and a doctor. If the latter were unavailable, then a certificate could be issued for temporary detention in the asylum for one week. This blueprint appears to have offered safeguards against wrongful certification and detention but the reality of Fiji's administrative and physical environment could mean lengthy delays in communication and the inability to follow legal processes (for more, see chapter 3). Fiji is spread over three hundred islands, from the capital Suva, to Rotuma, 646 kilometers to the north, and Ono-i-lau, 409 kilometers to the southeast. The necessary European medical personnel were few and NMPs had no authority to commit a patient to the asylum.

Fiji's governor could order a prisoner deemed a lunatic to be examined by the medical superintendent and committed indefinitely to the asylum. Involuntary confinement was the normal channel into the asylum, though a provision allowed for voluntary admission if two doctors certified the person. Michael, a trader from the Ellice Islands, was one of the few patients who pursued this option when in 1895 he sought admission to the asylum with delirium tremens from alcohol withdrawal. Michael told a minister in Suva that Roman Catholic priests had coerced him into marrying a woman against his will. This was his third marriage. His worries included unemployment in Suva, but he was also afraid that he would kill his children.[61]

Voluntary admission was not then a feature of English, Australian, or New Zealand legislation. It was part of Scottish legislation, and the insertion of this provision in Fiji's legislation possibly reflects MacGregor's influence.[62] The Scottish practice of "boarding out" patients to care outside the asylum was also not adopted in Fiji. Otherwise, Fiji's lunacy legislation followed general developments in Britain after the 1845 Lunatics Act, and similar legislation in the nearby settler colonies of New Zealand and Australia, and in other British colonies.[63] Lunacy laws in Fiji were introduced during a period of contradictory agendas regarding the constraint, isolation, and moral management of the mentally ill. Andrew Scull's assessment of management as repressive—incorporating "structural tensions

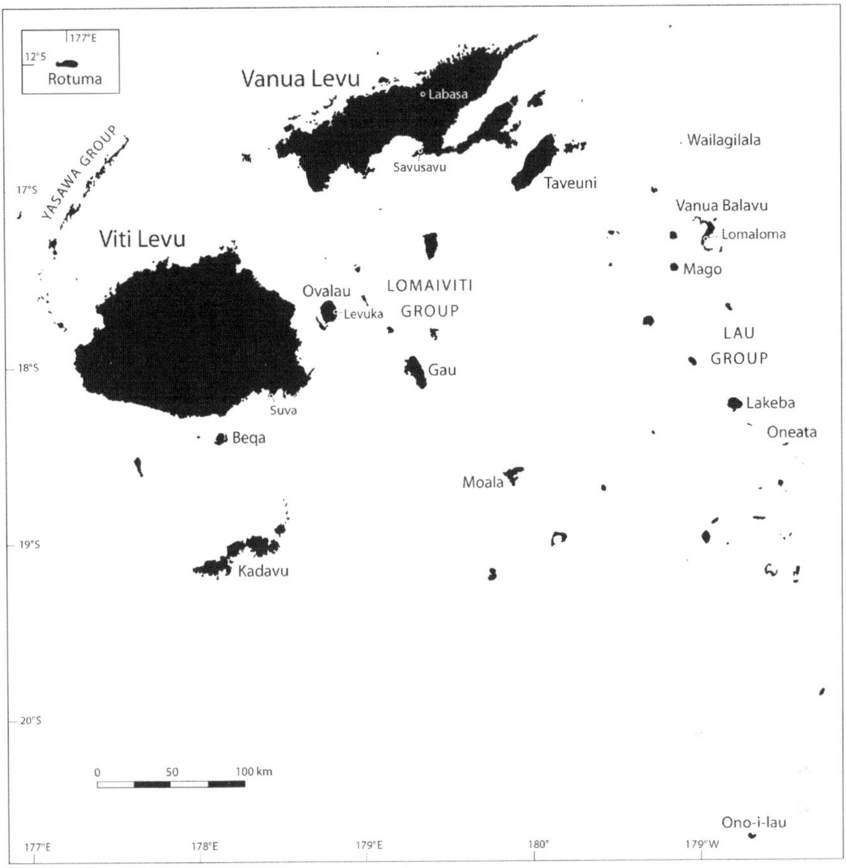

Map 2. Fiji Islands. Source: Les O'Neill.

between repression and rehabilitation, between the imposition of moral discipline and the development of self-government and self-control"—was well suited to colonial settings.[64]

Similarities in lunacy legislation and asylum management between Fiji and other British colonies extended to the accumulation of quantitative information concerning insane subjects. A community of the insane was developed by amassing information about minds and bodies and their institutionalization and relegation into legal categories. In colonial Africa, Vaughan argues, medical classification systems and practices were intrinsic to the operation of colonial power. Sally Swartz stresses the discursive nature of colonial regulations: "it aligned humane care with order, discipline, and statistical tables, and cleanliness with civilized standards."[65] Colonial knowledge gathering projects and discursive power, through definitions, such as normal and abnormal and racial classifications, inscribed rule over indigenous bodies and minds.[66] This equally applied to Fiji, where the paper trail tracing the insane began with certification papers, in which an individual became a case, "an object like a branch of knowledge and a hold for a branch of power."[67] Case notes can also be read to uncover the production of lunatic patient identity, which also "exhibited practices and forms of knowledge about colonial populations" as Coleborne has done for Australian and New Zealand colonial asylums.[68] This book adopts that methodology.

Doctors assigned patients to modern Western categories of mental illness (see chapter 5) that were neither objective nor static. Case notes included lay and medical observations relating to the evidence and causes of insanity. Some notes were copious, especially those of Europeans and prominent Fijians, but documentation concerning destitutes was often minimal.[69] The medical superintendent was the asylum's overseeing "eye," though his gaze was distant. Regulations stipulated that he should visit daily, but visits were probably less frequent; by 1928, he was required to visit three days per week or more often as needed.[70] Sketchy details of patients' behavior and moods were entered in the medical casebook.[71] The medical superintendent submitted an annual report on the asylum to Fiji's Legislative Council. The Board of Visitors—appointed by the Legislative Council and colonial secretary, and comprising the attorney general, CMO, and three gubernatorial appointees—was required to visit the hospital at least every three months but could make unannounced visits at other times. The board reported on patients, staffing, management, and conditions. Statistical documentation presented a semblance of pervasive efficiency, order, and legitimacy to the management of madness in Fiji. Yet missing and contradictory data between sources meant that official data did not always present an accurate picture of the patient population or how the hospital functioned; any depth about the social context could be piecemeal. Veronika Lipphardt and Alexandra Widmer remind us that colonial medical categories were "often ugly placeholders and poor witnesses of an extremely rich and troubled history of relationships between human beings."[72]

Colonial lunacy legislation was derived from metropolitan precedents, but legislature in other colonies was important. An 1858 parliamentary act for the Indian states set the standard for many British colonies.[73] Britain's Colonial Office may have issued guidelines for asylum building and management, but local practices circulated through informal and institutional networks between colonies.[74] Lunacy law in Fiji was also mediated by the colony's exigencies, such as the reliance on indentured labor. Employers were responsible for the costs of *girmitiyas* and indentured immigrants from the Pacific Islands committed to the asylum during their contract; however, after an amendment in 1885, the costs of maintaining lunatic indentured laborers were shared among the employer, the colony, and the Lunatic Immigrants' Fund.[75] Indigenous Fijians and Rotumans remained the responsibility of the Native Administration, a separate entity combining colonial and customary authority. The province from which a patient originated was legally responsible and covered expenses of care, including confinement in the asylum.

Lunacy legislation and asylum building in Fiji were also distinct from those in many other colonies because separate asylums for Europeans and natives were not established, as they were in India, for example.[76] Nevertheless, racial segregation was present in many institutions in Fiji, including formal employment, schools, social clubs, and residential areas. During the early twentieth century, racial, gender, and class boundaries were reproduced in the asylum's structure: separate wards for European men, European women, native men, and native women. Native meant all non-Europeans, including Indo-Fijians, indigenous Fijians, and others, such as Chinese. European embraced Europeans of diverse nationalities, including the Fiji born.[77] Part-Europeans were usually accommodated with Europeans, although family connections or class could determine their allocation to the European or native wards. The racialization of madness discourse and the implications of this raises the vexatious questions of social control and the construction of the colonial subject.

Power, Social Control, and Colonial Madness

Michel Foucault set the groundwork to link the social construction of madness, asylum building, and the history of psychiatry in the modern European state with power and social control.[78] Frantz Fanon was equally pivotal in critiquing colonial psychiatry and its role in the construction of the colonial subject in Northern Africa.[79] Control was real—asylums confined bodies and psychiatry tried to silence the mind—and control was discursive, internalized by subjects to constitute a hegemonic framing of madness and normality in the modern, civilized, and colonized subject.

Historians have debated whether medicine was an "agent of empire"[80] and psychiatry an "extension of social policing."[81] Vaughan clearly regards colonial medicine as part of the constitution of "the African" as an object of knowledge and a colonial subject. Mad colonial subjects were problematic to colonial control because they were insufficiently Other: they were feared because they broke "barriers of difference and silence."[82] This challenge posed by some indigenous leaders labeled as mad is explored in chapter 3. Was the institutionalization of madness in Fiji an extension of colonial oppression, as several historians and anthropologists argue in studies of asylums and colonial psychiatry? For example, Lynette Jackson sees the Ingutsheni Lunatic Asylum, established in Southern Rhodesia in 1908, as "a microcosm of an oppressive social order" because the colonizer had the power to control space, assign place, and define normality and abnormality.[83] Michael Goddard considers the introduction of psychiatry into Papua New Guinea after World War II as complicit in the institutionalization of colonial social control.[84] James Mills questions whether the patients in the Indian colonial asylums he studied were actually mentally ill or instead had been incarcerated for political and social reasons—medical and state authorities or family and community members using the asylum to negotiate behavior deemed deviant or threatening to them.[85] Richard Keller and Leonard Smith also see the asylum in colonial French North Africa and in the Caribbean, respectively, as providing new spaces for mentally disturbed people "whom family and communities could no longer care for, tolerate, or control."[86] In colonial Nigeria, Sadowsky takes a slightly less instrumental approach—as I will show—to stress community-defined madness: "in many cases these people were understood as mad by their kin and neighbours and not only by a colonial state."[87]

The link between the asylum and the community is a theme throughout this book, pointing to a more nuanced approach than simply dismissing the asylum and lunacy legislation as monolithic state control. Mark Finnane introduces this insight into the madness historiography with his study of the insane in nineteenth-century Ireland and New South Wales. Families and communities were complicit in using the insanity law and were active in the admission process to the asylum to "address very localised social problems caused by the disruptive and the dependent."[88] David Wright challenges the pervasive power that medical superintendents had in nineteenth-century England and Wales over confinement and emphasizes the role of families to care for and control dependent and violent relatives.[89] This pattern of care was common within Pacific cultures. New Zealand and Australian scholars have extensively explored casebooks to uncover the role of the family and other colonial institutions in the admission and discharge process to the asylum.[90]

Like Waltraud Ernst, I reject "any single homogenizing influence or of an all-pervasive, focused, colonial or psychiatric gaze" in the colonial context, or simplistic binaries of colonial hegemony and resistance.[91] Ernst argues that in India institutions like lunatic asylums were also symbolic, "a marker of colonial rule . . . aimed at impressing indigenous subject peoples and at justifying the imposition of colonial rule by virtue of the alleged good which institutions *per se*

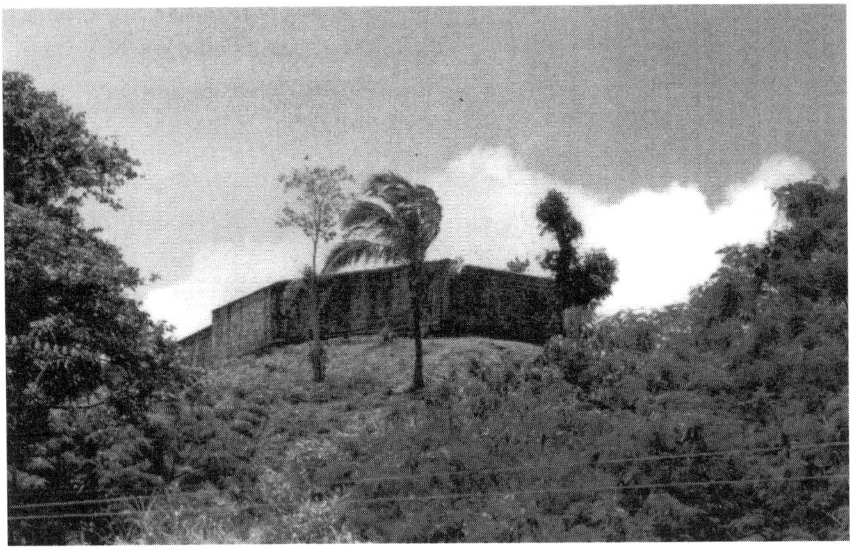

Figure 1.3. High wall near St Giles Psychiatric Hospital, 1965. Source: National Archives of Fiji, Neg. G7247.

were seen to endow."[92] In Fiji, St Giles was never considered a grand colonial institution and was represented uneasily as a prison rather than a hospital. It still signified the exercise of colonial power over bodies and minds, a site where bodies and minds were incarcerated. Locals referred to it as "*vale ni mate*" (place of death) or the "tin shack." It was mostly starved of funds,[93] a predicament also found in many African colonies.[94] This neglect and marginalization reiterate how an emphasis on hegemonic colonial power may overlook the messiness of many colonial projects and the minor place of professional psychiatry within wider colonial agendas.[95]

Reevaluations of Foucault and Fanon within colonial studies have moved beyond a hegemonic construction of the colonial subject to interrogate the contested nature of colonialism, the ambiguities in power relationships between the colonial masters and the ruled, and the agency of the colonized. One alternative perspective is to consider the messy entanglements of colonialism in the framing of colonial madness.[96] Edward LiPuma's concept of encompassment contextualizes colonial power, modernization, and the colonial subject and connects exogenous and indigenous structures and concepts of mental abnormality.

In Fiji, the colonial state imposed extensive laws regulating intimate details of subjects' lives and minds.[97] The institutional symbol of this—the asylum—appears to have represented an extreme in colonial social control, but only a small proportion of Fiji's mentally disturbed were incarcerated in St Giles. As several studies of psychiatry in African and Caribbean colonies reveal, asylum building did not constitute what Foucault argued was a "great confinement" within modern Europe.[98] Although kin normally took responsibility for mentally ill family members, communities began to negotiate their limits of care and control after the asylum was established. To a limited extent, this change reflected the normalization of the asylum and the hospital as a destination for the insane, as Joseph Melling and Bill Forsythe find in Devon, England, by the late nineteenth century: "The integration of the idea of the asylum as the necessary destination of the mad and the wayward had been absorbed by the public mind and into the memory of those who required treatment."[99] Similar evidence in the Fiji archives reveals shifts in the boundaries of acceptable behavior, introduced medical concepts of mental abnormality becoming entwined with local cultures. The outcomes of encompassment—the colonization of madness—were entangled with and shaped by local communities.[100]

The Community Within

The asylum was more than a repository of madness: it was also an institutionalized site where the "insane" and the "normal" met. This could be a brief encounter, such as between a visiting psychiatrist and a patient, or, more commonly, a relationship enduring several decades between warders and patients. To some extent, the patients and staff who lived in Fiji's asylum mirrored the outside world, but insanity created a unique community by throwing together groups usually segregated spatially and socially. Until 1906, all patients lived in one ward but had separate rooms. Among the twelve patients in 1896 were two European males and one European female.[101] Europeans accounted for around 18.6 percent of total admissions during the asylum's first decade and thereafter the proportion declined (table 1.1), though it was still higher than the proportion in Fiji's wider population.[102] Some European families could afford private nursing and custodial care or to send their mentally ill members abroad. In 1896, three Fijian females and one Indian were also admitted, as were native males from outside Fiji, including a New Hebridean, a Polynesian, and a Tongan. Most native patients that year were indigenous Fijians, but in subsequent years a growing number were *girmitiyas*. This increase replicated the rising proportion of Indians within Fiji's population. The ethnic patterns of Fijians and Indo-Fijians in the asylum soon became disproportionate to the wider population. In 1921, Fijians made up 53.7 percent and Indo-Fijians 38.6 percent of Fiji's total population.[103] In the asylum between 1919 and 1923, however, Indo-Fijians made up approximately 66 percent of first admissions, Fijians around 21 percent. Chapter 2 examines the role of destitution in this alarmingly high statistic among Indo-Fijians during the transition from plantation labor to the consolidation of family farm social and economic networks.

The asylum community comprised patients and staff, who had to be onsite for nursing and other essential services, such as cooking, cleaning, laundry, and security. From the beginning, the primary care and custody of patients at St Giles were entrusted to warders, also called attendants, and by the 1970s some were designated as mental health assistants and nurses. Warders had a huge responsibility: they not only constrained violent patients such as Qaqa but also assessed, managed, and cared for (with very limited resources) patients from diverse cultures who had wide-ranging mental and neurological disorders. Warders had little contact with doctors or the medical superintendent, who, along with a European female nurse from the Colonial Hospital, visited the asylum every few days. Warders were responsible for the care and control of a growing number of admissions and inpatients, from forty-five at the end of 1915 to 235 by the end of 1960.[104] Many of these patients were admitted as malnourished and destitute, having physical injuries or other signs of bodily neglect, such as scabies, lice, fleas, or tropical ulcers. Several patients had serious illnesses, such as tuberculosis, anemia, or tertiary stage syphilis, or contracted life-threatening sickness, especially influenza, in the asylum. A number of female patients suffered from severe mental conditions exacerbated by childbirth or from physical and mental abuse.

A permanent medical officer, Dr. Isaac Karim, was not appointed at St Giles until 1962. Two years later, Dr. Duncan Macgregor became the hospital's first psychiatrist and full-time medical superintendent.[105] A psychiatric nurse was appointed only in 1970. Although regulations governed the asylum's operation—for example, regulations were in place concerning restraints, bedding, clothing, diet, work, and visitors—in practice, these things were negotiated between patients and warders. Warders, as much as their charges, forged a community within the asylum. Until the 1960s, Samoan staff were pivotal to the asylum's functioning and identity.[106] It is not clear why Samoans were the preferred carers. The official reason was "the special aptitude of the people of those islands for the duties of attending to people of unsound mind."[107] Samoans were positioned to work across the two main "races" of Fijians and Indians; Europeans cared for their own kind. Ethnic and kinship networks were important in hiring Samoan employees. The St Giles community of warders and their families became more ethnically diverse as Fijians were hired and developed into a Kailoma community, with intermarriage between Samoans, Fijians, and others.

For several decades, the warders shared the substandard conditions of the patients, including poor sanitation. In 1927, forty-six patients were in the male native ward and thirty-one were in the female native ward; each ward had only one bath and two bucket-closets.[108] The same year, approximately forty-five native attendants and their families lived in the asylum's compound, sharing only one bucket-closet and one bath. Following the death of a patient from dysentery, Dr. Philip Harper, the acting CMO, complained to the colonial secretary about the inadequate sanitation for both attendants and patients, "with a consequent high mortality from dysentery, the Samoan attendants have been grossly overcrowded with a consequent high morbidity and mortality from lung diseases."[109] Dr. Montague, the CMO, refuted these claims.

The Chapters

This book goes beyond statistics and official reports to examine individual suffering and survival under the label of madness to uncover the interplay between community and asylum in understanding madness in colonial Fiji. It explores features within the colonization of madness in Fiji that were unique to the localized historical and cultural context but also locates these patterns against the global and colonial history of madness and psychiatry. The main source has been surviving patient records from the colonial era—primarily admission certificates—held at St Giles. The 3,866 certificates of varying physical quality offered qualitative detail and a unique insight into Fiji's medical and social history.[110] I read papers that had not been opened since they were filed well over a century ago, after a patient's death in the asylum or discharge into the community. I compiled a database from these certificates along with supplemental data from the Mental Hospital Register and the asylum returns in the *Blue Book of Fiji*. Several tables were generated from the qualitative data. These tables indicate general patterns only and do not represent precise statistical validity because of gaps in the data on the admission certificates and the register and discrepancies in data between different sources.[111] Data could be ambiguous, given that linguistic and conceptual meanings differed in the past and between cultures. For example, during the indenture period, many Indians were not legally married or their spouses may have been in India, so the meaning attached to the marital status recorded on the certificates could be ambiguous. Age was a notoriously vague category because births were not always registered for indigenous Fijians. Often information about destitute patients was scant, or, if provided, was often surmised.

Chapter 2 traces how mental disorder impinged on Fiji's communities of Indian descent, of whom the majority were 60,965 *girmitiyas* (indentured laborers). Displacement and destitution is a theme in this chapter so it is not surprising that the largest number and proportion of patients throughout most of the asylum's colonial history were Indo-Fijians (see table 1.1 and figure 1.4).[112] Stigma, frustration, and neglect toward those with mental illness did not evaporate when indenture ended. This chapter traces how such attitudes and suffering reflected economic and social pressures within the community.

Indigenous Fijians and Rotumans were the second largest group of patients at St Giles.[113] Chapter 3 considers indigenous understandings of madness and healing and their entanglement with colonial institutions and biomedicine. It discusses prominent Fijian religious and political leaders—Nacolauli Draviundrai, Sailosi Nagusolevu, Pita Turaganivalu, Ratu Penioni Ravoka, and Emosi Saurara—to determine whether colonial authorities used the asylum to incarcerate and suppress dissident Fijians. It interrogates colonial hegemony and the construction of madness to examine indigenous responses to Western medical institutions and community acceptance of the extreme space of an asylum. As British notions of orderly society and modern concepts of mental abnormality became entwined with local constructions, boundaries of acceptable behavior shifted.

Table 1.1. Total admissions by ethnicity per decade

			Ethnicity		
Decade	Fijian	Indian	European	Others	Total
1884–1893	27	28	16	15	86
1894–1903	49	36	19	14	118
1904–1913	66	64	23	20	173
1914–1923	90	221	20	20	351
1924–1933	77	162	22	20	281
1934–1943	108	188	14	39	349
1944–1953	121	237	35	49	442
1954–1963	293	680	27	105	1105

Source: Author's database from patients' admission papers, St Giles Hospital, *Blue Book of Fiji*, Mental Hospital Register. Patient data incomplete.

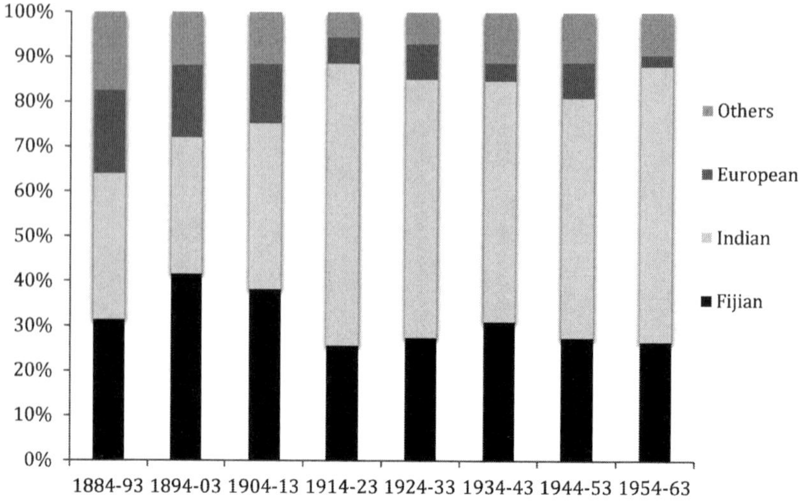

Figure 1.4. Percentage of admissions to St Giles by ethnicity, 1884–1963. Patient data incomplete. Source: Author's database from St Giles patient admission papers, *Blue Book of Fiji*, Mental Hospital Register.

The common articulation of indigenous, immigrant, and colonial constructions of normality and madness is possibly most evident through gender. Because men's voices and experiences dominate in many of the other chapters, chapter 4 focuses on women with mental illness.

Chapters 2, 3, and 4 investigate mental illness from the perspective of particular communities in colonial Fiji during the colonial era. Chapters 5 and 6 shift more to the asylum. Chapter 5 examines the discourse of madness through reported symptoms, causes (etiology), and shifting diagnoses and classification (nosology). The colonization of madness unfolded from the entanglement of the local with Western biomedical frameworks, but analysis of the local context reveals some strikingly different patterns to those found in asylums elsewhere, especially with general paralysis of the insane. Chapter 6 focuses on the struggles within the asylum community. The contestation over confinement, daily routines and controversial treatments, and the broader arena of biomedicine is revealed through traces of patient and staff voices.

Race and ethnicity thread throughout this book. I was reluctant to write ethnically exclusive chapters because such an approach can overlook how common conditions such as health, illness, stigma, suffering, and care can cut through racial divides. Indo-Fijians and Fijians made up the overwhelming majority of patients, but more detailed archival material was available for the far smaller number of Europeans. The voices of European doctors and others with colonial power dominate the archive but I did not want to foreground European patient narratives. Although no chapter discusses only Europeans and madness in Fiji, such stories feature in chapters 4, 5, and 6. Narratives of patients from other regions, such as China or Japan and the Pacific Islands, do as well. Among the latter group were indentured "Polynesians," most of whom originated from outside Polynesia, from Solomon Islands, New Hebrides (Vanuatu), Tokelau, New Guinea, and Gilbert and Ellice Islands.[114] Although the archive resonates with the discourse of race, I consciously use the term "ethnicity" rather than "race" to prioritize self-identified ethnicity over fixed, innate, and discriminatory concepts of race. The Fiji state nevertheless allocated ethnic identity to rigid subject positions. As in most aspects of life in colonial Fiji, race and gender were the primary criteria for classifying asylum patients, even if, as chapters 4 and 6 outline, the practice of racial separation within the asylum was occasionally fluid. Class also operated, such as in divisions between paying and nonpaying patients.

The final chapter concludes with efforts to decolonize the ways of the old asylum—parallel to Britain's colonial withdrawal from Fiji in 1970. How did the promise of the modern management of madness align with postcolonial development in Fiji? The community was expected to play a more active role in mental health care but the community could also fail in this. Chapter 7 asks whether new initiatives to reform mental illness and mental health suggest a recolonization of madness. The entanglement between the asylum and the community in managing madness in early colonial Fiji continues to be replayed in postcolonial Fiji. Disorders, diagnoses, and drugs may change but suffering and living with madness continues.

In 1936, the asylum was renamed the Suva Mental Hospital because of the stigma associated with the old name, which was considered "too redolent of Bedlam."[115] During the early 1960s, the name St Giles Psychiatric Hospital was adopted. Although it is widely known as "St Giles," the term "asylum" is still used.[116] St Giles has confined and cared for Fijians of all ethnicities, classes, and gender, many of whom were considered too bizarre or violent to be confined in jail, too disorderly to remain in their villages, too incapable to sustain paid employment, or too beyond the extremes of normal behavior. But what is "normal" within a colonial society of many cultures, where Western conceptions of civilization were entangled with Fiji's indigenous and immigrant communities?[117] The "mad" were incomprehensible souls, irrational not only to colonial authorities but also within their own cultures. The asylum was a microcosm of Fiji's wider colonial, indigenous, and immigrant communities. We therefore turn now to the colonization of madness among the *girmitiyas*.

CHAPTER 2

Displaced Minds

Indo-Fijians and Mental Distress

When, in 1884, Dr. William MacGregor referred to Fiji "as a great sufferer from the arrival here of insane persons," he was pointing to Fiji as a hub within the colonial Pacific.[1] Fiji was a nexus for indentured migrants, the majority being *girmitiyas* from India, though some were from other Pacific Islands. This chapter focuses on Indian immigrants and their descendants in colonial Fiji because more of them were patients in the asylum than members of other ethnic categories were during the colonial era.[2] The same year that he gloomily described Fiji as a destination for mad migrants, MacGregor was part of a rescue operation when the Indian immigrant ship *Syria* was wrecked on Nasilai reef. Fifty-six *girmitiyas* and three lascars drowned. In 1884, he recalled "people falling, fainting, drowning all around one, the cries for instant help, uttered in an unknown tongue, but emphasized by looks of agony."[3] His words equally evoke how he may have encountered those with mental illness in his medical career. MacGregor's intervention with the *Syria* parallels his efforts to rescue "wrecked minds," given that during the same year he was pivotal in introducing lunacy legislation into Fiji and opening the Public Lunatic Asylum in Suva.

Immigrants were displaced in Fiji, not only by physical dislocation from migration but also by profound shifts in their cultural worlds. The impact and length of this displacement varied, and, for a minority of immigrants, migration exacerbated or caused behavior that contemporaries interpreted as evidence of insanity. Freed from indenture, a small number of former indentured laborers became destitute. Their inclusion in admissions to the asylum during the early twentieth century speaks to the connections between disease and mental illness as well as to the profound social and economic dislocation wrought by indenture. Some migrants already worn down by their physical and social dislocation were also tormented by their mental condition and sought release. The most extreme consequence was suicide, but institutional confinement or repatriation could also be a form of death.

Despite the dislocation of migration and the social upheaval of the indenture system, Indian communities began to be reconstituted in Fiji. The family was pivotal in the care of mentally ill members, but kinship, economic, cultural, and gendered tensions could exacerbate mental stress, resulting, in extreme situations, in suicide. Traditional methods were applied to treat mental illness, but when families reached a "breaking point" they might seek external intervention, such as from the police and doctors.[4] Such interventions were increasingly adopted from the 1950s in Fiji as biomedicine became more established.

Girmitiyas and Madness

The arrival of the *Leonidas* off Levuka on May 14, 1879, signified more than the first indentured laborers coming to Fiji from India.[5] It also marked a defining trajectory in Fiji's development that would bring around 60,965 Indian laborers, recruited mainly for the sugar industry, which became the foundation of Fiji's modern economy. Two of the immigrants on the *Leonidas* were declared to be of unsound mind on arrival and so were not indentured. They were women: Ozeeari, a Muslim age twenty-eight; and Sukudaia, age twenty-four, a Hindu Bania originally from Dhollpur village in Sultanpur zillah.[6] Ozeeari had a daughter in India; Sukudaia's five-year-old daughter, Ramsomjh, accompanied her on the ship.[7] Ozeeari died just a year later, on June 2, 1880.[8] By October 1881, Sukudaia and her child were destitutes in Suva.[9] The *Suva Times* reported that she "daily squats herself with her child in the front verandah of the principal hotel hoping no doubt to excite pity and exact Baksheesh."[10] She gave "vent to her lamentation in songs of the most heartrending strains. Strains which not only affect herself to tears but which cannot but affect others."[11] Sukudaia was issued with partial rations from Suva Hospital and provided with a hut to live in, but this accommodation was destroyed in a gale in December 1881.[12] On February 18, 1882, Dr. Corney informed the agent general of immigration that, although Sukudaia suffered from mania, it was impossible to ascertain whether she would ever be sane enough to take up indenture over the following seven years. Sukudaia thus became the first woman to be committed to Fiji's newly established Public Lunatic Asylum. Her story resumes in chapter 4.

In 1916, the last indentured laborers arrived in Fiji. On January 1, 1920, all remaining indentures were canceled. Contracts had been for five years, but most *girmitiyas* reindentured for another five because they were not entitled to a free return passage until they had lived in Fiji for ten years unless they were declared rejects or incapables.[13] However, during the early twentieth century, many former *girmitiya* patients could not be repatriated; some were admitted to the asylum as destitute. Physical destitution or poverty exacerbated mental illness, but mental illness also precipitated the destitution of some migrants. The mentally fragile were less able to secure employment and accommodation after their contracts finished.

Sami was twelve years old when he left his father in India to be indentured in Fiji. Nine years later, in 1919, he tried to drown himself in the Navua River, refused to eat, speak, or move, and then was committed to the asylum as insane, diagnosed with severe melancholia—he "lays down as though dead . . . intensely miserable." He died there in 1940 with neither property nor known relatives.[14] Sami's case reflects how by 1920 an increasing number of Indian immigrants spent longer periods in the asylum because they could not be repatriated to India and did not have family to support them in Fiji. Sami was young when he left India, so it is unlikely that he would have been identified as suffering from severe melancholia. Was this melancholia subsequently induced by his experience as a *girmitiya*?[15] At what stage during migration and resettlement did mental illness become evident? Although the recruitment process involved various checks, including medical inspections, there were clearly loopholes through which mentally ill *girmitiyas* were recruited.

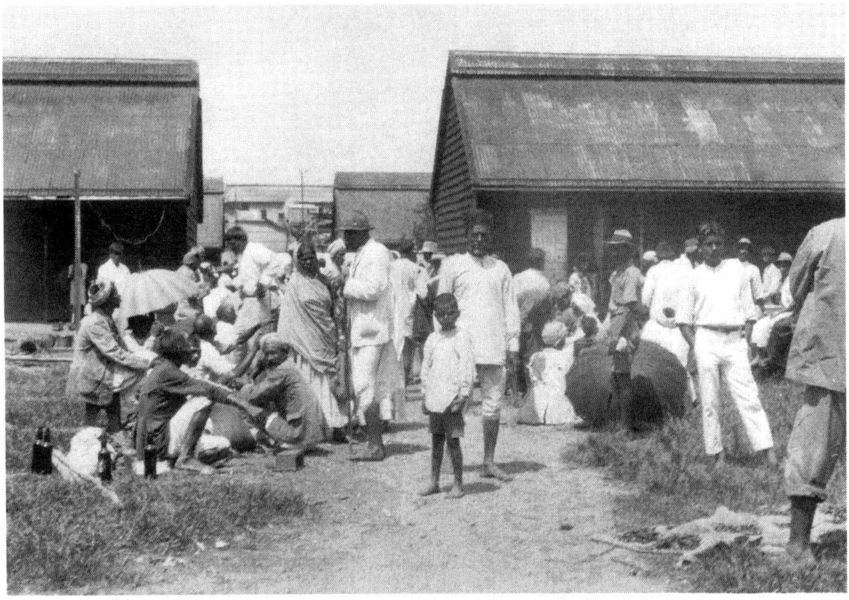

Figure 2.1. Labor lines, Fiji. Source: Photographer, Reverend John Burton, Methodist Church of Australasia Overseas Mission, used with permission by the Uniting Church in Australia—National Assembly. Ref: PXA 1137—Photo 809, no 49 PIC.CC.7061 MOM 236, State Library of New South Wales, Australia.

Displaced Minds and Recruitment

Although Indo-Fijians were the largest ethnic group of patients admitted to St Giles during the colonial era, briefly from around 1889 to 1904, Fijians made up a higher percentage of admissions (see figure 1.4). Thereafter, the number of Indo-Fijian admissions increased until Indo-Fijians outnumbered patients of other ethnic backgrounds. After about 1914, admissions of Europeans and Others (neither Fijians nor Indians) each fell from around 12 to 5 percent of total admissions, despite slight subsequent fluctuations. Before 1920, almost all Indo-Fijian patients in the asylum were *girmitiyas*. Some were mentally ill before they were recruited to Fiji; others deteriorated during the voyage; or illness was induced by the severe conditions on Fiji's plantations, which included the harsh realities of labor. Long working days and physically demanding work was compounded by extremely low pay; employers increasingly squeezed as much labor as possible from workers within a set time frame and paid at "task rates" rather than "time rates." Living conditions on the "labor lines" were cramped, and an authoritarian and violent culture pervaded the plantation.[16]

Historians Kenneth Gillion and Brij Lal documented the filtering process through which prospective laborers were accepted or rejected for indenture to Fiji.[17] Recruiters might find a mentally insecure person easy prey, but recruits underwent medical inspection at ports in Calcutta and Madras. When Fiji became a destination for indentured labor, the process of medical inspection was, on paper, more regulated than that for earlier destinations, such as in the Caribbean. Emigration passes had to be completed at the port of embarkation, and needed to include certification from the surgeon superintendent, the depot surgeon, the protector of emigrants, and the colonial emigration agent at the port that the emigrant "is free from all bodily and mental diseases."[18]

Despite these checks, mentally and physically impaired workers were recruited. This reality speaks to the rapacious demand for plantation labor, though it was in the interests of the surgeon superintendents to reject those who presented with obvious illness, because the surgeon superintendents were paid a gratuity for each *girmitiya* who disembarked alive. However, mental illness is not necessarily overt, so laborers with previous episodes of insanity could have passed through the recruitment process. Thakur, for example, was certified as free of mental disease when he was accepted as a *girmitiya* for Fiji. At the Calcutta depot, he probably would have presented as an ideal laborer because he had completed six years' indenture in Mauritius. He had also worked as an opium collector. In Fiji, his history of mental illness emerged after he tried to kill his wife and children and attempted to assault others. He spent six days in jail, but five days later another attack, which lasted fourteen days, precipitated his confinement in the lunatic asylum. Thakur's admission papers record several attacks during a period of sixteen years, including frequent hospital admissions while he lived in Mauritius. It is unlikely that this history was raised when he was examined in Calcutta. This example shows the episodic and changing nature of mental illness and how a person could lead a productive life despite suffering from it. Thakur was forty years old when he was admitted to Fiji's asylum. Two weeks later, he was repatriated to India along with his wife and a child.[19]

It is conceivable that emigration officials, including surgeon superintendents, were oblivious to existing mental distress because of cultural and language differences. Gajadhar's peers said that he had "manifested signs of mental alienation in India" before indenture in Fiji in 1885. Two years later, Koronivia estate's manager signed Gajadhar's papers when Gajadhar was admitted to the asylum with mania. But Gajadhar claimed that he was the estate manager, as well as the inspector of immigration, and a great Brahmin who desired to be worshipped but could not allow anyone near him because he was "too pure and too sacred" to have "woman contact."[20] His delusions reflected his emigration experience and his cultural background.

Into the *Kala Pani*

The phrase *kala pani* (black waters) encapsulates cultural and religious taboos (as well as the uncertainty of the journey) for some South Asian migrants venturing abroad. Colonial officials recognized the trauma and despondency that could set in on a long voyage of eleven to eighteen weeks that also entailed, for many, severing numerous kin and community ties. Surgeon Superintendent James Laing advised,

> I *know* that many people die from Nostalgia . . . can it be wondered at with all their caste prejudices, their leaving their native land, perhaps never to see it again, and being thrown among people strange in habits, language and even colour? The excitement of the newness of everything keeps them up for a time, but soon dies away, and is followed by depression when they realise what they have done; and to prevent this I would urge their being employed as much as possible while on board, and encouraged in every available means of entertainment.[21]

Despite efforts to keep *girmitiyas* occupied during the voyage, serious mental distress was evident. Some *girmitiyas* tragically attempted or committed suicide or harmed others. Less clear is the despair they suffered during the long voyage to Fiji. Hubraji jumped from the *Avon* in 1899. She also defecated in and destroyed her clothing, was violent toward other passengers, and sang, cried, or laughed. When examined in Suva, she refused to answer questions and was briefly committed to the asylum before being returned to Calcutta.[22]

Jahaji bhai or *jahaji bhen* (men and women together on a ship) might have considered a *girmitiya*'s behavior bizarre, but this opinion did not necessarily convince medical authorities in Fiji that an immigrant was insane. Rajani was so disruptive that the ship's surgeon had to confine her in handcuffs many times during her voyage to Fiji in 1892, and her shipmates called her a *pugali* (probably *pagaali,* or mad woman). The asylum's medical superintendent did not accept this as evidence of insanity, but saw it instead as "violence of character, or rather deportment . . . disorderly and not insane." He considered reports of her shipboard behavior as "riotous conduct . . . but . . . insufficiently weighty proof of insanity to turn the scale."[23] Rajani was still discharged from her indenture and repatriated to India along with another patient, Lalmokur. Other migrants were severely disturbed on the ship, but this problem ceased after disembarkation, and they worked for many years before being certified as insane. One *girmitiya* had an attack aboard the *Iman* in 1885 but lived in Fiji for twenty-three years before being admitted to the asylum from Suva prison.[24]

Disembarkation and Physical and Mental Displacement

Indentured migrants were again medically examined after disembarking, usually on Nukulau Quarantine Station. Madness induced on the voyage might have become evident in this examination, such as when Lalmokur "acted foolishly," absconded from the Immigration Depot, and was then briefly committed to the asylum.[25] Migrants who were rejected for work had to be repatriated, but it might be several months before a passage that included adequate supervision could be guaranteed on a ship to India. Delays created problems over where insane immigrants could be securely detained while awaiting repatriation. Prisons were not deemed humane, but mentally disturbed migrants might be too disruptive to be confined in a hospital or at the Immigration Depot. As outlined, this dilemma had been a reason for establishing a lunatic asylum in Suva, and the asylum could be a place of observation to ascertain whether a migrant was genuinely insane.

Once the asylum opened, a rejected *girmitiya* who was certified as insane could be admitted as a private patient. In 1900, the agent general of immigration signed admission papers for a *girmitiya* who had been highly disruptive in hospital, "vociferous and raving," smearing his body with boiled rice, exposing his genitals in public, and experiencing hallucinations. After two months in the asylum, he was repatriated to Calcutta along with his wife and family.[26] A female *girmitiya* classified as a "reject immigrant" had suffered a "continuing attack since arrival in colony" in 1913. She had been noisy and quarrelsome or morose and hurting herself during three months as a patient at the Colonial Hospital before admission to the asylum. She too was repatriated to India.[27]

Narak and Mental Breakdown

For Indian immigrants, the biggest environmental factor in mental breakdown was the physical and mental stress they endured as indentured laborers. The *girmitiyas* in Fiji referred to the exploitative and miserable experience of plantation work as *narak* (hell). Although the majority of *girmitiyas* developed coping strategies, high suicide rates among Indo-Fijians indicate how many *girmitiyas* resorted to this extreme solution to end their mental, social, and physical distress.[28] Other laborers did not end their lives but exhibited crazy behavior on the plantations. At Naleba estate in 1915, three years after he had arrived in Fiji, Ali leaped naked on to his employer's horse and "rode madly around." He spent about six months in the asylum but seven years later was readmitted for twenty-one months. His later admission papers state that he was "not violent and on several days 'quite normal', but without reason breaks out again."[29]

Indian nationalist supporters Charles Andrews, Reverend W. W. Pearson, and Florence Garnham of the London Missionary Society, Calcutta, campaigned about the high rates of suicide among male Indo-Fijian indentured migrants in Fiji relative to India and other colonies where indenture was practiced.[30] The *Register of Deaths of Indian Immigrants* recorded 291 suicides, of whom 259 were male and thirty-two female.[31] State officials such as Agent General of Immigration A. R. Coates attributed this discrepancy to "sexual jealousy and disappointment" resultant from the disproportionate number of women to men on the plantations.[32] Lal summed up these assumptions about indentured men:

> Unable to obtain or, worse still, keep their women, who supposedly exploited their sexuality to promote their own material interests, the men—so the argument ran—descended into despondency and melancholia and committed suicide. Or, alternatively, they murdered their women first and then took their own lives.[33]

One such case was Venkatewa Reddi, who complained of illness to the plantation overseer and was ordered to the hospital. Rather than going there, he walked nineteen miles to the sugar mill at Lautoka, where he threw himself into the shredder. The mill was stopped but his remains were unrecognizable. The death inquiry could not find any reason for Reddi's suicide but intimated that the cause was that a woman he had been cohabiting with had left him for another man.[34]

Historians elsewhere have critiqued the attention to high suicide rates among *girmitiyas* and the correlation with sexual jealousy. Julie Parle argues that the settler state in Natal and Zululand largely blamed the epidemic of suicides among Indians on their cultural makeup. Similar assumptions about cultural dispositions to suicide can be found in Fiji. Parle contrasts the emphasis on Indian suicide rates with a lack of comparable evidence of suicide among whites and Africans. She also suggests that suicide within the latter categories may have been underreported.[35] Likewise, data concerning suicide among those who were not *girmitiyas* in early colonial Fiji are incomplete, but evidence exists of suicide among indigenous Fijians and Europeans. Even less reported and documented were attempts at self-destruction and self-harm, especially among women.

Mental breakdown and suicide need to be considered in the context of the indenture system. Lal identified how indenture disrupted the "integrative institutions" of kinship, marriage, caste, and religion, significantly contributing to suicide among *girmitiyas*.[36] He asserted that suicide was both a cry of despair and an act of protest directed at the indenture system: "suicide was a rational and understandable response to a terrible and alienating situation."[37]

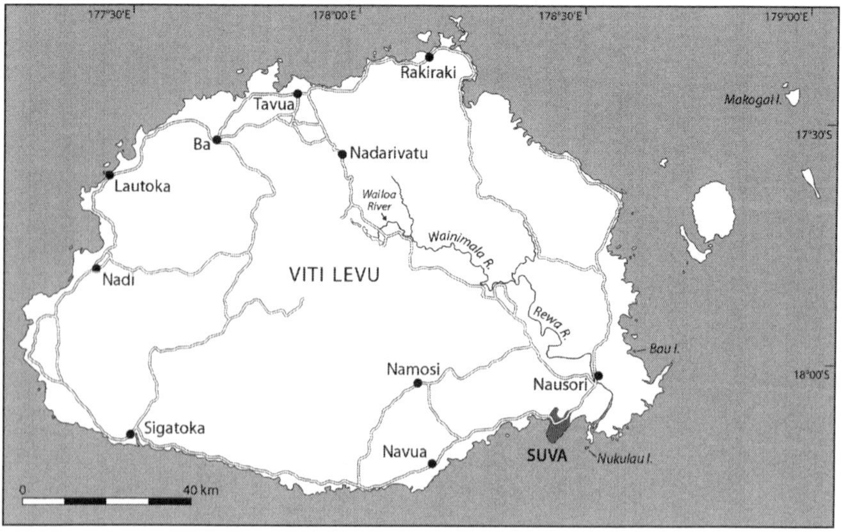

Map 3. Viti Levu and Makogai, Fiji. Source: Les O'Neill.

The relentless labor process that *girmitiyas* in Fiji endured was another cause of physical and mental stress. Lal reiterated that most Indian immigrants were accustomed to hard physical labor, but in India labor would have been punctuated with breaks, such as for the wedding season, monsoons, and religious festivals. He observes, "the sudden realization that an intended sojourn in Fiji would in all likelihood become permanent exile could have been unbearable for some immigrants."[38] Contemporaries drew similar conclusions, such as when the manager at the Lautoka Refinery reported Subbarayan's death: "Deceased probably despaired at what confronted him in the shape of work. He only arrived at the estate from the depot on the 4th and suicided on the 11th."[39] Unless they qualified for a paid return passage after ten years, *girmitiyas* found the cost of a passage, between five and ten pounds, prohibitive, especially given that many of them accumulated debts or fines. It was also shameful and not practical to return to India without earnings. Lal suggests that the small number of migrants of higher caste may have been more sensitive to displacement and the harsh realities of unaccustomed physical work.[40] Such tensions were revealed at the enquiry into Manesa's death by hanging from a tree on Navuso plantation. Manesa was a *rajput* (warrior caste) and was remembered by a workmate as a "great reader and writer and a high caste man." A hospital servant testified that Manesa had been in a melancholy mood before the suicide and had said,

> I do not feel inclined to work any longer at Navuso as the work was hard. . . . He said he was unaccustomed to hard [work] . . . here a man with a small amount of knowledge is made a Sirdar [overseer} while another with good education has to do hard manual labour, like myself.[41]

Lal further interrogated the disproportionately high number of suicides by *girmitiyas* from South India—56.9 percent of all Indian suicides between 1911 and 1920.[42] Authorities put this disproportionate number down to inherent attributes among South Indians: "a tendency to suicide, it would appear, among this class of immigrant," "a temperament easily depressed,"[43] given to despondency and homesickness,[44] "peculiarly prone to suicide on apparently slight grounds."[45] Lal rejected these comments as the primary explanations and outlined the considerable stress South Indians faced from environmental and structural factors.[46] Emigration from Madras to Fiji started after 1903, much later than that from Calcutta. By then, new laborers were more likely to be sent to isolated areas to break in land and establish plantations. Their loneliness was compounded by demanding labor conditions, where they could be under the tyranny of unsupervised overseers and *sirdars.* A *sirdar* in "the habit of kicking and cuffing the new arrivals" was berated by the Immigration Office after this violent action was linked to Bosanna's suicide in 1905.[47] Lal also suggests that Dravidian South Indians may have been subjected to ethnic prejudice and social oppression from Aryan North Indians.

Contemporaries and historians offered different explanations for the high suicide rates among *girmitiyas* in colonial Fiji. Some labor historians have regarded suicide in the workplace as an extreme form of resistance or agency.[48] Contention persists over whether it was "a rational and understandable response to a terrible and alienating situation."[49] The stipendiary magistrate of Rewa believed that Manesa "committed suicide and was sane at the time."[50] A more recent arrival, indentured to Vuna estate on Taveuni, who committed suicide in 1915 was considered "temporarily insane," however.[51] These cases point to how mental conditions, especially depression, could be temporary or reactive as well as more prolonged and end in suicide. A twenty-two-year-old male who hanged himself in 1915 "while in a state of mental depression" had been in Fiji since 1910.[52] As some mental disorders progressively worsened, suicide may have offered the only relief, such as when a *girmitiya* described as "half-witted" and suffering from epilepsy "was found hanging in his room in the lines."[53]

Melancholia

Although suicide is an extreme response to the labor process, a greater, unspecified number of *girmitiyas* reacted with chronic sadness or severe depression. Chapter 5 discusses how in the past, both lay and medical observers applied the terms "depression" and "melancholia" to a wide array of conditions.

Doctors diagnosed *girmitiyas* with melancholia from classic signs, such as refusing to eat or drink, sadness, lethargy, and crying, but the archive provides only limited understanding of the background to this condition. Imprisonment might precipitate depression or suicide attempts, such as when a woman with "slow speech; refuses to answer questions; memory deficient; very little idea of time or place" had spent a lengthy period in custody.[54] What trauma may have led to the "acute melancholia" of Daleepa, a former indentured laborer admitted in 1910 with aural hallucinations, who had to be fed but "was frightened of anybody who comes near him and seems to be continually apprehensive of some impending danger"? He died ten days after his admission.[55] Similarly, when a *girmitya* was admitted with melancholia in 1895, she was clearly terrified as she covered herself with a cloth and tried to hide from anyone in the room.[56] Melancholia often coexisted with other mental conditions classified within the nosology of the era, such as mania. Suffering from "melancholia puerperal," Jamuni was sometimes "depressed, at others very violent constantly talking & endeavouring to throw off all her clothes, then falls down on the ground & rubs her loosened hair in the earth."[57]

These cases show how the hidden signs of depression on plantations have received less attention in the historical literature than suicide. Refusal to work could reflect workers' agency, but it might also indicate depression or a mental or physical inability to perform tasks. Colonial authorities who sometimes dismissed this inability as malingering acknowledged the impact of displacement.[58] An estate manager sought Dhurma's repatriation in 1884: "This woman is not right in her mind, and only works when she chooses."[59] Dhurma had undergone profound upheaval. Age thirty-six, she was comparatively mature and—contrary to gender norms within her Brahmin caste—unmarried when she emigrated from Calcutta, left her son in her village, and enlisted as a laborer for faraway Fiji. Some asylum admission records cited an inability or refusal to work. In 1882, Chuni was indentured to a Taveuni copra estate in 1882 but four years later was certified as a lunatic. According to the plantation overseer, for nearly eighteen months Chuni

> refuses to obey all orders and answer any questions put to him; talks to himself, wants to wander away and if stopped resists the person in charge of him and on several occasions attacked him with stones. Has wandered away from estate on several occasions.[60]

Three years later, Chuni and four other "incapable" *girmitiyas* from the asylum were repatriated to India.[61] Chief Medical Officer Dr. Bolton Corney considered two of them to be "quiet and orderly men though in a condition which renders them quite incapable of earning a living in this colony or of properly conducting their own affairs." One patient, Khorlur, was convinced that he had offended the goddess Kali in Calcutta and to propitiate would fast, remain mute, and hammer his head on the floor.[62]

The Violence of Madness and Indenture

Most cases of mentally distressed *girmitiyas* are replete with violence to self and others, or from others. Contemporary experts named sexual jealousy as the cause of suicide among *girmitiyas*, but officials also recognized that Fiji's plantations could be enclaves of violence, where vulnerable migrants might be driven to suicide. One official wrote, "several suicides were reported during 1905 of indentured immigrants, in most cases they were recent arrivals, and it appeared that in more than one case, ill-usage by a Sardar [overseer] was alleged as the cause."[63] The correlation between institutional violence and suicide or mental illness remained ambiguous, with the victim's testimony usually being questioned. In 1909, a *girmitiya* working on a plantation near Labasa made a "very determined attempt at suicide; cut his throat very severely completely severing windpipe. Will never be able to speak above a whisper and will always have to keep tube in throat to breathe through." Before he died, he accused his employer of assaulting him, but Macuata's stipendiary magistrate dismissed the accusation.[64] Later, in 1919, an inquiry into another suicide—that of Soman—suggested that this was precipitated by a violent attack by five men. Although a medical examination had confirmed that Soman was in "great pain all over the body wherever touched," an overseer denied the attack.[65]

Soman's story points to the intersection of the plantation system, violence, and displacement. According to Constable Khan, Soman spoke in unintelligible Madrassi to Calcuttans and Fijians, though it is unclear from the records whether this communication breakdown was indicative of Soman's madness or of linguistic barriers. Soman was diagnosed as melancholic and, like several Indians admitted to the asylum, appeared to be severely depressed.

Displacement through migration can be considered a dominant factor in the mental illness of *girmitiyas*. Depression compounded the problems of those who had left close family in India. In 1887, a married woman was admitted to St Giles. She had "thoughts of her children in India" and was diagnosed with mania; she died in the asylum six months later.[66] The loneliness and longing for family left behind, so common among migrants, could lead to self-harm.[67] Nizar was admitted to the asylum after attempting to slit his throat in the cane fields on December 25, 1921. His testimony was translated by a police officer from Hindi into English and then transcribed by a doctor. It revealed that Nizar had been plagued by dreams and hallucinations in which his parents asked, "What did you leave your house for and go to another country?" He answered, "Because it is God's wish." Nizar said that his father had been crying every day since he left and wanted him to return to India.[68]

The violence of some *girmitiyas* toward family or coworkers or while a patient in a plantation hospital might also be implicated when they were certified as insane. Prior to his committal to the asylum in 1906, a laborer from Lautoka estate "cut down his woman with a knife," bit the hospital superintendent on the shoulder, and threw stones at people.[69] Ramgulam from Vucimaca plantation in Rewa had frightened the other workers at night in the crowded barracks. When he was admitted to Nausori hospital, he threatened patients and warders. Ramgulam attacked two patients because a *pari* (fairy) told him to do so.[70]

Destitution

A striking feature of the asylum records from the early twentieth century is that many patients had "destitute" written on their admission papers. Several of these patients were Indians, although indigenous Fijians as well as a few Europeans and those of other ethnicities were also admitted as destitutes or vagrants. Sixty-four admissions between 1904 and 1913 were Indo-Fijians, versus 221 between 1914 and 1923 though not all were destitutes (see table 1.1).[71] In 1915, Acting Magistrate R. Greene remarked that Suva was "reeking" with vagrants.[72] While indentured, Indians were more likely to have received rudimentary medical care, either in plantation hospitals or in a district hospital established by the Colonial Sugar Refining Company. These treatments were usually under the care of a European attendant who was not a qualified doctor.[73] Table 2.1 presents approximate patterns of death and discharge according to ethnicity, suggesting that approximately three-quarters of Indo-Fijians admitted between 1909 and 1913 died in the asylum.

Table 2.1. Known final patient outcomes

Admission Year	Fijian				Indian				Others			
	Number		Percentage		Number		Percentage		Number		Percentage	
	Death	Discharge	Death	Discharge	Death	Discharge	Death	Discharge	Death	Discharge	Death	Discharge
1884–1888	4	7	36.4	63.6	2	12	14.3	85.7	1	17	5.6	94.4
1889–1893	3	13	18.8	81.3	1	12	7.7	92.3	3	9	25.0	75.0
1894–1898	8	12	40.0	60.0	2	12	14.3	85.7	7	5	58.3	41.7
1899–1903	9	15	37.5	62.5	4	14	22.2	77.8	6	13	31.6	68.4
1904–1908	12	21	36.4	63.6	10	15	40.0	60.0	10	10	50.0	50.0
1909–1913	18	13	58.1	41.9	26	8	76.5	23.5	10	12	45.5	54.5
1914–1918	36	22	62.1	37.9	46	46	50.0	50.0	4	11	26.7	73.3
1919–1923	20	11	64.5	35.5	56	71	44.1	55.9	9	14	39.1	60.9
1924–1928	19	20	48.7	51.3	33	51	39.3	60.7	9	9	50.0	50.0
1929–1933	16	20	44.4	55.6	32	45	41.6	58.4	5	16	23.8	76.2
1934–1938	28	32	46.7	53.3	29	63	31.5	68.5	6	20	23.1	76.9
1939–1943	22	25	46.8	53.2	34	53	39.1	60.9	5	21	19.2	80.8
1944–1948	15	34	30.6	69.4	18	64	22.0	78.0	5	24	17.2	82.8
1949–1953	6	62	8.8	91.2	19	130	12.8	87.2	7	44	13.7	86.3
1954–1958	10	82	10.9	89.1	21	210	9.1	90.9	6	43	12.2	87.8
1959–1963	4	194	2.0	98.0	14	423	3.2	96.8	5	77	6.1	93.9

Source: Author's database from patients' admission papers, St Giles Hospital, *Blue Book of Fiji*, Mental Hospital Register.
Note: Patient data incomplete and approximate figures only. Figures calculated from known patient deaths or discharges within a five-year band of admission dates. The numbers do not include admissions where the outcome was unrecorded. Known outcomes that occurred outside the five-year band are included in these figures.

During the indenture years, new community ties and alternative livelihoods to plantation labor emerged.[74] Some Indians, however, including those mentally unwell, were not supported by these networks or any charitable or state provision for the poor. Ken Gillion found that destitutes were not a serious problem before 1920, but asylum records indicate otherwise, and that among the destitute, some were seriously mentally and physically ill.[75] Not all poor *girmitiyas* were cared for by the government or charities. Before his admission to the asylum in 1918, Chitanki, a male lunatic who had been living in the bush in Macuata, was described by police as having a "wild appearance; neglected sores on body; disconnected stories; delusions as to devils persecuting him; clothes torn up."[76] During the same year, Seoraji, a female with the appearance of being "mentally deficient," was found crawling along the road near Vuna on Ovalau.[77] Within eight months, both Chitanki and Seoraji died in the asylum. In contrast, a former *girmitiya* lived for twenty-six years in the asylum after being admitted as a destitute in 1919 with mania and hallucinations that the devil had pushed him into a ditch, before which he had lived for five years in the "bush" in Navua.[78]

That patients were admitted as destitutes or transients raises questions about how they came to the attention of authorities and entered the custodial or medical system.[79] Restrictions on spatial mobility applied to almost everyone in colonial Fiji. Indentured workers required a written "ticket of leave" to be absent from their workplace.[80] Indian women's mobility was further constrained by cultural restrictions. Transient people, however, were often left alone or ignored unless they were a persistent nuisance to others or considered a threat. Contravention of legal and cultural spatial boundaries, in association with strange, especially indecent or violent behavior, could constitute evidence of insanity. Jeoshi, a widow said to have no family or friends, walked about Navua town, sometimes naked. Like Sukudaia, she annoyed shopkeepers by asking for "charity" and sitting and crying on their verandahs. When she was admitted to the asylum in 1906, Jeoshi was certified by Dr. Halley as "wandering at large/not under proper care and control."[81] The same year, Jokhu was also "wandering at large in Navua" and exhibiting "wild excitable behaviour especially towards European ladies." However, it was only after he threw himself in front of a locomotive and tried to drown himself in the Navua River that he spent sixteen months in the asylum.[82]

Displaced and destitute new arrivals from India—such as Sukudaia—might wander Suva's streets. Once their indentures ended, more Indians flowed into Fiji's urban centers, and some were extremely disorientated. One male Indian "found in Suva" in 1902 would not talk but laughed, shouted, and cried. His other behavior was described as indecent, and, when locked in a cell, he smeared his body with feces. As with so many Indian patients before 1920, his time in the asylum was brief (a month in his case) and the archive reveals no trace of his life after he was discharged.[83]

Some narratives of the path into destitution and into the asylum include more details, especially when patients were able to communicate with medical authorities. In 1899, Ravi was apparently driven to wander by business worries and a fear of being killed by Fijians. He wandered several kilometers away from his small store in a Fijian village in Ra Province and "into the bush," going as far as Nadarivatu.[84] One of a smaller number of *girmitiyas* in Fiji from the Punjab, Ravi had arrived in Fiji at the age of sixteen. He told the district medical officer (DMO) that he had been persecuted by Fijians who cut firewood near his house; their blows, he said, were aimed at him. What he actually heard, however, was apparently *mekeing* (Fijian dancing). For some time after this, Ravi stopped feeding himself properly and neglected his business. He would spend a year in the asylum.

The asylum records shed little light on what happened to discharged destitutes, either in Fiji or in India. By 1901, a rule stipulated that "lunatics may not be repatriated to India" unless discharged from the Public Lunatic Asylum and cured for at least twelve months before the ship set sail.[85] Even then, some were unable to be repatriated during World War I because fewer ships were available. Gillion painted a despondent picture of most repatriated *girmitiyas*. The outcome was undoubtedly even more bleak for the "incapables," including former asylum patients with no money or family.[86]

St Giles was only one end point for *girmitiyas* in poverty and experiencing mental and physical distress in colonial Fiji. During the course of 1897, Musai was treated for melancholy and dementia at the Colonial Sugar Refinery's Labasa hospital. He was considered too weak to undertake the journey to the asylum, yet about six months earlier he had been sent to Labasa from Ba. Authorities in Labasa wrangled over the cost of keeping him in the hospital at Labasa, and, despite the earlier assessment that he could not travel to Suva, he was sent to the Indian Depot at Korovou, located close to the asylum, to await repatriation. While there, Musai revealed the cause of his destitution and illness. He said that he had been swindled out of thirty pounds by Mr. Potts, the manager of Yalalevu estate at Ba, who had been entrusted with Musai's savings for safekeeping. Musai denied that he was sick; he said that he was instead "distracted about my money . . . I am quite well and do not wish to leave Fiji."[87]

The Indian Depot was also known as the Poor House. Patients admitted to the mental hospital from there tended to be in a very weak physical condition, such as a sixty-year-old male in 1934, in a "religious frenzy . . . helpless and dirty . . . could not assist himself in any way."[88] By the 1930s, more elderly Indians were admitted to the asylum than before, which was only to be expected given the growing number of older people within Indo-Fijian communities. Some elderly Indians lacked family ties and had not been cared for, such as an eighty-year-old vagrant who required constant care in the asylum from 1943 until his death in 1946.[89] A seventy-five-year-old woman was admitted from the Indian Depot in 1941. She originally emigrated to Fiji as a "passenger emigrant" and was probably from Gujarat.[90] She had been abusing others in the depot and wandered at night. We know nothing of what led her to the depot; Gujarati families were close-knit, and destitution was unusual, especially for an elderly married woman. This "very wasted and frail" patient, who could do nothing for herself, died six months later.[91] A seventy-year-old Muslim beggar was the father of two sons, but this detail was not known when he was admitted in 1948 after attempting to hit a Muslim "priest" over the head with a stone. While in hospital, he "always appeared depressed" and in 1960 committed suicide by tying a loin cloth to the iron bar on his door and hanging himself.[92]

Destitution and mental disability also affected the very young. In 1947, Philip Snow, the district officer for Nadi, sent an eleven-year-old, known as Baby, to the asylum. He wrote, "this is a bad case. The girl is at the moment living in filthy conditions. The mother, who is a widow, and has her living to earn is unable properly to look after the child, who is thus neglected." Baby had been born with microcephaly, a neurodevelopmental disorder characterized by a small head circumference, and had subsequently suffered the effects of poor nutrition. She was "totally blind," had an underdeveloped eye and a deformed foot, had never learned to speak, and was unable to stand properly. Despite her condition, she was collected from the asylum by her mother five months later when they were due to return to India.[93] A twelve-year-old "destitute" admitted in 1917 was said to have "hereditary insanity" because his father had been a patient who had died in the asylum in 1910.[94] Some children were admitted from Dilkusha Orphanage in Davuilevu. One was a fourteen-year old diagnosed as an imbecile in 1919 and discharged from the asylum to Dilkusha but later readmitted in a weak condition suffering from dementia mania and epilepsy. Six years later, she died in the asylum from pellagra.[95]

Disease

Malnutrition and poor health were linked with many accounts of insane Indians who were living "rough." Chitanki and Seoraji were suffering from "general debility" when they died, and their poor physical state was evident on their admission in 1918. Debility was a vague term, referring to weakness and cited as the cause of approximately 6 percent of deaths in the asylum between 1885 and 1940 (table 2.2). Among Indian patients, about 9 percent of deaths were attributed to debility; among Fijian patients, only 2.4 percent were. Although more cohesive Indo-Fijian communities developed after indenture ceased, sick destitutes were still common among admissions to the asylum; for instance, in 1941, a sixty-year-old cultivator was described as "almost a skeleton."[96] Several new patients in 1938 were emaciated and so were administered cod-liver oil and a "liberal diet" to build up their weight and resistance to disease. That same year, the asylum's medical superintendent confidently reported that patients were free of any diet-deficiency disease, although it is unclear which diseases this statement accounted for.[97]

Table 2.2. Causes of asylum deaths: Percentage by ethnicity and gender, 1885–1940

	Total	Female	Male	Fijian	Indian	European	Others
Heart	18.36	18.18	18.42	14.40	20.26	28.89	17.19
Exhaustion	14.03	13.64	14.17	15.20	13.50	11.11	14.06
Other	11.64	14.77	10.53	14.40	9.65	13.33	9.38
Dysentery	10.00	13.64	8.70	10.80	9.97	4.44	10.94
GPI	8.21	5.68	9.11	11.60	4.82	6.67	12.50
Debility	5.97	6.25	5.87	2.40	9.00	4.44	6.25
Tuberculosis	5.97	6.25	5.87	5.60	7.40	2.22	3.13
Pneumonia	5.52	5.11	5.67	7.20	4.18	4.44	6.25
Renal	3.58	3.41	3.64	2.80	5.47	0.00	0.00
Senility	3.58	4.55	3.24	2.80	3.22	11.11	3.13
Brain	3.13	0.57	4.05	2.80	2.25	4.44	7.81
Meningitis	2.69	0.57	3.44	3.20	1.61	2.22	6.25
Anemia	2.24	3.41	1.82	0.40	4.50	0.00	0.00
Dementia	2.09	1.70	2.23	2.40	1.93	2.22	1.56
Influenza	1.79	1.14	2.02	2.80	1.29	0.00	1.56
Unknown	0.75	1.14	0.61	0.40	0.96	2.22	0.00
Suicide	0.45	0.00	0.61	0.80	0.00	2.22	0.00

Source: *Blue Book of Fiji* and patients' admission papers, St Giles Hospital.

Note: Figures refer to listed causes of death and are not the actual numbers of deaths. Many patients had more than one cause of death. The patient's form of mental disorder was usually listed but this might also be recorded as a cause of death. Unknown refers to five patients who died before the end of 1940 but were not recorded in the *Blue Book*. The ethnicity of two patient deaths during this period is unknown.

Other causes listed less than eight times are not subsumed under the above categories. These causes are: accidental burns, asthenia, asthma, atrophy of pancreas, bedsore bulbar cyst, cancer, cellulitis of arm, cholecystitis, chronic suppuration, colitis, coma, congestion of lungs, dementia inanition, diabetes, dropsy, drowning, edema, emaciation, emphysema, endarteritis, epilepsy (as specific cause of death), fever, filariasis, fraction of femur, gastritis, hemiplegia, leprosy, mania (as a specific cause of death), marasmus, melancholia (as a specific cause of death), ovarian cyst, paralysis, paraplegia, pellagra, peritonitis, pleurisy, septicemia/toxaemia, syphilitic cirrhosis of liver, tubercular liver abscesses, volvulus.

Symptoms such as seizures, mania, psychosis, and depression could be directly caused by malnutrition, especially a severe vitamin B12 deficiency. A B3 or niacin deficiency (also linked to a lack of the amino acid tryptophan) might result from no meat, fish, dairy, or legumes in the diet. This deficiency could cause pellagra, one symptom of which is dementia.[98] The five cases of pellagra I traced between 1884 and 1964 were all Indo-Fijian women—four were admitted between 1915 and 1921 and pellagra was given as a cause of death.[99] We do not know whether they suffered from pellagra on admission or their mental illness caused them to refuse food in the asylum, thus leading to pellagra. Ankita was not destitute but married and a resident of Suva when she was transferred from the Colonial War Memorial Hospital (CWM) to the asylum because pellagra was causing her to hallucinate visually. She had pernicious anemia and hookworm; however, by the 1940s, because doctors had a much clearer understanding of vitamins, she was treated with nicotinic acid, vitamin B, and iron and given a blood transfusion for the hookworm.[100]

In some cases, the mental effects of dietary deficiencies were soon alleviated if the hospital provided nourishment and rest; some patients thus required only a brief admission. In most instances, the relationships of physical illness, mental illness, debilitation, and destitution were far more entwined, and one factor compounded the other.[101] Regardless of their ethnicity, many patients who had a severe illness or malnutrition when they were admitted died soon after, sometimes within days or a few weeks. Between 1885 and 1939, approximately one-third to one-half of all deaths in the asylum were among patients who had been admitted the same year.[102]

The cause of death was not always precisely the one listed on a patient's death certificate but instead, or in addition, was also from more general factors, such as lack of immunity and a lifetime of poor diet. During the nineteenth and early twentieth centuries, medical knowledge was limited, including in scientific understanding of the links between diet and health; it is problematic to equate earlier medical categories with contemporary usage. For example, before World War II, some asylum patients had phthisis listed as a cause of death, but this term is no longer in use and has generally been replaced by tuberculosis.[103] As table 2.2 suggests, between 1885 and 1940 tuberculosis was a significant cause of death for Indian (7.4 percent) and Fijian (5.6 percent) patients, but accounted for only 2.22 percent of deaths among European patients and 3.13 percent among other ethnic groups. Another now-redundant term, asthenia (which referred to "wasting," weakness, and loss of muscle strength) was listed as a cause of death for five asylum patients (three Indo-Fijians) before 1940. Few death certificates explicitly stated the patient's psychiatric disorder as the cause of death, with the exception of general paralysis of the insane

(GPI), though the illness was often considered inherent in the recorded cause. This practice accounts for the high proportion of patients who died from exhaustion (approximately 14 percent of causes between 1885 and 1940) or debility.

Table 2.2 makes it clear that multiple causes of death were often given. Thirty-nine-year-old Mahadeo, for example, died from dysentery, toxemia, and heart failure in 1932.[104] Four years earlier, he had been admitted in a very poor state of health and claimed no family or property in Fiji. Like many patients, over the years he would have contracted several illnesses that lead to his debility, which in turn lowered his resistance to infectious diseases and weakened his overall health. He likely had a poor diet and resultant severe dietary deficiencies that also made him susceptible to illness and reduced his ability to heal. His poor physical state was made worse by severe epileptic attacks that most likely weakened his heart. In the hospital, he depended heavily on care and needed to be fed and carried.

Hygiene was always problematic in psychiatric hospitals, especially in Fiji, where the asylum had inadequate sanitary facilities. Poor hygiene facilitated the spread of infectious diseases, such as diarrhea, dysentery, influenza, meningitis, and tuberculosis—common causes of death for asylum patients just as they were among *girmitiyas* outside the hospital (table 2.2).[105] Yet non-infectious diseases were significant among causes of death, heart-related conditions being at the top (about 18 percent). Cardiac-related causes accounted for approximately 20 percent of Indian deaths and 29 percent of European.

Anemia stands out as a cause of death among Indian patients (eleven deaths relative to one Fijian before 1940), but it coexisted with other illnesses.[106] It was a serious health problem among *girmitiyas* and persisted among Indo-Fijians, especially women.[107] Anemia compromises the body's immune system, making the person more susceptible to infection and reducing the body's ability to fight diseases. Pernicious anemia is especially linked with vitamin B12 deficiency, which can be manifested through neurological symptoms or worsen existing psychiatric conditions, sometimes causing severe and irreversible damage to the brain and nervous system.[108] Anemia would have accounted for some of the physical and mental illness among *girmitiyas* and contributed to overall physical debilitation and morbidity, including in asylum patients. Diet is not the only cause of anemia. In Fiji, hookworm infection (*ancylostomiasis*) could lead to iron deficiency anemia, but this condition was exacerbated if the person already had low reserves because of their diet. Hookworms were widespread in Fiji's plantations, thriving especially in the wet areas of Rewa and Navua.[109] During the 1920s, Dr. Sylvester Lambert of the International Health Board of the Rockefeller Foundation spearheaded the campaign to eradicate hookworm in Fiji. In 1932, he inspected the asylum and found a low incidence of hookworm there.[110] This finding was significant, because insanitary conditions, such as around latrines, could promote the spread of hookworm, and sanitation was a continual problem at the asylum.

Syphilis invoked the most direct and feared link between physical disease and madness. In Europe, it was entangled with moralistic judgments about sexuality, and in Fiji this connection fed into racialist and gendered discourse about the degraded nature of the Indian race. As discussed in chapter 5, syphilis was implicated in the causes of GPI. Syphilis was specifically linked to *girmitiyas* in Fiji, as D. M. Wilson, the DMO for Ba, summed it up: "one of the many evils arising from the small number of women recruited in comparison to the number of men."[111] Before 1940, it was listed in the records of twelve Indo-Fijians in the asylum but not mentioned in those of any indigenous Fijians (see table 5.3). A further twelve Indo-Fijians had GPI, probably caused by syphilis, even if that was not recorded. A few Europeans and patients of other ethnicities also suffered from tertiary stage syphilis; however, because some of these patients were possibly treated privately in Fiji or sent overseas, the numbers may have been underestimated. As outlined in chapter 5, by 1906 doctors were certain of the links between syphilis and GPI. Fijians were considered to have immunity from syphilis because of the prevalence of yaws (*coko*), a nonvenereal treponemal infection, among their people. Some Indians, however, also contracted yaws. Yet, as we will see, more Fijians had GPI than Indo-Fijians did, suggesting that the distressing prognosis and deadly outcome of this disease did not distinguish between patients on the basis of ethnicity or causative factors.

By the time Indo-Fijians reached the asylum and were diagnosed with tertiary stage syphilis or GPI, their mental and physical condition could be severe. Death might occur within a year, but they might live in the asylum for several years as their condition deteriorated even further. Mahabir, who first arrived in Fiji in 1901, was admitted to the asylum in 1922 as a destitute, diagnosed with GPI. This condition is associated with delusions of grandeur, and Mahabir proclaimed that he had great riches. He was filthy and smeared himself with feces. His physical and mental state weakened for eight months until he died.[112] Ganga, also destitute, was admitted in 1917 but lived much longer in the asylum than Mahabir. During the last five years prior to his death in 1936, said to have been caused by "syphilis of the brain," he was "almost helpless."[113]

Communities and Care after *Girmit*

Despite the rending of family and community ties and the profound disruption to cultural identity, Indo-Fijian communities and new cultural expressions took root during the *girmit* era. Although many *girmitiyas* continued to work on plantations, others were able to establish small family farms, especially after 1920.

Land was leased from indigenous Fijians via the Native Lands Trust Board or the Colonial Sugar Refining Company, which also controlled much of the production process and milling. Some former *girmitiyas* established small businesses as hawkers or shopkeepers. This sector was added to by a small but significant number of non-indentured "passenger" immigrants from Gujarat and Punjab, who also worked as artisans and dairy farmers.[114] Emigration was entrenched and acceptable within these communities, and kin and caste networks usually provided support on the journey to Fiji and during settlement there. Nevertheless estrangement from family and familiar surroundings could be traumatic. Although the first wave of such immigrants usually left their wives and other close family in India, they expected to return to them. Mohan, from the Punjab, probably sailed to Fiji via New Zealand, as he was a passenger on the *SS Navua*. Two days before disembarking in Fiji, he became violent, tore up his clothes, writhed on the floor, and talked ceaselessly. He then broke the door of the cabin he was confined in and tore down and twisted a lifeboat rack. He spent sixteen months in the asylum but was much calmer on his return voyage to Calcutta: the ship's medical officer reported that Mohan was "lamblike" and did not require any constraints.[115]

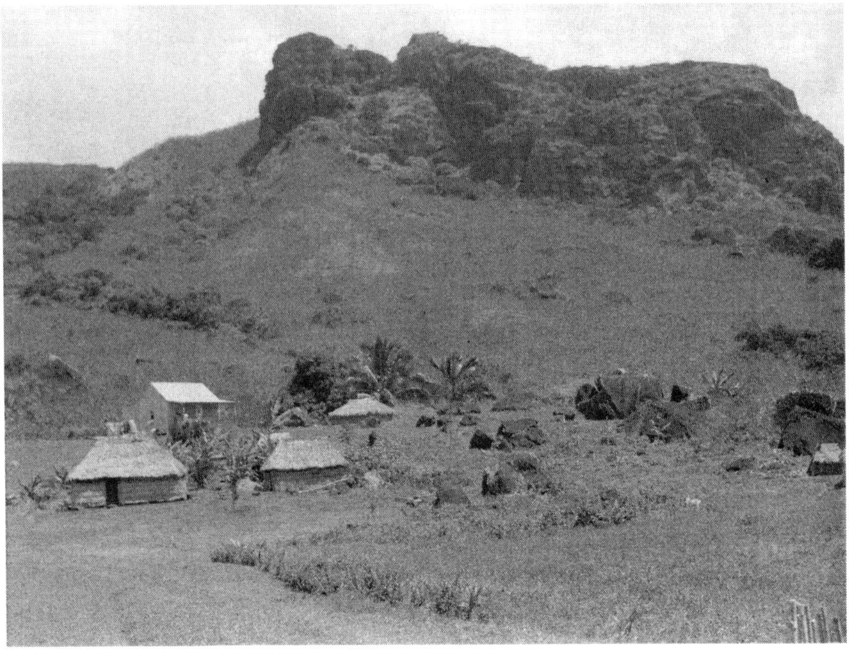

Figure 2.2. Indo-Fijian settlement, Ra Province. Source: William Hall Raine. Ref: 1/4–020921-F, Alexander Turnbull Library, Wellington, New Zealand.

By 1946, Fiji's growing Indian communities made up more than half the national population.[116] Most Indo-Fijians were located in southern and western Viti Levu and in Macuata Province on Vanua Levu. They lived in relatively dispersed rural settlements where social connections were not usually as traditional as those in villages in India. This situation may have enhanced a sense of isolation within households but could also have encouraged Indo-Fijians to seek support outside the local community. During the first half of the twentieth century, an increasing number of Indo-Fijians settled in urban centers, especially as employment opportunities opened up in businesses, industries, and the civil service.

These shifts in the demographics and social dynamics of the Indo-Fijian population brought with them challenges for health provision and how mental health was perceived and treated. The proportion of Indo-Fijian patients in St Giles continued to be high (see figure 1.4) between 1949 and 1969—some 55 to 61 percent of all admissions. Between 1944 and 1953, 237 Indo-Fijians were admitted; between 1954 and 1963, Indo-Fijians made up 680 of the total 1,105 admissions. The number of Indo-Fijian admissions was more than twice the number of Fijians (293) and well above that of other ethnicities (105) and Europeans (27). The sharp increase in all admissions during these years corresponded with the introduction of new drug and shock therapies, when patients were admitted for shorter periods and then discharged. Death rates within the asylum were also much lower than earlier in the twentieth century.

During the twentieth century, an increasing number of patients were long term.[117] Some of the long-term Indo-Fijian patients were first admitted during the indenture years, such as Sheobaran, admitted in 1905, only six years after his arrival in Fiji on the *Ganges*.[118] He had assaulted another Indian, threatened a European overseer, and tried to hang himself. He remained at the asylum for thirty-six years until his death in 1941, apart from escaping for several weeks in 1908. Sheobaran apparently was never able to speak while in the asylum, though he had been able to before being committed. In 1927, a stroke left an upper arm paralyzed and he was "helpless" during the last three months of his life. By then he was elderly, like several other long-term patients.[119]

Like Sheobaran, some patients remained at the hospital because they had no family to care for them, but even those who had family in Fiji might be abandoned after they were committed. In 1917, for example, Jamuni's husband's name was recorded on her papers when she was admitted as a destitute after childbirth. He never visited nor made enquiries about her during her years in the asylum, however, even when he was informed of her death in 1934.[120] The problem of patients being abandoned in St Giles by their families did not go away. It raises broader questions over understandings of madness, the kind of care the mentally ill might have been given, and the choices available to families within Indo-Fijian communities.

Illness and Healing

Very little information is known about the concepts and practices of health and illness among the *girmitiyas* or within the longer span of Indo-Fijian history.[121] As noted earlier, Rajani's shipmates and the medical superintendent differed over whether she was *pagaali* or mad. This term could range from being a slang term for foolish, silly, or strange behavior to meaning insane. Like its Fijian equivalent, *lialia,* the Fiji Hindi term *pagla* was used as slang for crazy or to connote madness.[122] *Pagaali* was used for a crazy woman and *pagalaa* for a man.[123] Similar terms include *jhak maar* and *dimaag kharaab hai. Buddhuu, ulluu, muurkh,* and *gawaar* are terms for idiot that could be derogatory or refer to a person with an intellectual disability. The words *dam, muurkh,* and *bhong* can mean stupid, and *bholaa bhaalaa* means simple, as in having little sense.

During the 1980s in Sigatoka, Kuldip Gill undertook one of the few ethnographic studies on illness and healing among Indo-Fijian communities.[124] She found that *pagla* embraced a wide range of culturally recognizable behavioral disorders.[125] Under indenture, the scope for cultural misunderstanding would have been far greater when workers were fragmented by culture, region, caste, and language but forced to cohabit and work together under oppressive and stressful work conditions. Murmurings of unacceptable behavior that was considered mad come through only occasionally in the archive, and traces of how individuals understood their depression or mania are very few indeed.

In Fiji, as in India, many people believed that illness was caused by spirits.[126] Like many other mental patients, some Indo-Fijians believed that spirit possession had provoked their madness, though the underlying cause was often thought to be wrongdoing by an individual, family, or the community or witchcraft by others. In 1917, Sudesh, an Indian storekeeper, said that he had been bewitched by another Indo-Fijian. Because he believed this, Sudesh threw himself into the Rewa River and shouted at imaginary people in Fijian. He was twice admitted to the asylum; the second time he thought he was God. He had also begun beating his children though he was usually very devoted to them.[127] Mentally disturbed Hindus might attribute their madness to malevolent and powerful deities, such as Kali. One female patient, who was admitted twelve times between 1914 and 1928, thought that the devil entered her and made her violent.[128] In 1950, Shaitan (the devil) was said to be persecuting an eighteen-year-old delusional Hindu male.[129] A few Indo-Fijians believed that they were the victims of Fijian *draunikau* (spell, curse, or witchcraft).[130] "Fijian devis" were knocking inside Kalidas's head, body, and limbs and asking for tobacco, but it is unclear whether these devis were Fijian *tevoro* or Indian goddesses or both.[131]

Spiritual and magical intervention could be part of the diagnosis and cure for the ill and those with aberrant behavior. Such intervention would have been important in the treatment of the mentally disturbed in earlier Indo-Fijian communities, but evidence is scant of how and when this form of treatment was transferred from India to Fiji or how widespread it was. The diversity of ritual healing on the Indian subcontinent was reinforced by the diverse origins of the *girmitiyas* and other Indian migrants to Fiji.[132] Very few among the *girmitiyas* were religious specialists, such as *pandits* (Brahmin scholars), *pujaris* (Hindu temple priests), or *maulvis* (Islamic scholars), and there were no known *vaidyas* (Ayurvedic physicians). *Girmitiya* Totaram Sanadhya observed, "The religious situation of our people is very unstable. . . . As a result, the Fiji Indians are like an unsteady boat caught in a whirlpool."[133] Once religious specialists became established in Fiji, they offered healing, which embraced those suffering from mental afflictions. Religious provision and practices, including those linked with healing, became more widespread with the growth of settled Indo-Fijian communities, the post-indenture immigration of traders, teachers, and religious experts, and the institutionalization of Hindu faiths and Islam in Fiji. Earlier Indian immigrants may have turned to traditional remedies or magical intervention as these methods were often transmitted through families, and some *girmitiyas* may have had such magical knowledge. Traditional midwives (*dais*) practiced in the labor lines of Fiji, and they would have had knowledge of folk medicine.

Gill suggests that magical healers or *orjahs* (also called *ojha*) began to practice in Fiji in the 1930s or possibly the 1920s.[134] *Orjahs* sometimes practiced sorcery (*jaddu*) or witchcraft to treat spirit possession. According to Ram Narayan, doctors, including psychiatrists, were critical of the ambiguous power that Indian and Fijian healers had, because this power could heal as well as harm.[135] In their diagnoses, *orjahs* and other Indian healers looked to the social causes, which was pertinent in addressing mental disorders. Gill observed that illnesses were regarded as arising "out of antagonisms due to envy, spite, kinship relations, property disputes or other social disorders," and this observation applies to some of the cases in this chapter. Illness could be diagnosed as *hawa,* caused by *setan* (an evil wind or malevolent spirits) or by *nazar* (evil eye). *Hawa* could be manifested through unease, insecurity, headaches, loss of appetite, and general aches and pains. Gill reported that "disordered behaviour, behaviour out of character for the person and social settings," may be caused by possession by *hawa.* She found that young married women were especially prone to this diagnosis, possibly reflecting their anxiety. Stress, such as relocating and living with their husband's family or the pressure to conceive, could lead to mental distress, self-harm, and suicide.[136]

Indo-Fijian healers primarily intervened spiritually, but they also used herbs, medicines, massage, fasting, and diet to treat those mentally unwell. Dr. Ram Narayan listed treatments for mental illness that included prayers, worship, holy scriptures, talismans, and drinking the washings of sacred writings.[137] *Pandits* and *pujaris* might consult astrological charts while making their diagnosis, and treatment might require the sufferer to undergo penance and the family to perform *pujas* or to propitiate a deity. *Maulvis* often told the ill to wear amulets (*tabiz*) with Islamic verses in them.[138] Healing was often syncretic, embracing Hindu and Muslim Indian practices, while Fijian healers might also be consulted.[139]

An outbreak of "mass hysteria" in 1968 among eighteen girls between eight and fourteen years old at Qawa Indian Primary School near Labasa illustrates how an Indo-Fijian community turned to biomedicine as well as Hindu, Muslim, and Fijian traditional healers.[140] When rumors of "mysterious epidemics were rife," the medical superintendent of St Giles, Dr. David Sell, was sent for. A local doctor, R. G. Randall, described the schoolgirls' symptoms as hyperventilating, twitching hands and arms, fainting, and "exhaling with a musical wheeze." Five girls were examined at the hospital. One was given Largactil intramuscularly.[141] Randall identified her as the "trigger girl," who had a past history of unstable emotional behavior. Sell later had Eysenck's body sway test administered to her to confirm a diagnosis of hysteria.[142] The girl's parents consented to treatment with Largactil tablets because they had already exhausted various traditional options to cure her distress and possible spirit possession. Other parents also believed that their daughters had become possessed by spirits as a result of humans previously disturbing normally benign spirits that lived near the school, including those in a sacred pool of the local *yavusa*, Qawa-i-ra, Davuiyaliyali. First, Hindu healers were consulted; parents then took their daughters to Amina, an Indo-Fijian Muslim healer. She applied Fijian forms of healing by rubbing coconut oil on the girls' throats, praying, and calming them, but their "hysteria" returned when they left her compound. Amina suggested that the school committee should ask the Fijian landowners to appease the spirits of the pool by presenting *yaqona*. When this move failed to "cure" the girls, the parents requested that Mara Sirdar, the main *pujari* of the Vunivau Hindu fire-walking *mandir*, cleanse the school of *shaitan* (evil spirits) to reduce the young women's anxiety and to seek forgiveness from the pool's spirits. This *puja* of Hindu and Fijian offerings calmed the girls' distress. The girls also wore talismans that Mara

Sirdar had prepared for them as protection from evil spirits. A week later, the girls and their parents participated in a bigger *puja* that another priest organized to exorcise the *shaitan*.

Spiritual and traditional remedies offered relief to the schoolgirls and their families at Qawa, but in other instances similar forms of intervention were not always effective. Indo-Fijian families turned to the state and biomedicine for solutions when dealing with more severe mental disorders, especially if the illness seemed to be uncontrollable or beyond their capacity to care. This was the option Biman's family tried.

Family Care at Breaking Point

Like other families in Fiji whose members suffered from mental disabilities, Biman's family reached a point where they were unable to cope with his behavior or its consequences. They had come to live in fear of what he might do to others and himself. Biman had had epileptic seizures since he was seventeen, and, as his illness progressed, his behavior became more bizarre and frightening. Dr. Girij Mukherji wrote, "He is liable to be a danger to himself and to others."[143] Biman's father, Pratap, had first reacted by insisting that his son rest from work for six months, despite this loss of labor on the family cane farm in Nadi District. Biman's seizures continued with increasing violence. In 1949, he attempted to hang himself, and this attempt was reported to the police. Although charged with attempted suicide, the onus of control and legal responsibility for Biman's actions were placed on his father, which did not stop Biman from attempting suicide again. Pratap warned Biman that, if he made another attempt, he would be sent to prison. Pratap became afraid of Biman's "constant exhibitions of temper"; in one such instance, Biman was annoyed with someone in his house, so he grabbed a rooster and wrung its neck. Pratap asked "the police to do something about his son as he was not capable of caring for him any longer." Assistant Superintendent Lovell declared Biman normal, but a month later Biman plunged headfirst into a well in an attempt to drown himself. Pratap saw Biman's legs protruding from the well and that his head was under the water and managed to pull his son out.

Pratap's next strategy was to send Biman to Savusavu and place him in the unpaid employment and care of another farmer, Mahesh. Biman stayed there for two months but was easily annoyed by others and reacted with violence. He assaulted Mahesh's son and two workers, threatening one of them with a knife. Mahesh retaliated by beating Biman and forcing him to work. Some days later Biman announced that he was quitting work and going home to Nadi; a fight broke out between him and Mahesh, but afterward Biman resumed work.

Mahesh's wife then caught Biman cutting a rope, in preparation for what appeared to be another suicide attempt. After a struggle, Mahesh stopped him and telephoned the police; Biman was arrested and charged with attempted suicide, which was contrary to section 240 of the penal code.

While in court, Biman had a seizure and the court had to be adjourned. His father testified, "We live in fear of him, particularly just after he recovers from a fit." Biman was ordered to serve part of his sentence at St Giles, where he was treated with electroconvulsive therapy and probably also medication. The medical superintendent deemed his treatment successful—evidence being that he was a "good worker"—so Biman was discharged to the prison in November 1951 to serve the remainder of his sentence on the condition that he continued his treatment.

Biman's father and his guardian had tried to cope with his epilepsy and violent outbursts toward himself and others, but they reached a point where they sought police intervention. When Lovell initially assessed Biman, the police may have believed that the family was responsible for Biman's care. This same course was followed by the district officer for Ra when seventeen-year-old Nand came twice before the court for "abnormal behaviour," including threatening people with iron bars and stones. Nand was "consigned . . . to his parents, that they might look after him and keep him under proper control." Like Biman's family, Nand's family was unable to do this, so the district officer ordered Nand to the mental hospital on the grounds that "he should not at the present time be allowed to roam free." Nand was diagnosed with manic depression, said to be caused by "adolescent insanity." He was discharged after eight months but later readmitted five times, his diagnosis changing to being a mental deficient. The local doctor reported that Nand was still not under proper care and control, wandering about and annoying females and children. After he was back in the hospital, he stopped speaking, became unable to care for himself, and lost control of his bodily functions. Ten months later, his father received a letter informing him of his son's death.[144]

It seems that some families, such as those of Biman or Nand, reached the limit in their ability to care for mentally disordered children when they became adolescents. Until then, families may have coped by watching the children closely, relying on restraints, using traditional medicines and healers, and consulting doctors or nurses. After World War II, as more families accessed medical institutions and possibly with more state intervention, increasingly more children—both Indo-Fijian and indigenous Fijian—were treated at St Giles. When fourteen-year-old Vitendra was admitted there in 1948, he was unable to hear or speak but cried and did not seem to sleep. He was unresponsive and had mostly refused food when living with his family. His brother said that Vitendra had tried to run away, so the family had tied him up with a rope and left him at home. On admission, Vitendra was unable to stand unsupported. He died in the CWM eighteen months later.[145]

Most families would not have wanted to physically restrain their children. However, as the children matured, it became more difficult to prevent them from wandering outside their home. Parents worried that mentally subnormal girls were especially vulnerable to sexual abuse and could become pregnant, which was especially shameful among Indo-Fijians. In 1962, a probation officer from the Education Department wrote to the medical superintendent at St Giles about Ayesha, age eighteen, who had secondary dementia. Her condition had been caused by meningitis when she was about three years old. Her parents were concerned about her behavior, such as when she wandered into a Fijian village. The letter detailed that "in desperation" they had "requested us if we could help them. . . . Because of her age and mental condition, the parents thought it best to bring her here for admission."[146] Parents found it challenging to control adolescents whose violent episodes could have serious consequences. The father of one seventeen-year-old said that he had to restrain his daughter at home because she was very violent.[147] Many mentally disabled children were not violent, but some families did not have the resources to care for them. One family had thirteen children, including an eighteen-year-old who was "silly all his life." When he became worse for a few months, his family admitted him.[148]

Conclusion: Displaced Minds

Much of this chapter focuses on *girmitiyas* who experienced enormous environmental and cultural displacement when they emigrated to and settled in Fiji. Although only a tiny percentage were certified as insane, many more *girmitiyas* experienced severe mental distress outside the asylum. They may have received some relief from traditional and religious forms of healing, but such support was quite limited during the indenture era and was only partially established in later years. Indenture offered Indians in Fiji access to Western medicine, and, although it could be rudimentary, biomedicine was an important resource within Indo-Fijian communities.[149] *Girmitiyas* were still susceptible to many forms of disease, and disease compounded with poverty and destitution could contribute to serious mental illness.

The other Dr. Macgregor—Duncan Fleming Macgregor—appointed in 1964 as St Giles's first full-time psychiatrist saw a correlation between the rise in Indo-Fijian admission rates after World War II and another form of migration and displacement—urbanization. By 1951, he argued, Indians had established "preeminence in all business matters" and as "Commercial folk in any country tended to be acquisitive, litigious, and hypochondriacal." In contrast, "the peace of mind of Fijians might be due to their unwillingness to enter the commercial 'rat-race.'"[150] These ethnic generalizations were curious because, although Macgregor had noted that many Fijians resisted the urban and commercial pull, the numbers of Fijian patients were increasing and, as chapter 3 reveals, mental distress was hardly absent from Fijian villages. Certainly Indo-Fijians were becoming prominent in business, but Europeans—both in Fiji and through foreign interests—continued to be dominant in Fiji's economy after World War II. Several Indo-Fijians were tenant farmers and laborers, and patients at St Giles continued to be drawn from these backgrounds as well as from urban and peri-urban communities. Suicide among Indo-Fijians continued at high rates during the mid-twentieth century, as it had during the *girmit* years.[151] As discussed in chapter 4, the striking difference between the two eras was the high rates of suicide and reports of attempted suicide among young Indo-Fijian women after World War II. Many Indo-Fijians lived in rural settlements and suffered very different pressures from the businessmen that Macgregor described. Moreover, the stresses of urbanization and modernization, as well as community, religious, and other tensions, affected other ethnic communities in Fiji.

CHAPTER 3

Lialia? *Indigenous Fijians, Community, and "Madness"*

In 1885, Adolph Joske, the stipendiary magistrate for Colo East, accompanied by a police posse, made his way up the swollen Wainimala and Wailoa Rivers to the interior of Viti Levu to arrest Nacolauli Draviundrai, a chief and former native magistrate who had crossed into land outside his village and "taken possession of Mbuethandra" (Nabuecadra).[1] Joske found Nacolauli inside a *bure* (indigenous house) handcuffed by Sergeant Naikasau. Nacolauli was also of interest to Joske because he was a priest within the outlawed Tuka movement, a movement that first emerged during the 1870s, offered immortality to its followers, and envisaged a world overturned when foreigners would be driven out by a return of the ancestral gods.[2] To Europeans, Tuka was an irrational cult, even collective madness. After his arrest on February 26, 1885, Nacolauli was committed to the newly established lunatic asylum.[3]

The confluence of Nacolauli's dissident activities, madness, and incarceration indicates colonial control of a prominent Fijian and the exercise of colonial power through the construction and disciplining of mad subjects. Closer reading reveals that Nacolauli was regarded as *lialia* or mad by villagers, and it was a Wesleyan teacher who had complained about this to Joske because Nacolauli was "waging a war on us" through his violence and slaughtering of livestock. By the time Joske reached Nabuecadra, all the villagers except a few elderly men had fled. As Joske later recalled, Nacolauli's "rank and insanity had frightened the villagers, so they ran and relied on me to put matters right." Joske applied reassurance rather than coercion to convince Nacolauli "that he would have to come on a visit with us to Vunidawa, where he might be assured he would be kindly treated." Joske also appealed to Nacolauli's "sense of gentlemanly behaviour" and employed "a certain amount of diplomacy to get it done without hurting Nathola-uli's feeling and invoking a display of violence." Nacolauli still made a great show of his madness after being arrested, "prancing and capering about the village square, yelling out that he was a steam engine and required pigs, fowls and sugar-cane with which to keep up steam." This madness performativity was reenacted at other villages on the journey to the asylum. His madness drew ambivalent reactions from villagers as well as from colonial and medical authorities. Sergeant Naikasau respectfully addressed Nacolauli as his elder brother, and after the arrest "the women wept and mourned for him."[4] Joske treaded lightly because this arrest took place amid a potentially volatile situation. The account also shows how the path to the asylum was not necessarily overtly coercive and could involve the negotiation of various relationships between the subject and other agents.

Unlike most patients, Nacolauli's stay in the asylum was brief. The medical superintendent did not consider him "sufficiently out of his mind" to be committed.[5] This was an exceptional assessment, as were the conditions of his discharge. Nacolauli was placed under surveillance at Fort Carnarvon, where the commissioner instructed the Buli Nadrau to appoint a "competent person" to be constantly with Nacolauli.[6] These instructions were not always followed, and in 1899 Nacolauli burned two *bures* and threatened to club anyone who intervened. This convinced Colo West's commissioner that Nacolauli was "undoubtedly mad and at times dangerous," so he was committed to the asylum for eleven months.[7]

Nacolauli was not the only Fijian patient in the asylum of political interest to the colonial authorities. The most well-known was Sailosi Nagusolevu (known as

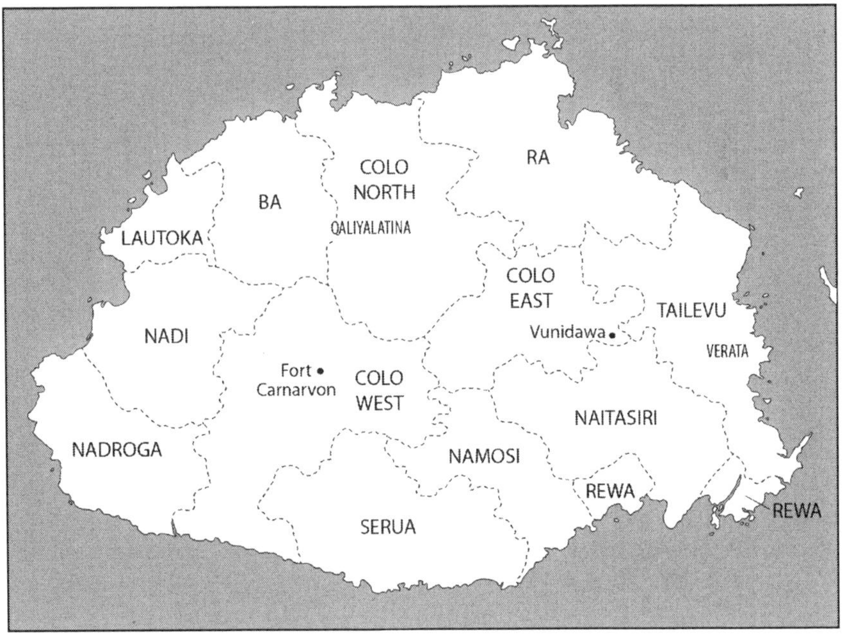

Map 4. Viti Levu Provinces before 1945. Source: The Australian National University, College of Asia and the Pacific, CartoGIS; Les O'Neill.

Sailosi Ratu), a Tuka priest during the 1890s who was later, during World War I, involved in the Viti Kabani (Fiji Company). His moves to establish a breakaway church caused the most alarm—as did the religious activities of Fijian leaders Pita Turaganivalu and Ratu Penioni Ravoka during the early twentieth century and of Emosi Saurara after World War II. The stories of these colorful i-Taukei leaders thread through this chapter because they raise concerns over dubious incarceration in the mental hospital.

The interface and tension between asylum and community has therefore been linked to the colonial control of dissident Fijians. Nicholas Thomas suggests that Fijians who resisted colonial, chiefly, and religious authority, such as Sailosi, and circulated "false positions," according to the British colonial imagination, could have their names erased from history through relegation to institutions, such as the asylum.[8] Yet sometimes the community pressured officials to remove leaders, such as Pita, who they insisted were mad. Other Fijians, and some Europeans, such as Joske, questioned the need to commit these men.

This chapter explores the complicated path into the asylum for indigenous Fijians. It also highlights how non-Christian and Christian spiritual beliefs were entwined within lay and medical understandings of madness in Fiji. Fijians also considered transgressions of cultural norms and expectations, excessive violence, and indecency as signs of an unhinged mind. Along with the more well-known dissidents incarcerated in the asylum were other indigenous Fijians. Separately, an indeterminate number living in the community were considered *lialia* (mentally ill). As is the case in studies of madness elsewhere, families and communities were active participants in the admission process of their members.[9] Indigenous meanings and treatments of madness persisted and became entangled with Western biomedicine and the institutionalization of madness in Fiji. A small but growing number of mentally ill Fijians were destitute. Their madness may have precipitated their physical isolation and impoverishment, or these material circumstances may have pushed them further into mental alienation.

Indigenous Concepts of Madness

Nacolauli reacted violently to being called *lialia*. Today this colloquial term is used in jest in all Fiji communities to refer to silly, childish, or crazy behavior, but it is also an all-encompassing term for madness. Reverend David Hazlewood's dictionary listed terms relating to *lialia* such as foolish, absurd, crazy, out of one's mind, or an idiot; Arthur Capell included madman and *vei-vaka-lialia-i*, meaning derision or mockery.[10] Regional synonyms for *lialia* are *sauvou* (spoken in Colo East) and *riva* (in Lau and Western Viti Levu). *Cavuka* is slang that can be used humorously or more seriously to refer to going, "into a mental fit, have a nervous breakdown, go crazy, lose one's mind, be out of touch with reality."[11] *Matiruku* was a figurative term for someone periodically insane usually when the tide was low in the morning.[12] During this period, they might be manic, loquacious, short on sleep, and up on libido, but otherwise were considered normal. Psychiatrists in Fiji attempted to identify *matiruku* as a culturally bound mental syndrome (as discussed in chapter 5). Another contemporary Fijian term for mental illness is *kaci yalo,* which stems from traditional concepts of mental disturbance associated with the spirit or soul (*yalo*).[13] Capell recorded that *yalorua lialia* was a person entirely insane (rather than episodically).[14] *Yalololoku* or *yalolailai* referred to depression, a different state to *vakaloloku,* which means to sit quietly, to be low, or melancholy (often, as in mourning).[15] In 1896, a native police superintendent observed a Fijian woman "to be of unsound mind '*yalo levu*' for about a year at Bau."[16] This points to how indigenous concepts of mental illness were linked to the spiritual, although Fijians did recognize neurological disorders such as epilepsy, which was known as *manumanuisoni* and sometimes *laquiqui. Mateulu* referred to a disease of or pain in the head.[17] *Mate ni vakasama* (thought illness) is another contemporary term for mental illness—indicative of the link to sickness or even death. Jan Rensel and Alan Howard identify Rotuman concepts for various forms of mental disabilities from retardation to violent outbursts, including *filo' raksa'a* (bad head), *jaurara* (half witted, silly, stupid, delirious), *koko* (foolish, silly, mad, naughty), and *huag hapa* (of unbalanced mind, simple, not all there).[18]

Fijians also had terms for suicide. Hazlewood listed *vakamatei koya vakai koya* and *rika i savu* (translated by Capell as "to commit suicide by jumping from a precipice").[19] Hazlewood identified *kukuna* as "to strangle or hang one's self," but contemporary dictionarist Ron Gatty asserts that *sa domo-dali ko koya* (he or she hanged himself or herself), was a form of suicide that never existed in ancient times and that suicide was traditionally rare among Fijians.[20] The period that Gatty referred to is unclear. In 1892, however, the Council of Chiefs demanded a regulation to prevent attempted suicide because it was becoming so common among Fijians. Causes were attributed to sexual jealousy, lovers' suicide pacts, revenge, coercion, avoidance of consequences, and women disobeying their husbands or chiefs.[21] Hazlewood had also stressed suicide as being "mostly done to be revenged on friends who have given offence."[22] The cultural meaning and acceptance of suicide during different historical eras and cultures is hugely variable.[23] Explanations of suicide among Fijians in the past, though, are based on decidedly limited evidence. Any link between mental disorder and suicide was not recognized in the early records concerning indigenous Fijians.

Missionary and colonial accounts emphasized the malevolent side to Fijian concepts and the causation of illness—the anger of the *vu* or *kalou,* the ancestral spirits or gods.[24] Although European terms such as witchcraft or sorcery feature strongly within patient, community, and doctors' discourse about madness, these were contextualized within indigenous beliefs and practices, notably *draunikau.* This practice was criminalized under colonial rule, along with other "heathen practices" such as *luveniwai* and *kalourere.*[25] Anthropologist Naoki Kasuga distinguishes between an older form of witchcraft, where powerful witches used leaves and other items, especially the victim's personal items, and a newer form of *draunikau,* according to which nonspecialists invoke a *tevoro* and place a curse usually before a bowl of *yaqona.*[26] A patient in 1962 said that he was subjected to *draunikau* because he had claimed he was from heaven, and that he had speared the person who had inflicted this curse in order to stop it.[27] In New Zealand in 1965, psychiatrist Laurie Gluckman treated Salote, a Fijian patient with anxiety and depression who had been subjected to *draunikau* in 1948 in Fiji. Gluckman observed that *draunikau* victims, who had a minor physical illness attributed to *draunikau,* often developed an emotional reaction with depression, weight loss, and hopelessness. He also reported patients who said that they were victims of *luveniwai,* "a form of Fijian black magic," but that they knew little about it apart from the name.[28]

Spirits, ancestors, and the community were entangled with illness, including that of the mind. Fieldwork by Dorothy Spencer during 1935 and 1936 in Nasaucoko village in Viti Levu's interior and by Laura Thompson in southern Lau was pivotal in documenting indigenous Fijian concepts of disease causation (*mate ni vanua*), including "disease of the head" (*sulua*) and madness. Thompson described mental illness as *lialia:* "The patient shows symptoms of mental disturbance and accompanying physical disability. He loses touch with reality and becomes absorbed in the spirit world."[29] Illness was traced to a disturbance of the ancestral spirits (*vu*), but, according to Spencer, the underlying cause was a failure to fulfill social obligations or conform to cultural norms.[30] Later anthropologists, such as Anne Becker, further interrogated interconnections between illness and community and spirit or ancestral worlds:

> In many cases, the spirit articulates moral transgression or disorder in the community; alternatively, the community is pressed to fathom the social etiology of the illness by searching for conflict or disruption within the village or *mataqali.* Thus spirit illness or possession is a social rather than a personal event. . . . What is often conceived of as private and personal in Western experience—whether secrets,

> reproductive choices, dreams, or illnesses—is appropriated for community purposes in Fiji.[31]

Patients and the community therefore have often attributed madness to the supernatural, either directly or through a spell being cast. Medical Superintendent Dr. Ram Narayan observed in 1974 that such beliefs about disease were common among "traditional" indigenous Fijians and Fiji Indians: "illness is the result of the work of noxious agents such as the evil spirits, the sorcerers, or the result of punishment by the gods."[32] Talei, who suffered "attacks" in her village in Colo East, had appeared before the court and was hospitalized prior to a brief admission to the asylum in 1921.[33] She knew she was ill but told a native medical practitioner (NMP) that "a devil was the cause of her illness." The NMP's diagnosis was translated into English: "My opinion is that she is a lunatic. She talks like one." Talei was discharged to the Colonial Hospital, where Dr. Mildred Staley observed her "acute mania with delusions that devils are chasing her." Although belief in supernatural causes of illness persisted within Fijian communities, they did not tolerate when this spilled into disruptive violence. In 1948, Waisiki attacked his brother and accused him of causing his sister's recent death through *draunikau*.[34] Waisiki claimed that the spell was cast because the sister had stopped the naming of her granddaughter after the brother had chosen the name. Waisiki also threatened others and stole a boat. The villagers seized him, and he was taken to the Colonial War Memorial Hospital (CWM), formerly the Colonial Hospital, before being diagnosed with manic depression.

Community and Treatments

Fijian communities have long embraced a variety of treatments and methods for managing mental illness. Although contemporary indigenous healing practices provide insight into the past, treatments have changed over time, especially with the impact of Christianity and Western medicine. Early European accounts of Fijian care for the ill, including those mentally impaired, must be treated with caution. Not only is there a lack of written sources, but late nineteenth-century European accounts were preoccupied with the decline of the indigenous population.[35] Tropes of the brutal "savage" extended to accounts of the ill treatment and neglect of mentally disordered Fijians:

> Families had such a repugnance to having deformed or maimed persons about them, that those who met with such misfortunes were invariably destroyed. . . . If sick persons had no friends, they were

> simply left to perish. Among friends they were cared for until they became troublesome, or, through weakness, offensive; whereupon they were usually put out of the way.[36]

During the late nineteenth century, the state in Fiji attempted to ban native healing.[37] Native Regulation no. 10 in 1888 imposed penalties of twenty-five pounds or up to three months imprisonment: "It shall be unlawful for any person not registered as a Government Medical Officer or Nurse to administer drugs or herbs to a sick person or perform any operation whatsoever on any person." Only certain elements of Fijian medicine were illegal, though; it was not until the late 1940s that prohibition was complete.[38] Traditional healing rituals and medical remedies secretly persisted, before and after the ban.[39] This secrecy may have also been because such practices were associated with a heathen past or the time of darkness (*tamata butobuto*),[40] beliefs in witchcraft and devils, and were condemned by the main Christian churches. Vina's husband said she had been successfully treated in her village in the Yasawa Islands for a mental disturbance some time before she was admitted in a noisy and restless state to Lautoka Hospital in 1948.[41] She had seen devils in her village and they visited her in hospital before returning to the village.

Fijian healers (*vuniwai vakaviti*) primarily applied spiritual intervention and offered *yaqona* to ask the ancestral gods to exorcise an evil spirit, but they also used herbs, medicines, massage, fasting, and diet to treat the mentally unwell.[42] Kasuga found that the Christian god was often invoked, along with prayer and the use of a Bible, to "strengthen this cure or to mitigate uneasiness about taking part in *tevoro* worship."[43]

Thompson documented how Kama, the "best witch doctor on Kambara," treated Suma during the 1930s.[44] Suma had lost his memory and "power of thought," wandered about the village, could not eat, sleep, or work, and was tortured by dreams of evil spirits. He lived with Kama for two months, during which time he was treated with herbal medicines, diet, and massage. Kama also spent a considerable amount of time talking to and soothing Suma, which Thompson implied was similar to psychoanalysis. Suma appeared to recover when he revealed the spirit's name and it was released. He returned to his village, but his symptoms presented again and he grew steadily worse. Suma confessed that he had stolen money from the church. Soon after, he died.

Women have played a key role in administering traditional medicine in Fiji, but research on this role in relation to mental disorders has been scant.[45] The focus in earlier accounts on spirit possession among traditional Fijian healers possibly accounts for the lack of documentation on more mundane healing practices that were often the preserve of women.[46]

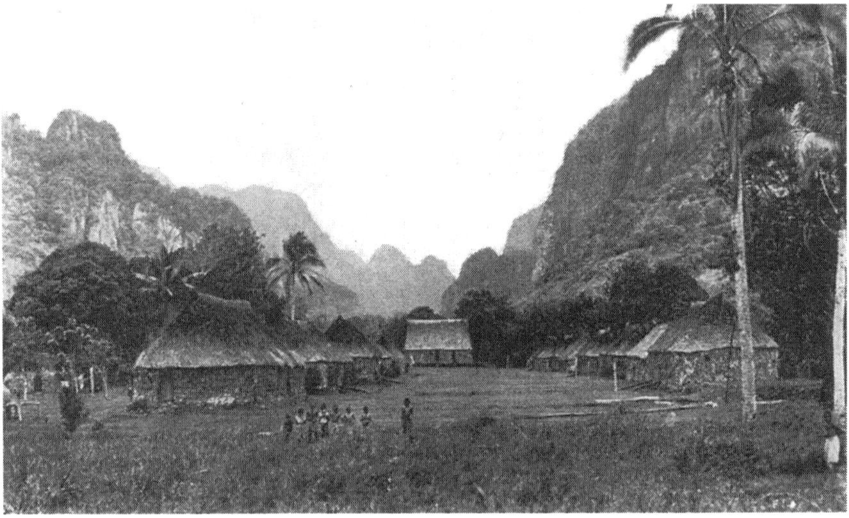

Figure 3.1. Namosi village, interior of Viti Levu, possibly during the 1920s. Source: Henderson 1931.

Close supervision was possibly the most common way to manage those considered mentally ill in villages in colonial Fiji. Before Suma was treated by Kama, other villagers watched him in case he burned or cut himself, set fire to a house, or committed suicide.[47] As noted in reference to Nacolauli, supervision was not always maintained. Nor was it always feasible, especially at night. In 1897, a Fijian from the Ra district was "supposed to be watched, but gets away at night, gets into houses and frightens people. . . . witnesses say he wanders at night, breaks into neighbours' houses; dances and sings; occasionally violent."[48] Kasinoro in 1936 had "frequent brain storms" (probably epilepsy) and before admission had needed constant watching "as he wanders aimlessly."[49]

Physical restraint was used in more severe cases, to control or punish those with aberrant behavior. Families may have resorted to this as a final option or if they were unable to offer alternatives, such as supervision. One woman behaved in such a "wild manner" that she had to be locked up at night.[50] Villagers sometimes urged local police to restrain mentally ill kin. On Rotuma in 1947, NMP Erasito reported that a mentally unwell villager kept running away from his house and was therefore put into custody at the police station.[51] Restraint could be abusive. In 1936, a Fijian widow was admitted to St Giles in a very weak condition with numerous septic sores; in addition, her hands were swollen because her relatives bound her with rope to prevent "nocturnal wandering."[52]

Communalism, Tolerance, and Colonial Intervention

Indigenous Fijians recognized madness and used various methods to manage it. Only a few were admitted to the asylum, but these numbers were not indicative of the extent of mental illness in the community. Dr. Philip Harper reported that he had seen several probable cases of general paralysis of the insane (GPI) in his medical district but that cases were sometimes difficult to diagnose.[53] Harper's estimates did not include those suffering from life-long mental disabilities. Neither did they include those with periodic or sudden mental episodes of depression or psychosis.

Medical notes suggest that, by the time many Fijians were admitted, their mental illness may have reached a severe stage and was often accompanied by serious physical illness. Many of the deaths among indigenous patients were during the same year as admission (see table 3.1). Further, with the exception of a spike in deaths among mentally ill Indo-Fijian patients admitted around 1909 to 1914, Fijians were marginally more likely than Indo-Fijians to die than be discharged after admission to the asylum (see table 2.1). A high percentage of patient deaths between 1885 and 1940, and especially before 1920, were Fijians (figure 3.2). Putting these numbers in perspective, Fijians never made up more than 40 percent of all admissions (see figure 1.4). In some instances, Fijian deaths in the asylum may have reflected organically based mental illnesses, especially GPI. Indigenous Fijians were often reluctant to access state medical services, frequently

Table 3.1. Fijian patient deaths showing length of stay in asylum since admission

Year	Total	Same Year	Two to Three Years	Four to Ten Years	More than Ten Years
1885–1889	4	1	3	0	0
1890–1894	1	0	1	0	0
1895–1899	12	5	5	2	0
1900–1904	11	3	4	4	0
1905–1909	11	6	5	0	0
1910–1914	23	13	7	3	0
1915–1919	32	14	17	1	0
1920–1924	25	14	9	1	1
1925–1929	14	7	6	0	1
1930–1934	17	7	7	3	0
1935–1939	26	7	16	2	1

Source: *Blue Book of Fiji* and patients' admission papers, St Giles Hospital.
Note: The ethnicity of two patient deaths during this period is unknown.

avoiding medical stations or hiding from the NMP when he visited villages, partly because of the association of medicine with coercion and penalties.[54] Even when administered, Western medicine fared poorly in rural Fiji before the advent of curative medication. Villagers might have considered it a burden to take a family member to a medical station if they lived some distance away and would have to be responsible for feeding the patient in hospital. The inculcation and acceptance of Western medicine varied between Fijian communities and changed over time, and some NMPs were more accommodating in regard to indigenous medicine and concepts of disease.[55] In other instances, villagers requested colonial intervention and the removal of mentally ill or troublesome people. The relationship between indigenous Fijians and Western medicine was complicated and ambivalent, especially when the destination was the mental asylum.

As outlined, Fijians recognized and treated madness but were less likely than Indians to use state medical facilities. When in 1959 visiting psychiatrist Eric Berne learned that fewer mentally disturbed Fijians were hospitalized than mentally disturbed Indians, he assumed that this reflected cultural differences toward tolerance of the severely mentally ill:

> People in the Fiji Islands are sent to the mental hospital when they become "nuisances". The communal villages of the Fijians have a very high tolerance for "nuisances" and label people as "lunatics" or refer them to the mental hospital only as a last resort. The Indian households . . . have a low tolerance for "nuisances," which is reflected in the admissions to the general hospitals as to the mental hospital.[56]

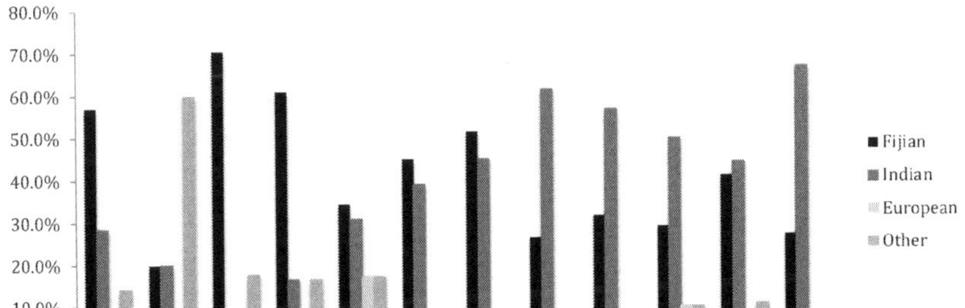

Figure 3.2. Percentage of deaths at St Giles Hospital by ethnicity, 1885–1940. Ethnicity is not known for two admissions during this period. Source: Author's database from St Giles' patients' admission papers; *Blue Book of Fiji*.

This quotation requires scrutiny. As noted in chapter 2, far more complex factors were behind the hospitalization of Indo-Fijians than just regarding a mentally ill family member as a "nuisance." Berne, among others, assumed that living in a communal society offered Fijians caring and protection from mental stress. In contrast, Indo-Fijians were considered to be more individualistic and to lack the communal support found within Fijian villages. As we saw in Biman's story, Indo-Fijians used extended kin in caring for their mentally ill, even if they were also more likely to access medical facilities than Fijians.

Berne was correct in that *veiwasei kei na veikauwaitaki* (sharing and caring) is a primary value in Fijian society.[57] This value undoubtedly provided protection to mentally vulnerable members, but an idealized representation of Fijian communalism overlooks significant qualifications. The terms "communal" and "communalism" have been extensively interrogated in ethnographies, especially the tensions of hierarchy and individualism.[58] Fijian culture and village life were never immune to tensions and change. A review of the Lau Islands during the early twentieth century, for example, shows that the communal system was neither cohesive nor static.[59] By the eve of World War II, the colonial secretary and the director of medical services noted the growing tendency among Fijians, as well as Indo-Fijians, to "depend more and more upon Government to maintain their sick, needy and helpless."[60]

The St Giles archive contains ample evidence of Fijians caring for mentally vulnerable kin. In 1889, the chief medical officer declared seventeen-year-old Losiu to be an "incurable" epileptic. His father urged that his child be returned to his village on Taveuni where friends would care for him.[61] Tina, a thirty-two-year-old sole parent, never returned home after admission to the asylum in 1929.[62] Her illness had developed during the previous year, following childbirth. Her elderly brother in Rukuruku had tried to care for her, the baby, and their elderly parents. When Tina died in the asylum two years later, her brother continued to care for the family.

By the early twentieth century, clearly, not all Fijian communities were able or willing to care for the mentally ill. Lunacy records indicate that some Fijians were considered different, possibly because of their mental illness, or pressured to leave their communities. Some were teased, or, like Sireli, "natives in his village encourage[d] him in his foolishness."[63] In 1912, the hospital's Board of Visitors recommended that Fijian native patients "should remain under care, [rather] than . . . be discharged to be neglected by their relatives and friends."[64] The ability of families to cope with mentally ill members could depend on available resources, community support, and family demographics. For example, elderly parents might find it difficult to care for a mentally disabled adult. Adolescence could be the turning point in a family's capacity to cope, especially when it was no longer possible to physically control violent behavior. Inoke was admitted three times during 1914 and 1915 when he was between fourteen and fifteen years old. His father said he had "quite suddenly stopped working well, without reason." Inoke started wandering at night, annoying and wanting to fight villagers, including the *roko* (a chiefly rank).[65] By 1928, the parents of a sixteen-year-old Fijian male, who had suffered "fits" for six months after falling from a tree, were afraid to leave him in his village any longer because they considered he was dangerous to children.[66] Families in desperation might resort to tying their children or using other restraints to prevent them from running away or hurting themselves or others.[67]

Some Fijians who were admitted to the asylum appear to have been banished from their homes. Their mental state and moods would have tested the limits of tolerance to their behavior, but occasionally the community pressured families to expel a difficult person. A doctor in Suva refused to sign a reception order for Ratu Mele because he was unconvinced of any "noticeable derangement of mind," although Ratu Mele had "a very bumptious and overbearing character." Both Europeans and i-Taukei from Tubou village, Lakeba, had "induced" the Roko Tui to have Ratu Mele incarcerated in Suva because he had terrorized local people, paraded around the town with a gun, attempted to impose military law on other Fijians, and threatened to shoot a trader because of his loose morals. Ratu Mele told the Suva authorities "that the people of his Province want to get rid of him 'because he will not allow certain abuses to go on.'" He was returned to his village.[68] Ananaiasa from Sabeto, Ba, was also ousted by fellow villagers in June 1905, but it is unclear whether his manic behavior precipitated their rejection or this response exacerbated his illness. Sydney Smith, the stipendiary magistrate, was convinced that Ananaiasa had been "more or less driven to insanity by his brutal fellow-people who have taken pleasure in teasing him; and the probability is a short respite from their annoyance will suffice to return his equanimity." This was not the outcome. Ananaiasa died in the asylum in December 1906, diagnosed with religious mania and GPI.[69]

In 1939, the secretary for Native Affairs claimed that not a single Fijian was destitute or homeless,[70] yet destitution and poverty crept into Fijian communities during the early colonial years. A few destitute indigenous Fijians, often both extremely physically and mentally ill, ended their days in the asylum. The archives reveal little of their lives, partly because some were unable to speak, such as a forty-year-old Fijian found wandering in the highlands inland from Nadi in 1898. He died a month later in the asylum.[71] In 1892, a Fijian from Moala Island in Lau was found on the street in Suva throwing stones. Described as having a "loss of flesh to a marked degree," he said he was dying of hunger even after being fed in the asylum. His sanity appeared to be restored after he ate regular meals, and he was discharged after only a week.[72] More details were provided of Isikeli's remarkable journey before entering the asylum as a destitute in 1922. He was found (without any food or water, incoherent, and "apparently without purpose") in an open boat at Lavena, Taveuni, after drifting approximately ninety-seven kilometers from Vanua Balavu in the Lau island group. A Fijian officer on Taveuni said that Isikeli was known as a person of "mad mind" in his home village on Lakeba.[73]

Indigenous Fijian women were also admitted as destitutes. Sala, age fifty years, was found living alone in the bush on Kadavu in 1918. Villagers finally sent her to the asylum after two months of "attacks," in which time she attempted to set fire to houses and assault people. She had been considered "feeble minded" since birth. Kadavu had no medical officer at the time, and doctors in Suva discharged her from the asylum after a week there.[74]

The Committal Process

When Joske remarked that "To get a man committed to a lunatic asylum is a long, difficult and complicated process," he was referring to doctors questioning lay assessments and "the reluctance of the doctors to certify them as mad."[75] He could also have been recounting the environmental challenges faced in Fiji. During the colonial era, most indigenous Fijians lived in villages, many located on Fiji's largest island, Viti Levu. Vanua Levu and Taveuni were the next largest land masses, and several other smaller islands were home to patients in the asylum. Colonial and native regulations attempted to limit Fijian movement to villages, but many disregarded these regulations.[76] Fijians lived and worked outside their village in urban or semi-urban locales. After World War II, urbanization slowly developed and, by the end of the colonial years, a number of Fijians had permanently settled in towns, especially in Suva.[77]

The asylum was a vast distance from most villages in Fiji, and reaching Suva could be an arduous journey, possibly by boat or trekking on foot or by horse through the mountainous reaches of Viti Levu. Not all potential patients were as acquiescent as Nacolauli, and neither were those accompanying them as tactful as Joske suggests he was. Inclement weather and moving and feeding violent, manic, or severely depressed patients compounded the journey's hurdles. It would have been deeply confusing for those already mentally unsettled to be

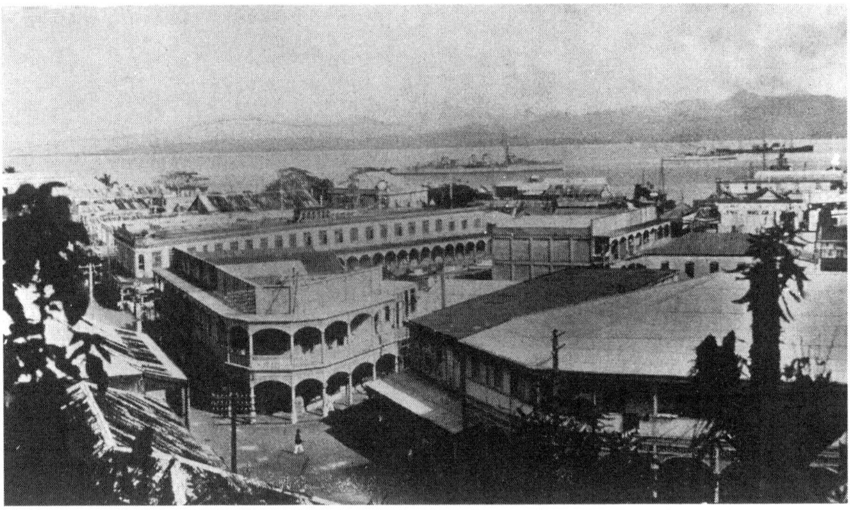

Figure 3.3. Suva and the harbor, about 1936. Source: Photographer, A. E. McMicken. Ref: H96.46/2, McMicken Collection, State Library of Victoria, Australia.

wrenched from familiar places and people. Authorities in Suva were often aware of Fijians deemed insane in their villages only after they arrived at the asylum under police escort. Medical officers in Suva despaired at these procedures. On admission to the asylum in 1896, Veresi from Rewa had scars on his wrists from having been detained in handcuffs for days. Dr. Bolton Glanville Corney, the medical superintendent, advised the colonial secretary that Veresi should have been brought before the district magistrate when he showed signs of lunacy rather than being ill-treated and forwarded to the asylum.

> Natives should be informed through the "Na Mata" of procedures re sending lunatics. At present ship them off to Suva with village constable, no evidence/history of their disease; results in delay & possible public danger as they are kept at large.[78]

Many parts of Fiji remained outside the reach of telegraphic and telephone communications until after World War II. Postal communication could take weeks.[79] Local doctors and *bulis* (government district chiefs) often had no one to consult with and had to make the decision when to "ship off" a mentally disturbed Fijian to Suva. Such action may have been delayed or rushed because of the availability of a boat sailing to Suva, which was how Taniela ended up in the capital in 1895.

In 1895, the Buli Lomaloma on the island of Vanua Balavu in the Lau archipelago noticed that Taniela "gave strange wandering answers and looked and wandered about in a dazed fashion."[80] Although he did not suspect "mental disease," the *buli* ordered Taniela to Suva for further examination by a European practitioner. An opportunity to transport him arose on a boat sailing for Suva; on board was a group of Lauans also being sent to Suva for medical treatment. Taniela's peculiar behavior was revealed when the boat stopped at Mualevu, en route from Lomaloma to Suva, where he killed and boiled a cat, kept the skin on, and ate it. He was admitted to the Colonial Hospital on February 22, 1895. Dr. Pound treated Taniela for epilepsy and anemia, although he initially considered Taniela "stupid" and surmised that he had only come to the hospital to be with fellow Lauan patients and students. Taniela sneaked out of the hospital and was soon reported to the police as "an insane man" wandering in the bush near Vatuwaqa in Suva. He was returned to the hospital. Pound learned from Lauan patients that Taniela had wandered and disappeared for a few days in Lomaloma but later was unable to recall doing so. Taniela "himself said that his 'spirit' left him and a devil took him away. He was very quiet. No one suggested that he was insane (*lialia*)." This statement indicates how Taniela's behavior was framed within indigenous cosmologies and not by mental illness. Pound remained uncertain about diagnosing Taniela as an epileptic and therefore discharged him on March 29.

Taniela was supposed to join the Lauan patients on their return home but moved to a house near government buildings. The house-owner recalled that Taniela did "seem off . . . morose" and had spent a night "with a devil in the Indian town." Taniela then went to near Cumming Street, where he had a sleepless night. On Sunday morning, he attacked a laborer from Malaita with a club. The victim later died, and Sergeant Ulaiasi, who tried to capture Taniela, was severely wounded. The police reported that the assault seemed "to be the act of a mad man." Taniela was charged with murder and detained for twenty-four hours in the asylum before spending eight days in jail. He was acquitted of murder on the grounds of insanity, diagnosed with "epileptiform melancholia," and sentenced to an indefinite period in the asylum.[81] He died in the asylum on Christmas Day the following year, 1896.

The fatal consequences of Taniela's ad hoc process of committal to the asylum probably prompted Corney's warning about the delay and danger to the community posed by mentally ill Fijians being transferred from their villages to the asylum with inadequate supervision and documentation. This confusion came in part from the limited authority that Fijian doctors and native officials had in the committal process and their ambiguous role in the provision of health services, the extension of Western medicine, and the imposition of colonial

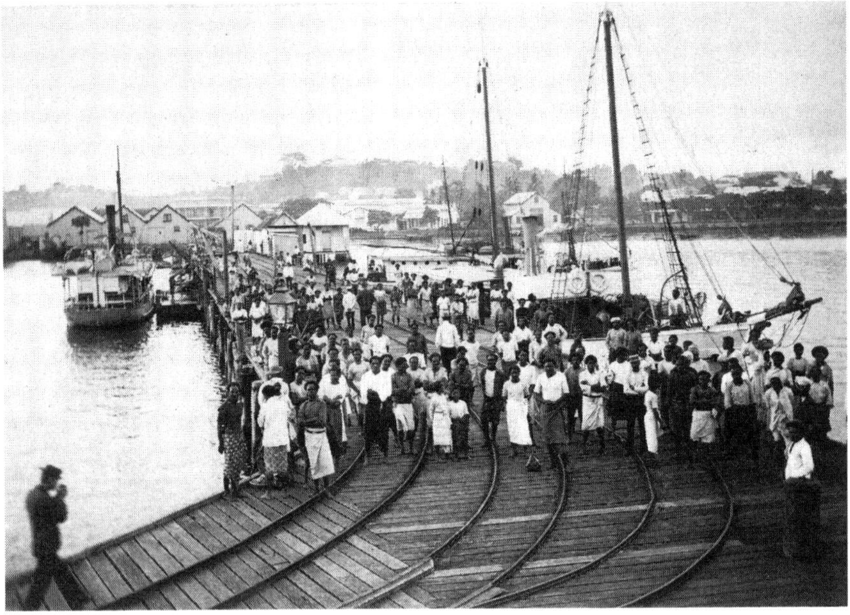

Figure 3.4. Suva wharf, 1900 when New Zealand Premier Sir Richard Seddon visited. Source: Ref: PA1-0-461-16, Alexander Turnbull Library, Wellington, New Zealand.

authority. NMPs, along with nurses, were responsible for most of the primary health care in colonial Fiji but were expected to defer to European medical officers. Yet it was often the NMP that communities called on to make crucial judgments—not only in medical crises but also in community and family matters, such as dealing with a mentally disturbed member. NMPs provided much of the information on lunacy papers, derived from their personal or others' knowledge or from a medical examination. Seci's admission to the asylum shows a process stemming from the community and involving the *buli,* district commissioner, and NMP. The initiative for Seci's certification, like that of Nacolauli, came from villagers who were "all scared of him and his practices." The *buli* reported this to the acting district commissioner for Lau when he visited Oneata Island in 1923. Seci had beaten his wife and children and destroyed the walls of the *turaga ni koro's* (village headman's) house. He also collected roots, made "concoctions," and watered trees and plants with sea water. The *buli* was concerned about Seci's frequenting the cemetery and talking to "devils." The commissioner sent Seci to the hospital at Lakeba, where the NMP observed him and wrote two letters in Fijian confirming Seci's insanity. Because Lau had no European medical officer, the commissioner was responsible for documenting Seci's history. Seci spent only eighteen days in the asylum, which suggests that doctors were not fully convinced that he should have been sent there.[82]

NMPs were vital intermediaries in the extension and acceptance of Western medical provision among indigenous Fijians, but they also represented colonial authority. Their success as vaccinators, especially in the campaign to eradicate yaws, was applauded by officials. Their role was far more ambivalent in dealing with indigenous beliefs about illness and healing practices. Buell Quain, who undertook anthropological fieldwork at Nakoroka in Macuata Province between 1935 and 1936, observed the lengths villagers would go to to avoid the NMP.[83] Ill people would not attend the medical station on the coast because they were afraid of being detained against their will. When the NMP visited Nakoroka, the sick were hidden. Villagers distrusted the NMP, who was responsible for uncovering native healing practices. During the interwar years, some accommodation was made for traditional medicine in medical training.[84] Colonial officials, however, such as G. K. Roth, Rewa's district commissioner, still thought NMPs could exert influence in persuading patients to "overcome superstitions," and *draunikau*.[85] NMP Banuve Vakatawa found that "still a large amount of witchcraft [is] done in the various districts and it's the same whether a Native Medical Practitioner is stationed there or not. . . . This Fijian belief in witchcrafts [*sic*] is not only among the uneducated class, but even among those that are educated."[86]

Community and Cultural Transgressions

Naucolauli's account indicated the initiative taken by the community "to launch the process of casting out the undesirable from the community and into the asylum."[87] Andrew Scull emphasizes that in eighteenth- and nineteenth-century England, the decision to commit was a measure not of a patient's condition but of the family's economic and emotional resources to cope. In Fiji, customary officials, such as *rokos* (provincial heads) and *bulis*, had a pivotal role in providing crucial testimony and verifying what care was available within the village.[88] The state bolstered customary authority under the Native Administration (in 1944 restructured as the Fijian Administration).

The ability of Fijian communities to cope with mentally disturbed members was strongly influenced by customary limitations and tolerance of social transgressions. Fijian culture was not homogenous, varying regionally and changing over time. Asesala Ravuvu presented an essentialized account of Fijian culture, but key aspects resonate with common cultural transgressions recorded in the lunacy archives. Ravuvu stated that *vakaturaga* is the most important concept depicting ideal behavior for i-Taukei. It embraces expectations of proper comportment in the presence of a person of high status and should also be displayed with others.

> People who are *vakaturaga* in behaviour know their place in the community and act appropriately. They comply ungrudgingly with their various social obligations, they direct their services to others, respecting alike those who have defined authority over them and those who are either socially lower or with whom they have no known relationship.[89]

Disturbed, especially manic, individuals could easily violate important attributes, such as displaying respect for others (*veidokai*). This respect is also demonstrated by speaking in a quiet, hushed voice and never standing or sitting above a person of higher rank, showing deference (*vakarokoroko*), and maintaining a quiet demeanor (*yalo malua*).[90] Violation of customary norms could be considered abnormal even if it were not the only evidence of madness.[91] When a Fijian villager from Ra was committed to the asylum in 1903, he had both transgressed expectations of *veidokai* as well as committed theft:

> In presence of the Roko walked upright & spoke freely in defiance of Fijian etiquette . . . entered stores & helped himself to goods; entered before Bulis of their Roko & eaten food prepared for them.[92]

Other examples of severely mentally ill Fijians who were disrespectful toward chiefs and elders included Lepani and Setefano. In 1955, Lepani interrupted a chiefs' meeting and threatened them with a stick; in 1964, Setefano disrupted a *yagona* session and tipped the container upside down.[93]

The Violence of Madness

Villagers did not tolerate excessive violence, especially when it crossed over into the kind of unpredictable madness that Lepani showed, or was as depicted in the account of Nacoulauli's passage to the asylum. Repeated acts of unprovoked violence against people, especially small children, were abhorred. Lepani was not only disrespectful toward his chiefs, but also violent, chasing women and children, and alarmingly tried to cut off his daughter's nose and her hair. She would later be diagnosed with schizophrenia and be admitted to St Giles several times.

Persistent violence against animals, crops, or property was also unacceptable. Sireli admitted in 1891 that he had "savagely assaulted two natives, killed village pigs, stole from gardens and yam houses, burnt down a yam house."[94] The destruction of gardens was especially frustrating and added to the economic burden on families and communities. Sixty-year-old Enoki repeatedly chopped up plantations and set fire to houses in Savusavu in 1917.[95] He threatened to kill people and entered people's houses. He wanted to commit sodomy with women. Probably in an emaciated state on his admission to the asylum given that he had been refusing food for at least two weeks, Enoki died two weeks later from diarrhea. The *buli* reported that a villager, besides killing "animals quite aimlessly," threatened his wife with an ax, set fire to *bures* in his village on Kadavu, and stole and destroyed villagers' clothing.[96]

Indecency

In 1942, the Buli Vuna complained about Nemaia being "a general nuisance through digging up young *yagona* roots and other crops without permission," but more likely it was Nemaia's undressing and exposing his genitalia to women and others that caused more concern.[97] Fijians drew the line at what they considered indecent speech and behavior. Stereotypes of permissive attitudes toward sexuality and nudity in the South Seas had no place in Christian Fiji villages. Although bantering of a sexual nature could be considerable and extramarital sexual relationships occurred, Fijians maintained strict protocols about what was deemed immoral and where and when sexual joking was appropriate.[98] Mentally ill people did not always observe these boundaries. When a constable brought Karalaini to the asylum from Nadroga Province in 1905, he stated that she was "generally reputed to be mad" with a "disregard of surroundings and 'proprieties' . . . [and] behaved 'extravagantly' and indecently in village."[99] Children's safety was paramount, as when, in 1936, a Ratu and district commissioner in Ra reported Josefa's sexual acts on school children. This was diagnosed as sexual psychosis, though later Josefa's "angry melancholy" was recorded as manic depression.[100] One of the most extreme violations of Fijian taboos occurred in 1916 when a villager in Bua heard a corpse call to him from a grave and then dug it up for the "purpose of sexual connection." The village *buli* also reported that this patient had attempted bestiality with a dog.[101]

Gender appears to have some bearing in the admission of thirty-four patients between 1884 and 1935 on whose papers indecency or obscenity was explicitly mentioned. Eighteen patients were females, a higher percentage (53 percent) than the number of female admissions during this period. The representation of ten Fijian women and two "half-castes" among this group is striking. Salote's and Kara's indecent public behavior featured prominently in the evidence of their insanity when they were admitted to the asylum at the age of seventeen. Salote wreaked havoc along the banks of the Rewa River and in town in 1910, shouting obscenities and running about naked. Father Jullot of the Catholic Mission at Naililili complained to the Roko Tui Rewa about her disruptions to the convent, classrooms, church, and working parties on the plantations, where she chased "boys" away with her "indecent exposure." W. J. Chalmers, the stipendiary magistrate, was also worried that in her "present insane condition" Salote might seriously injure a woman or child.[102] The Buli Sawau on Beqa reported that Kara had wandered around town from the age of twelve with an "apparent want of consciousness" indecently exposing herself.[103] Kara spent seven months in the asylum in 1888 before being discharged into her father's care.[104] Salote, however, died in the asylum from phthisis (pulmonary tuberculosis), age twenty-three. Much later, in 1978, psychiatrists John Spiegel and Leah Davidson met a forty-six-year-old mentally disturbed woman who had engaged in embarrassing sexual behavior from the age of eighteen. The woman said that this occurred when a devil or Satan possessed her and that she had no control. Her behavior was considered damaging to the village's reputation, and thus she was socially isolated and subjected to severe teasing and shaming.[105]

Sese: Wandering Bodies and Minds

Wanderers, who had either a real or a perceived reputation for unpredictable violence, were a problem in villages. In all Fiji communities, madness was often equated with excessive energy, endless mobility, and the transgression of spatial boundaries. The Fijian term *sese* connotes wandering in a physical and mental sense; it is also a term for craziness or madness: "wandering about; astray; in error: hence used of the mind, foolish" or "to be lost."[106] Friends described a patient from the island of Beqa in 1899 as "always wandering about," "silly," "could do nothing with him."[107] A degree of physical mobility was tolerated within many Pacific communities but not when wanderers, such as Ratu Meli, became violent to people, animals, or property. Ratu Meli "wanders about the countryside from Koro to Koro and is a well known phenomenon."[108] He was sent to St Giles in 1951 after he assaulted a young man because the doctor, Lindsay Verrier, was concerned that Ratu Meli might commit an even more serious assault.

Most Pacific communities were hospitable toward the mentally and physically disabled, but this hospitality came with an expectation of respect from dependents. Unless they were closely related as kin, it was assumed that "disordered wanderers" would move on. Consequently, some mentally disabled people were, whether by choice or force, highly mobile. A NMP on Rotuma was concerned about the escalating insanity of Jimi, who "frequently loses sense of direction, going in the opposite direction to any village or house to which he set out." He broke the plates belonging to a family who offered him shelter, causing a resident to flee. On several occasions, he threatened villagers and was placed under the charge of a local constable.In 1938, however, the district officer sent him to the asylum:

> This man has his sane moments but I have observed him over a number of years and his insane condition has increased gradually, until recently he has shown such conduct as to warrant his being detained in the Public Asylum have no doubt whatever that he should be placed under proper care and treatment—which is not possible at Rotuma.

When Jimi finally was admitted, age thirty-eight, he was in a "filthy and very weak condition, almost blind, could do little to help self." He died six months later, demonstrating how mentally disordered wanderers were often in an emaciated state by the time they came to the attention of medical authorities.[109]

Wanderers transgressed colonial and native restrictions on mobility. When Nacolauli crossed over into another district, he was infringing on colonial demarcations of native spaces at provincial, district, and village levels.[110] Nacolauli's agitation, like those of some Fijians committed to the asylum, included concerns about the Lands Commission that sought not only to codify land but also to control Fijians by "ordering them ever more tightly into categories and bounds of identity."[111] Colonial limitations on mobility became entwined with tradition and were especially restrictive for women. Wandering female lunatics transgressed native and colonial regulations against women's absence from villages (see chapter 4).

Neglected Work

Another reason mentally ill villagers could become a nuisance was their inability or unwillingness to contribute to social and economic obligations. In his ethnography of the island of Moala during the mid-1950s, anthropologist Marshall Sahlins provided a detailed account of work obligations at the levels of family, kindred, extended kin, and village. In 1877, British rule through native regulations introduced the compulsory planting of a stipulated amount of specified crops with penalties of hard labor for defaulters. Communal village work included building houses, agricultural tasks, and maintaining the village. Labor defaulters could be taken to court by the village chief or *buli,* but exemptions could be granted because of illness. Those who were unable to contribute to village labor could still invoke censure. One of Sahlins's participants described "a poor idiotic (*lialia*) man" who had not planted his food and was dependent on his wife's family: "The people in the village hate him."[112]

Tolerance of not working was more likely to be tested when it was associated with violence, excessive or unpredictable disruptive behavior, or cultural transgressions.[113] Maciu not only destroyed his brother's house and village plantations on Lakeba but also had "consistently neglected all communal work for the last two years." His efforts at paid work in Suva as a laborer for the police had also been "VERY unsatisfactory" (emphasis in the original), and he had eight court convictions in 1922, including one for assault.[114] Family, peers, and even some employers were usually aware of episodic "attacks" and recognized that many mentally ill dependents could contribute through work at other times. As discussed in chapter 4, women's neglect of domestic duties and childcare usually featured in evidence of their insanity. The removal of mentally ill people who contributed to the livelihood and reproduction of communities was problematic, especially women who were mothers and caregivers.[115]

Religious Insanity

Religion is a dominant theme in the asylum records, not only for i-Taukei, but as well for all communities. Religious mania was a distinct diagnosis within Western psychiatry that was problematic in Christian Europe and even more so when transferred to Fiji and applied cross-culturally. Colonial Fiji was religiously diverse and included Christianity, Hindu faiths, Islam, other religions, and indigenous spiritual beliefs. As noted, many Fijians attributed illness or misfortune to supernatural forces, witchcraft (*draunikau*) or a devil (*tevoro*), even if they were receptive toward Western medical care. Although talk of a *tevoro* might be frowned on in certain contexts, such claims usually were associated with violent or bizarre behavior before the community regarded this as lunacy that required intervention. In 1913, Isoa from Lakeba was convinced that the angry shark god Dakuwaqa and a "friendly spirit" Vodii were struggling within his head. Vodii transformed into a four-bodied canoe, then into a stone. The spirit emerged from Isoa every few days to look after his coconut plantation and then would take on the form of a very small old man with gray hair. Vodii failed to expel Dakuwaqa, so Isoa tried to drag the god out through slitting his own throat and smearing himself with blood. Isoa also crept into a villager's house and attempted to slash his head with an ax before chasing him through the village trying to kill him.[116]

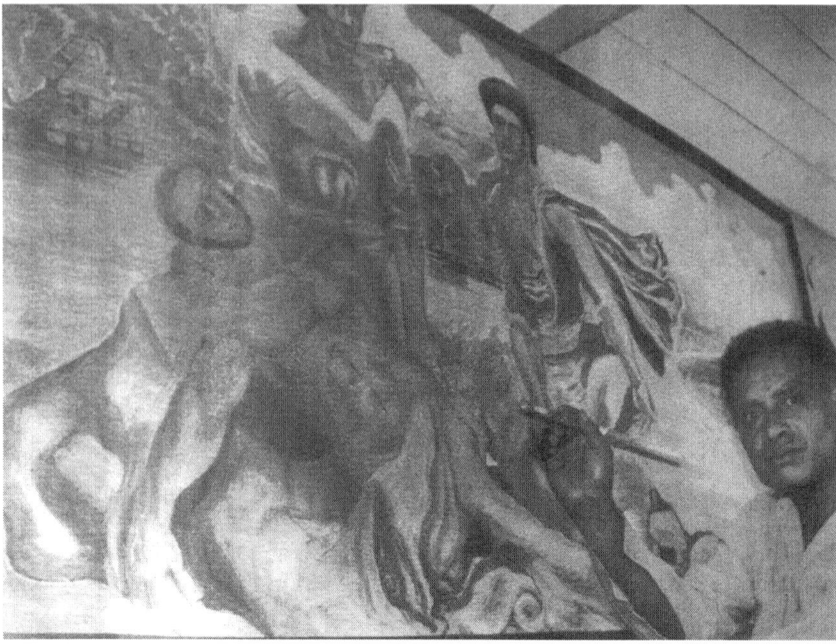

Figure 3.5. Setareki Veikosi, with a painting he did as a patient at St Giles Hospital. Source: Photographer, Dev Anand, *Fiji's Daily Post,* February 6, 1999.

Fijians who declared markedly Christian views and behaved in accordance with these were hardly abnormal, but communities might notice when this belief became obsessive, or was associated with what were deemed strange thoughts or behavior. Where a doctor might recognize delusions, the patient and others sharing similar beliefs might see the truth and visions. Even so, some utterances, could be unconvincing or unacceptable to other Christians. A Fijian woman living on Rotuma claimed to be Christ's wife and intended to join him in Auckland. Her mission, she said, was to inform the world that those who did not observe the Sunday sabbath would be slain and that she had God's authority to order Fijians and others to be her disciples. She threw herself off a precipice into the sea to drive the devils out of her.[117]

Religious experiences, visions, and teachings that challenged conventional churches were of far more concern to many indigenous Fijians, church and colonial officials. This was especially so when "mad fanaticism" attracted followers.[118] Joske summed up Navosavakadua and other prophets: "He and other Fijians are perfectly mad in the way they have mixed up their old stories with the Bible."[119] This remark referred to new religious movements during the late nineteenth century that incorporated indigenous cosmologies into Christianity, resulting in seemingly bizarre manifestations. Nacolauli, Sailosi Ratu, Pita Turaganivalu, Peni Ravoka, and Saurara, all public figures admitted to the asylum, were associated with outlawed religious activities and movements that challenged the Christian establishment. In Fiji, the Methodist church—estimated to embrace 80 percent of indigenous Fijians[120]—was closely entwined with indigenous and state authority, so undermining the church could be politically dissident. Doctors decided that the patients just mentioned were afflicted with religious mania, a diagnosis partly based on their behavior in the community, which was at times illegal, at times violent or considered insane, offensive, or intolerable to Fijian communities. Yet, as we have seen, communities were not always in agreement over their tolerance and acceptance of aberrant individuals. The cases of those religious leaders sent to the asylum revealed tensions among Fijian hierarchies and churches. Europeans were also entwined in this, especially when colonial and religious authority was challenged. The pressure to confine Sailosi Ratu to the asylum in 1918 epitomized such complexities.

Sailosi Ratu

Sailosi was convicted by Joske for being a Tuka priest in 1897.[121] A year later, he sent Joske letters containing prophecies and mystical signs. Although Joske did not consider him dangerous, he kept Sailosi nearby in Nadarivatu, partly because Tuka was gaining momentum in Qaliyalatina. As with Nacolauli, Joske was warmly disposed toward Sailosi, even taking him on district tours. But, as Joske recalled, Sailosi

> began to be a nuisance, moving about and disturbing the people's minds with his mad fanaticism. One Tuesday morning he marched into my office and said, "The Ranandi (Queen Victoria) died yesterday and she is to be buried on Thursday. It has been so revealed to me by the spirit."[122]

Joske opposed imprisoning Sailosi because of his ill health: "apart from his madness, [Sailosi] is, in my opinion, a most amiable person. I think a little seclusion & care in the Lunatic Asylum is what he wants."[123] While under observation at the Colonial Hospital in Suva, Sailosi informed Mary Anderson, the matron, "that he was the shrine of a spirit, whose absolute servant he was," and that if asked by this spirit he would kill her, the asylum superintendent, Dr. Corney, or Joske. Sailosi belonged to the religion of Marama and prophesized that

Navosavakadua—Tuka's leader, who had been exiled to and died on Rotuma in 1897—would rise from the dead and return to Fiji.

As in Nacolauli's case, medical specialists were at odds with colonial authorities over Sailosi's insanity. His admission papers stated that for years he had suffered from religious insanity, but influenza was recorded as the cause of this attack. Corney voiced his doubts:

> I do not feel justified in detaining him as a lunatic any longer, as he has never manifested any symptom of actual mental alienation since he was admitted. He is a man of distinctly nervous organisation & temperament; and, as such, is in no doubt easily impressed by the legends and superstitions amongst which he was brought up. He is also a hereditary priest of the ancient cult—enough in itself to stamp him as a not quite ordinary man.[124]

After nearly four months of observing Sailosi, Corney concluded "that he is now more likely to become really insane if kept among lunatics than if released to be among the common herd." Sailosi was discharged a fortnight later.[125]

On Sailosi's second hospital admission in 1918, authorities were in agreement that he was insane. By then his dissident activities were of greater concern, not only because Fiji was at war, but also because the Viti Kabani, founded by Apolosi Nawai in 1913, had amassed widespread support in Sailosi's home region of Ra and other parts of Fiji. This Fijian cooperative marketed Fijian produce, engaged in other activities and challenged colonial and chiefly domination.[126] Even before Sailosi was medically examined by the chief medical officer (CMO), Dr. Lynch, he was charged with behaving and speaking "as a Lunatic at a meeting of Natives."[127] The statements he allegedly made indicate how questions over his sanity were entangled with highly charged local unrest—spanning the war, the legacy of Tuka, Viti Kabani, and rivalries between Christian churches in Fiji.

Police vs. Sailosi Nagusolevu, Police Court, April 15, 1918, before Frank Spence D.C.

> **Charge:** Behave and speak as a Lunatic at a meeting of Natives assembled by the said Sailosi to wit that he was Jesus Christ's representative on earth on the 25th March 1918.
> **Pleads:** He says it is true.
> Witness's testimony: Representatives from all over Fiji were present at that meeting. I heard him make the following statement to the assembled people.

> 1. Great Britain had surrendered.
> 2. The appointments of the Government the foreman [Governor] Roko Buli Magistrate are finished.
> 3. That appointments of Managers, Overseer, Tola and Share holders were only to hold.
> 4. Taxes were finished once and for all this year 1918.
> 5. With reference to Na Vosa Vakadua who died at Rotumah after three nights rose from the dead reached Na Dari Vatu and this was the cause of the death of the Queen.
> 6. With regard to the Religion the Sabbath was now Saturday and nothing was to be given to Religion.
> 7. He was to be Christ. When God came he would give him a record of all the good men and bad men, the name of his book should be the "Buea Ko Viti".[128]

For Reverend W. Brown of the Methodist Mission, Sailosi's declarations that Britain had surrendered to Germany provided evidence of German agitators' infiltrating Fiji: "Sailosi's manifesto is too well drawn up to be the mere production of a mad Fijian."[129] Brown highlighted Sailosi's insanity in order to quash his leadership in the breakaway No. 8 Religion or "Religion Eight" (*lotu naba walu*), which had adopted a Saturday sabbath and boycotted contributions to the Methodist church. He wrote, "It is a shame that a mad man like Sailosi, and I look upon him as truly mad, should by a sweep of the hand charge the people to change the Sabbath Day."[130]

The forces to sequester Sailosi coalesced over his leadership in the Viti Kabani, which Brown condemned as a seditious movement. Frank Spence, Tavua's district commissioner, tried to have Sailosi arrested and placed under medical observation four days before Sailosi was due to convene a Fiji-wide meeting of the Viti Kabani at Tavua—the day he predicted that Britain would surrender. The meeting went ahead. Spence offered a solution to the colonial secretary on March 30: "I think this man should be dealt with as a lunatic. While he may not be dangerous in one sense he is dreadfully dangerous in his utterances."[131]

Sailosi appeared before Spence in the police court on April 15 charged with being a lunatic at a meeting. Commitment to the asylum could not be determined in this irregular and unprecedented way, however. Sailosi was instead arrested and charged under the 1915 Ordinance for the Suppression of False Reports and for the Better Preservation of Public Peace. This ordinance could cover a wide range of dissident activities, especially during wartime years and appeared to include the actions of insane public "nuisances."[132] But it was not the correct warrant for the asylum and so another had to be issued in Suva, charging Sailosi with being a lunatic at large, for remand under medical observation.[133] He was admitted to the asylum on April 24, 1918, diagnosed with mania.[134] Sailosi was probably suffering from severe mental illness, but the memo that G. Maxwell, the acting secretary for Native Affairs, wrote to the colonial secretary on the same day as Sailosi's court appearance indicates that the push to sequester him was to stamp out indigenous resistance to colonial and Fijian authority:

> Now that active steps have been taken by the Government against Sailosi and his principal disciples, I am confident that the movement will die out provided that Rokos and Provincial Commissioners keep a sharp look-out and rigidly enforce the Native Regulations.[135]

Joske recalled that the return of Sailosi to the asylum "speedily disabused" Sailosi's followers.[136] They unsuccessfully attempted to rescue Sailosi, but he died in the asylum from filariasis and influenza on December 12, 1918, when the global pandemic hit Fiji.[137] His followers tried to keep alive what authorities called the "Sailosi movement," including the No. 8 Religion, as "partly an effort on the part of the inferior tribes to assert themselves."[138]

Ratu Penioni Ravoka

Verata in Tailevu Province was one "tribe" that attempted to reassert itself up to the 1930s, especially against the dominance of Bau. A version of the No. 7 Religion (Adventist Church or *lotu ka vitu*) and No. 8 became involved in this attempt. So, too, did Ratu Penioni Ravoka from Ucunivanua in Verata, who was a patient at the mental hospital in 1932 and 1935, diagnosed with religious insanity and paranoia.[139] Tailevu chiefs alleged that, in 1915, Ratu Peni declared himself and Verata independent from the king. Ratu Peni subsequently incited acts of intimidation, all challenges to Bau. The Rokos of Cakaudrove, Bau, Ra, Macuata, and Lau warned the governor of "the insolence of the people of Verata," "a spirit of foolishness and the spirit of discord" toward the chiefs that would spread throughout Fiji.[140] At the Council of Chiefs (Bose Levu Vakaturaga) in 1923, it was suggested that Ratu Peni was insane and should be incarcerated, but this was not acted upon until 1932. By then other areas, as well as Verata, were standing up to Bau and the chiefly establishment.

Ratu Peni's admission papers cite his religious convictions ("delusional insanity") and his violence. The Buli Verata confirmed that people there were afraid of Ravoka. Indications of his insanity included his general appearance and manner of speech and his assertion that he was the real king of Fiji and the leader of a new church. Ratu Peni abolished the Sunday Sabbath (not surprising, as he had been a Seventh Day Adventist), and proclaimed that on Christmas Day *mangitis* (food) should be presented to him. He also stated that he would allow a man to have five or six wives. By his second admission in 1935, Ratu Peni's power proclaimed that he was "God and the Government all in one," and that all religions were wrong. It took the physical act of ejecting Catholic and Wesleyan mission staff from Verata to hasten his readmission to the asylum. He proved to be an exemplary patient.[141] H. C. Monckton, the acting secretary for Native Affairs, insisted that he should be advised by the medical superintendent when Ratu Peni's discharge was imminent and that he should not return to Verata, for Ratu Peni's "own sanity, and also for the good of his people."[142] This concern was designed to avert social and political disruption during a period when Tuka was resurfacing in Viti Levu's interior. Monckton wanted to curtail Ratu Peni's influence, writing, "His chiefly authority at Verata is such that his people will do anything he asks. Government and provincial authority are secondary matters to them."[143] Fijian authority was also brought in to ensure that Ratu Peni did not return to Verata. In a meeting that included Ratu Sukuna (Fijian high chief and then provincial commissioner of Lau), Monckton, Medical Superintendent Dr. Hoodless, the chief attendant, Anning, and Ratu Peni over cigarettes and *yagona,* Ratu Peni was persuaded to live on the island of Batiki. Hoodless recorded this as an amicable agreement but others have considered the conditions of his discharge as equating to the exile of a political dissident.[144]

Pita

Pita, in his early twenties, from Qelewara village in Nadogo, Northern Macuata, was at the center of a government inquiry into allegations of engaging in the illegal revival of spirit possession (*luweniwai*) in Nadogo on Vanua Levu during 1913.[145] He was the leader of a religious faction known as the Kingdom of God or the Kingdom of Jesus, and was alleged to have insulted the king, the governor, and the Roko Tui, and advocated a tax boycott at a meeting on March 23, 1913.[146] He said that this occasion was when the Holy Ghost had entered him and given him powers to cure the sick. NMP Wilisoni Qara asked Pita to prove this claim by healing an ill chief under Qara's care. Pita failed, was arrested because of other insulting remarks and behavior, and was carried by police overland to the Buli Macuata. He was then sent to the Roko Tui Macuata and the district medical officer, Dr. J. W. Hunt, to see whether he was mad, as Qara and other Fijians had claimed. Hunt could not sign him up "*on my own observation* [emphasis in the original]" as a lunatic because Pita appeared to be in a "normal state of mind," aware of what he was doing and rationally answering questions.

Soon after his release, Pita and about seventy Fijians decamped at Daku estate in Nadogo.[147] Later newspaper reports claimed that Pita had "lost his reason" because an evil spirit had entered into him.[148] The spirit could be exorcized by killing the planters, Oscar and Maurice Brown. They were absent when Pita's group arrived. Mrs. Brown met them and remained remarkably calm after the "raving mad" Pita forced his way inside the house. Events rapidly escalated after the brothers returned to Daku. According to Maurice's account,

> Peter screamed and yelled and handled Mrs Brown in a very rough manner pulling her about, in fact went on like a raving lunatic all the time telling Mrs Brown he was God, Jesus, the great war Chief etc and that there would be no more white men in Fiji after 10th June and that he would be King.[149]

After Pita left the house, serious violence broke out between the Fijians, who attacked the Brown brothers with clubs as Maurice brandished a loaded revolver. The Indian workers who came to their employers' rescue suffered the worst; one nearly died from head wounds. Other Indians informed Maurice that "the Fijians were coming back under orders from Peter to murder all the Coolies in the lines and then come up to the house and murder the white folk."

Pita was rearrested and this time Hunt had no difficulty "signing him up as a lunatic." Yet the Roko Tui Macuata considered that Pita was not insane but instead "an impudent impostor and that his seditious speech was only intended to deceive the credulous and superstitious people around him."[150] Pita, who was extremely manic in the asylum, was diagnosed with religious mania "with delusions of spiritual paranoia" and confined for seven months.

Meanwhile, the governor sent a Commission of Inquiry to Daku. Lynch, the CMO and superintendent of the asylum, admonished the district medical officer in Labasa for freeing Pita after the first arrest. Instead, Pita should have been more closely observed to disclose "the form of insanity from which he was suffering."[151] The native commissioner found fault with the Roko Tui Macuata for not being in direct contact with local developments and failing to report the sedition. The Buli Nadago was terminated from his post because of his "apathetic attitude" toward Pita and his followers and replaced by a *buli* who would stamp out *luveniwai* and "similar heathen practice."[152]

Ratu Emosi Saurara

This chapter began with Nacolauli, who was considered *lialia* but nonetheless was respected by villagers. His mental state was at times frightening and delusional, but, compared with the majority of patients, he spent relatively short periods in the asylum. Joske was ambivalent about Nacolauli's condition, an ambivalence shared by other medical and lay authorities about the few Fijian leaders certified as mentally ill. Certification might be considered a convenient channel through which to remove political and religious dissidents from society, but if so why were not more troublemakers, including Indo-Fijians, sent to the asylum? Considerable evidence of an unsound mind—in accordance with contemporary medical definitions of madness—was required for certification. Even when evidence was provided, diagnosing mental illness was both uncertain and ambiguous. Although NMPs and district officials may have been convinced that an individual was mentally ill, their judgment could be questioned by a senior official or doctor, as in Pita's and Taniela's cases. Nacolauli's narrative revealed the ambiguity over lay and medical assessments of insanity.

We end with Ratu Emosi (Amos) Saurara, another prophet who was hospitalized with mental illness. Like other Fijian leaders mentioned here, he too was responding to the impact of social and economic change on indigenous Fijians. Historian John Garrett argued that Ratu Emosi had a "sense of succession" from Fijian dissidence, following the likes of Tuka and Apolosi Nawai, and was a threat to the old order of the Methodist church.[153] Ratu Emosi's challenge was both an alternative model of village development and his prophetic visions. As "the self-confessed prophet—chief of a new Jerusalem on Fiji's soil, [he] was once a familiar sight in the streets of Nausori, in his red robe, staff in hand."[154]

Ratu Emosi's first admission to St Giles was in 1947 when he was forty. He remained there for five years.[155] This admission occurred after he was arrested for burning the houses of two of his family members who had refused to obey his orders. Colonial administrator Philip Snow provided other details: "having incited the people of Daku . . . to truss up some tribal opponents and deliver them like cannibal victims to the chiefly headquarters on Bau in the pre-Cession manner. He had gone off his head suddenly and with religious overtones."[156] Ratu Emosi informed Dr. Lindsay Verrier that he was still considering taking direct action after he was released. Verrier observed that Ratu Emosi was hallucinating and was hearing the commands of heaven coming direct to him.

Ratu Emosi was a patient in the European section of the mental hospital when shock therapies and psychotropic medication were introduced. It is not known whether he received these treatments, but soon after his admission it was reported that he had "settled down to the altered surroundings and has proved quite a tractable patient."[157] Initially, the director of medical services ordered that "for political reasons it is imperative that Emosi Saurara . . . should not receive *any* visitors" (emphasis in the original).[158] The hospital's Board of Visitors later recommended that these terms be changed to allow selected visitors but only in the presence of the district commissioner (southern), or a district officer.[159] Emosi asked to see Snow, who recalled being taken to a locked cell, where he was left "with this demoniac, in no way morose or disconsolate, inmate. The mad glint of triumphant exhilaration in Emosi's eye was new to me. He wanted me to present three crazy, nonsensical, scriptural scrolls crammed with biblical annotations to the highest authorities."[160] Emosi had been able to work on his scrolls while he was hospitalized. Snow took some scrolls, which might be the ones Garrett reported as having ending up in Scotland Yard. When Garrett viewed Ratu Emosi's charts at Daku in 1973, he interpreted them as "a quasi-religious schematization of history."[161]

Snow put Ratu Emosi's madness down to "the almost macabre religious frenzy of what I could only consider a 'Methodist Mission victim.'"[162] Garrett suggested that Ratu Emosi's "own people and many who know him have never regarded him as of unsound mind," but Nayacakalou recalled that when he spoke with Ratu Emosi in 1960 "he could not speak coherently and was almost stark mad."[163] Ratu Emosi was admitted to St Giles at least five times, where he was initially diagnosed with manic depression and later with schizophrenia. Doctors also considered him to be paranoid. In 1955, Australian Methodist missionary Alan Tippett warned the colonial government that Ratu Emosi and his work at Daku had the "potentiality of a cargo cult" and that Ratu Emosi should be kept under observation.[164] Ratu Emosi was arrested and readmitted to the mental hospital in January 1956 after expelling a group of Catholics from Daku.[165] A condition of his discharge, thirteen months later, was that he should not return to Daku, though he later did.

On one level, Ratu Emosi, along with Nacolauli, Sailosi, Pita, and Ravoka, represented a political challenge to the colonial and religious establishment, but at another level their words and actions became significant as part of the evidence in their committal to the asylum. These patients' politically inspired demands and visions for the future were dismissed as delusional. Also dismissed were the exaggerated utterances and performativity of lesser-known patients, who may have indirectly challenged colonial authorities or voiced tensions within society.[166] In 1896, a doctor examined a Fijian who "fancies that he is a white man and endeavours to talk English; says has been to London."[167] Suliasi, a village preacher, who saw Christ in "bodily form" and was diagnosed with religious mania, crawled and kissed a doctor's boots in 1904. In the Levuka courthouse, Suliasi lay on his back with his mouth open under a picture of the king and said he was "taking in words of wisdom which fell from the King's lips."[168] This might suggest harmless parody, but Suliasi was readmitted in 1907 after roaming during the night, exposing himself to women, and threatening to kill people with a knife and to burn a European's house. His medical certificate also stated that, because Suliasi was a Taukei, "he imagines he is a big landowner and Government surveyor."

Communities, Confinement, and Care

Much of this chapter has focused on indigenous concepts of mental disorder and healing and shifts within communities toward seeking state and medical intervention to deal with the actions and threats of crazy and "difficult" Fijians. The decision to seek outside help would not have come lightly because Fijian communities value caring and communal support. The transgression of customary and moral codes, or acts and threats of violence, may have been the tipping point in efforts to remove an individual from the community. As we will see in chapter 5, evidence also indicates that, until the 1950s, some Fijians had degenerative mental and neurological diseases that European doctors labeled as GPI.

Although the village remained the place of care for most mentally disturbed Fijians in colonial Fiji, the mental asylum was regarded as a place of detention. Many Fijians may have had this view because their attitude about medical institutions was ambivalent, and also because the asylum was a place of confinement, the end point when a "raving lunatic" was forcibly taken away by the police. The asylum was adjacent to Suva's jail and main cemetery and near the Colonial Hospital, sites that all evoked death. Although many Fijians had never seen these places, if the asylum captured the individual or collective imagination, it was likely to kindle fear and stigma. It is too easy to trace simplistically a unilinear shift from indigenous concepts of madness or mental disorder to the madness shaped by and within the asylum that was associated with biomedical discourse and interventions. Such a generalization overlooks continued care provided within Fijian communities for members suffering severe mental disorders, even when the option of medical intervention was available. Conceivably, care within the asylum was not devoid of Pacific-centered practices, as reflected, for example, in the work therapy discussed in chapter 6. Until the 1950s, the majority of asylum attendants were Samoans, who, as Pacific peoples, shared certain cultural values with Fijians. Indigenous and biomedical concepts of "madness" and treatment of the ill became entangled, albeit within a colonial framework.

However, the incursion of the biomedical model of psychiatry for severely mentally ill Fijians can be traced in the increasing numbers admitted to St Giles after World War II (see figure 1.4 and table 1.1). By the 1970s, parity in admission rates for indigenous Fijians and Indo-Fijians was higher.[169] Admission rates for young adult Fijian men trebled from 1951 to 1966 and for young adult Fijian women doubled between 1956 and 1966.[170] These patterns may have reflected a more youthful Fijian demographic as well as other transformations.

The late colonial decades brought intense social and economic change and mobility for indigenous Fijians. World War II was a catalyst for change for many Fijians, opening new horizons and enticing some, including women, into urban areas.[171] By the 1966 census, almost one-third of Fijians lived in expanding urban and peri-urban areas, a substantial increase from the 1956 census, when 24 percent of Fijians were living in urban areas.[172] The growth in urban settlement was due to increasing permanent migration, especially to Suva. Fijians were also increasingly dependent upon paid employment. Change impinged on villages on the periphery, increasing economic vulnerability, social problems, and mental stress.[173] As social and economic changes, including economic deprivation, within urban and rural Fijian communities intensified during the decades after World War II, the capacity of communities to care for those with mental disorders became stretched.

Psychiatric definitions of mental illness may have become normalized by medical oversight and intervention, though the extent to which this model affected lay understandings of "madness" and toleration for mental difference within Fijian communities is uncertain. Near the time of Fiji's independence, C. H. Gurd, director of medical services, stated that the rising number of Fijian patients "appears to be an indication that the Fijian attitude towards the Mental Hospital is changing: it is becoming for them not merely a place of detention as in the past but a place of cure and rehabilitation."[174] Attitudes among Fijians toward St Giles may indeed have shifted, given that new therapies allowed faster discharges from the hospital and appeared to offer the hope of cure. But Gurd also observed that, "despite being illegal, 'witchcraft continues to be practiced' in the treatment of mental disorders."

CHAPTER 4

Mad Women

Among the 498 Indian indentured laborers on board the *Leonidas* were 149 adult women when it sailed from Calcutta bound for Fiji on January 28, 1879.[1] The *Leonidas* docked at Levuka on May 15, but because cholera and smallpox had broken out during the voyage, the passengers were quarantined on the nearby tiny island of Yanuca Lailai. Among those quarantined were two women, Ozeeari and Sukudaia, who were declared insane.[2] In 1882, officials recommended that Sukudaia and two other mad Indian women, Janki and Montumi, be taken to Makuluva Island and left there.[3] As outlined in earlier chapters, Sukudaia and her child made their way to Suva, where Sukudaia attracted public attention as an insane vagrant. Montumi also lived in Suva but was able to accumulate more than thirty pounds by 1884 as a prostitute—considerably more than the two pounds, seventeen shillings, and ninepence she previously earned as a laborer on Deuba estate.

Sukudaia's mobility ceased in 1884, when at age thirty-one she was admitted as the second patient to the newly established Public Lunatic Asylum. Like Qaqa, she died there two years later, from tuberculosis. We do not know what drove her into indenture or anything about her journey from India to the Pacific; one sympathetic Suva resident commented, "Unfortunately, we cannot tell the burden of her ditty."[4] Sukudaia's few remaining case notes offer little detail about how she became the first woman to be committed. These papers, however, like those of most of her contemporaries, record the extremes of violence and depression.

Also a first is the gendering of admission and case notes. Observations about Sukudaia focused on her sexuality, transgressions of gendered morality, and embodied madness. Dr. Alfred Munckton observed,

> She had a wild manner and expression generally, and often refused to wear any clothes during my visit. The chief conversation is of sexual intercourse and the male sex. Her gestures are often of an indecent and lascivious character.

The chief warden, Mr. Ferris, reported that Sukudaia was sometimes extremely violent and "gave great trouble to the male patients who refused to have anything to do with her."

Decades later, in 1958, Lani, an indigenous fourteen-year-old Fijian woman, was admitted to the same mental institution. By 1987, she had been admitted eight times. Although they lived around a century apart, both Sukudaia and Lani were poor women with severe mental disorders, living in Suva. Lani's records reveal a turbulent sexual life, including possibly contracting gonorrhea from a close family member. By the 1960s, she was living with sex workers in Suva. One night, she was offered twelve pounds to have sex with twenty sailors in a Suva park. They left her lying on the ground with no payment. Soon after this, she was back at St Giles.[5]

Sukudaia's and Lani's madness records were infused with gendered discourse, sexuality, and poverty. Their circumstances represent extremes of struggles with mental illness in the asylum and living with this in the community in colonial Fiji. This chapter focuses on gender and madness in colonial Fiji, women's experiences in particular. Although delusional and corporeal worlds were blurred, mad women's testimonies offer insight into the stresses women faced and the contradictions of gender roles in the community. Women's transgression of gendered norms and roles were more likely than men's to be cited as evidence of mental instability. Gendered cultural and spatial boundaries intersected with ethnicity, hierarchy, and age and extended into the asylum. Women's madness was highly embodied, notably when reproduction was linked to diagnoses and treatments of madness. My research on gender and mental illness aligns with Catharine Coleborne's and similar analysis in colonial settings.[6] This approach stresses that gendered patterns within the asylum are both constructed by and form gendered and colonial identities. Within Fiji, gendered identities also strongly reflected indigenous and migrant cultures. The state and doctors did essentialize such identities, but so did members of different ethnic groups and religions, both with their own and other cultures. Fiji was not a white settler colony and, compared with asylums in New Zealand and Australia, patient numbers were far smaller, but the indigenous and Indian proportion was far greater. When comparing gendered patterns within Fiji and Australasia, it is important to remember that colonial rule in Fiji lasted until 1970.

Gendering Madness

The relationship between gender and madness, specifically, women's multiple subject locations as subordinate in society and their categorization and treatment as mentally ill, emerged in second-wave feminism and the antipsychiatry movement.[7] Both movements emphasized the social construction of madness and the repressive role of psychiatry and asylums. In 1972, Phyllis Chesler analyzed gendered constructs of mental disorder: "the 'norm violations' in madness-cum-deviance involved a transgression of the core male/female identity."[8] Where such transgressions were perceived as madness, Chesler identified agency in women's attempts to escape restrictive subject locations. Elaine Showalter developed these links between madness and gender through cultural history and literary criticism to link the representation of madness as a female malady with women's repression.[9] Joan Busfield further located women's committal to the asylum with female oppression and recognized the social construction of the mad female.[10] Chesler and Showalter's positions were extensively revised, most notably where colonial hegemony reinforced medical power, and the gender roles within migrant and indigenous cultures.[11] Coleborne's research reiterated that the greater numbers of men within colonial populations meant that they were more highly represented than women within colonial asylums in the Australian colonies.[12] However, in Fiji, the higher numbers of men in the asylum was not just a corollary of gender imbalance caused by immigration because until well after World War II indigenous men far outnumbered indigenous women in the patient population (figure 4.3).

"Women Rather Excited"

Dr. Lynch made a cursory observation—"women rather excited"—on his visit to the asylum on January 5, 1914. No reasons were given for the women's elation, or in other racialized remarks—such as "Natives as usual."[13] Such discourse homogenized and essentialized non-Europeans and women but was hardly unexpected given the racial and gendered frameworks that permeated colonial Fiji. Medical Superintendent Dr. Clunie, pointed out that, apart from the indenture system, racial segregation in Fiji had never been as rigid as it was in India, Africa, and the southern United States, where separate racially designated compounds were established to treat the sick.[14] Nevertheless, race and gender were integral to the spatial and administrative infrastructure of St Giles as well as constitutive of assumptions about managing mental illness within an ethnically complex colonial society.

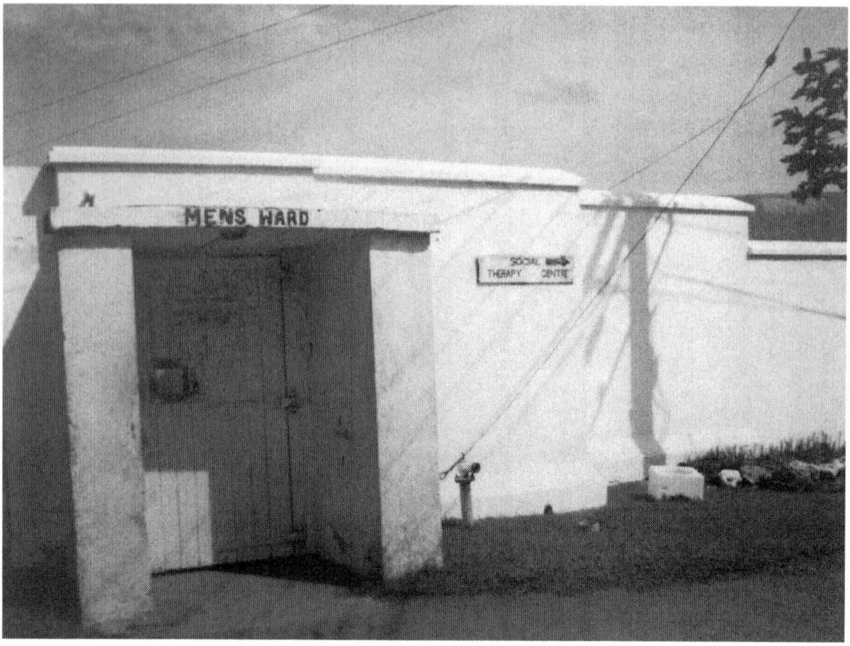

Figure 4.1. Men's ward, St Giles Hospital, 2002. Source: Author.

Gender remains the principal spatial demarcation for patients at St Giles.[15] This divide superseded the severity and categorization of mental conditions and, in the past, even racial locations. Initially, the need for gendered spaces threatened colonial racial hierarchies.[16] In 1892, a Fijian woman had to be confined in the European women's building "to save her from annoyance and physical danger caused by the male Indians and Fijians. This can only be done at the risk of the Europeans."[17] During the asylum's early years, inadequate resources made it difficult to sustain both gendered and racial boundaries. In 1914, the Board of Visitors complained about natives' being accommodated with Europeans overnight: "Native female patients in the female European Ward owing to insufficient accommodation could not under any circumstances be justified."[18] The increasing number of patients also necessitated native males sometimes sleeping in the male European quarters.[19]

Despite such racial discrepancies, racial boundaries were maintained with separate wards for European men, European women, native men, and native women throughout most of St Giles's colonial history. Natives included all non-Europeans (that is, Indo-Fijians, indigenous Fijians, other Pacific peoples, and other Asians). "Half-castes," who by the 1960s were termed "Part-Europeans," and today Kailoma, disrupted precise assignment to bureaucratic racial categories within the mental hospital. Some half-castes were accommodated with Europeans, and family connections were possibly decisive in allocating beds. Nancy, of European and Polynesian descent, was a patient at the mental hospital between 1934 and 1936 after she was diagnosed with mania following childbirth. Her husband pleaded for her release because "she is amongs[t] Indian Fijian Lunatics that is only making her worse."[20]

During the early twentieth century, separate wards were established according to gender and race. In 1906, a female "side," enclosed within a fence, was established.[21] By 1910, European wards had been established as well.[22] The European women's ward, which closed in 1962, had a separate entrance from the asylum's main entrance and was located away from the men's wards. Between the two was the native women's ward. Regulations also determined the style of accommodation and clothing according to race and gender. In 1914, Europeans were provided with considerably more clothing than natives, with separate clothing for day and night wear as well as shoes, socks, or stockings (see figure 4.2). Native women patients were allocated cloth to make jackets and *sulus*. It is unclear what clothing Indian women were expected to wear in the asylum. Native men were supposed to be issued with *sulus* and jumpers; in 1914, however, the Board of Visitors found that Indian men were often provided only with a loincloth, which was "totally insufficient."[23] Native patients were allocated blankets; Europeans, however, were also supplied with a mosquito net, pillows, sheets, mattress, and towels.[24] For several years, only Europeans had beds; natives were provided with mattresses that had been previously used by Europeans.[25] The number of mattresses available was inadequate and mattresses were often in appalling condition.[26]

Racial distinctions were initially reproduced through separate diets for Europeans, Fijians and Polynesians, and Indians. These diets differed with respect to quantity and content, but non-European diets could be especially monotonous.

Schedule of Diets, Public Lunatic Asylum, Fiji 1885:

Europeans

Breakfast: Bread 6 oz, butter 1/2 oz; Oatmeal 20 oz, or salt fish 2 oz, or bacon, 2 oz.
Cocoa, coffee, or tea, 1 pint; Sugar, milk.
Dinner: Soup 1/2 pint, vegetable 12 oz, fresh meat 5 oz, or salt meat 4 oz.
Bread 4 oz, water 1 pint; Cheese 1 oz.

Supper: Bread 8 oz, butter 1/2 oz or jam 1 1/2 oz; Tea 3/4 pint. Milk and sugar.
Additional: Salt, *ad lib,* Pepper 3/4 oz weekly. Ripe fruit occasionally at breakfast. Tomatoes and garden produce from asylum grounds.

Fijians and Polynesians

Breakfast: Yams 2 lbs or bread 8 oz or dalo 2 lbs or rice 3/4 lb; Coconuts 1 oz or sugar 1 oz or butter 1/2 oz; Tea with milk and sugar 3/4 pint.
Dinner: Same as breakfast with 4 oz fresh meat 5 oz; or 3 oz salt meat added. No tea.
Supper: Same as breakfast.
Additional: Salt, *ad lib,* Ripe bananas occasionally. Cooked bananas twice a week instead of yams or when the latter are unobtainable.

Indians

Breakfast: Rice 8 oz; mutton or salt fish 2 oz; Dhal 2 oz, curry 1/3 oz, ghee 1 oz, beans or tomatoes etc. from asylum grounds.
Dinner: Same as breakfast
Supper: Same but without meat or fish and 3/4 pint tea with sugar.
Additional: Salt, *ad lib,* Ripe bananas occasionally. Cooked bananas twice a week instead of yams or when the latter are unobtainable.[27]

In December 1887, diets were formalized according to two classes, which equated to the different fees levied on patients that usually corresponded to racial categories.[28] A first-class diet contained high proportions of fresh meat, dairy products, and carbohydrates, jam, milk, coffee, cocoa, or tea; the second-class diet was based more on carbohydrates, such as yams, taro, *kumala,* bread, and rice that included small quantities of beef or fish. In practice, these diets varied depending on the availability and cost of food and supplies, the number of patients, and the superintendent's prerogative to approve special diets. In 1914, the Board of Visitors condemned the practice of substituting more expensive yams or taro for bananas in the diets of native patients.[29]

Work and occupational therapy further reproduced gender and racial stereotypes. Men and some women worked in the food gardens, and by 1938 flower cultivation was a task for female patients, including some Europeans. That year, the female patients also remade the mattresses in the native female ward, sewed dresses for the patients, and wove Samoan baskets and fans.[30] Both female and

SCALE OF CLOTHING AND BEDDING, PUBLIC LUNATIC ASYLUM PATIENTS.

EUROPEAN MALE PATIENTS.

	£	s.	d.
6 Day Suits (coat and trousers), 36 yds. Scotch twill, at 9d.	£1	7	0
2 Night Suits (coat and trousers), 12 yds. striped twill, at 8d.	0	8	0
6 pairs Shoes, Canvas, at 3s.	0	18	0
6 pairs Socks, at 1s. 6d.	0	9	0
2 Blankets, at 4s. 10d	0	9	8
1 Mosquito Net	0	13	0
2 Pillows, at 3s. 5d.	0	6	10
4 Sheets, at 1s. 10d. yd. (6 yds.)	0	11	0
1 Mattress (fibre)	1	5	0
4 Towels, at 2s.	0	8	0
Total	£6	15	6

EUROPEAN FEMALE PATIENTS.

	£	s.	d.
6 Dresses, 36 yds. Scotch twill, at 9d.	£1	7	0
6 Undercloths, 18 yds. longcloth at 11½d.	0	17	3
6 Pairs Shoes, at 3s.	0	18	0
6 Pairs Stockings, at 2s.	0	12	0
4 Suits Night-clothes, 16 yds. longcloth, at 11½d.	0	15	4
2 Blankets, at 4s. 10d.	0	9	8
1 Mosquito Net	0	13	0
2 Pillows, at 3s. 5d.	0	6	10
4 Sheets, 6 yds. sheeting, at 1s. 10d.	0	11	0
1 Mattress (fibre)	1	5	0
4 Towels, at 2s.	0	8	0
Total	£8	3	1

NATIVE MALE PATIENTS.

	£	s.	d.
6 Sulus, 12 yds. Scotch twill, at 9d.	£0	9	0
2 Blankets, at 4s. 10d.	0	9	8
4 Jumpe s, 12yds. Scotch twill, at 9d	0	9	0
Total	£1	7	8

NATIVE FEMALE PATIENTS.

	£	s.	d.
6 Suits (jacket and sulu), 30 yds. Scotch twill, at 9d.	£1	2	6
2 Blankets, at 4s. 10d.	0	9	8
Total	£1	12	2

Approved,

BICKHAM ESCOTT,
Governor.

13th July, 1914.
M.P. 3839 14.

SCALE OF CLOTHING, PUBLIC LUNATIC ASYLUM STAFF.

RESIDENT FEMALE EUROPEAN ATTENDANT.

	£	s.	d.
8 Uniform Dresses, 48 yds. of longcloth, at 11½d.	£2	6	0

SENIOR NATIVE ATTENDANT.

	£	s.	d.
1 Suit (coat and sulu), serge, 4 yds. at 10s.	£2	0	0
2 Suits (coat), white duck, 8 yds. at 1s. 5d.	0	11	4
Sulu, longcloth, 8 yds. at 11½d.	0	7	8
Total	£2	18	0

NATIVE MALE ATTENDANTS.

	£	s.	d.
4 Suits (coat and sulu), 32 yds., striped, at 8d.	£1	1	4
12 Silver Buttons, large, at 2½d	0	2	6
4 Silver Buttons, small, at 2½d.	0	0	9
Total	£1	4	7

NATIVE FEMALE ATTENDANTS.

	£	s.	d.
4 Suits (jacket and sulu), 32 yds. striped, at 8d.	£1	1	4

TOTALS.

	£	s.	d.
1 Resident Female European Attendant	£2	6	0
1 Senior Native Attendant	2	18	0
6 Native Male Attendants	7	7	6
5 Native Female Attendants	5	6	8
Total	£17	18	2

Approved,

BICKHAM ESCOTT,
Governor.

13th July, 1914.
M.P. 3839/14.

Figure 4.2. Scales of clothing and bedding, Public Lunatic Asylum patients and staff, 1914. Source: CSO MP 6232/14, NAF.

male patients cleaned for patients and staff. Occasionally, some men performed more skilled work, such as painting, building, and tailoring. These patients included Europeans, who were not expected to do gardening or cleaning tasks. European women could participate in appropriate feminine activities, such as needlework, reading, or playing cards. The resumption of gendered and ethnic-appropriate activities was considered therapeutic and indicative of recovery. As Coleborne found in colonial Australia, work indicated the restoration of femininity.[31] This is noted in the record of Mrs. J.'s progress in 1896:

> [She] seems to be bright and cheerful, was employed in sweeping her room out . . . Actively employed yesterday (by her own request) in assisting the female attendant, in hanging out the Asylum washing . . . still doing well, went for a walk in the Gardens on Saturday, and again yesterday; reads a good deal now.[32]

The asylum's infrastructure defined gender, race, and class boundaries not only for patients but also for staff, setting different accommodation, diet, clothing, pay scales, responsibilities, and spaces for male and female doctors, male and female European and native attendants, and male and female servants. The 1914 regulations stated that "male attendants and servants [are] not to enter compound or wards of female patients except under order of head attendant." In 1952, a Fijian male and a Fijian female attendant were dismissed because they were found in a European compound.[33]

Gendered Patterns of Mental Distress

Feminist literature highlighted links between women and mental illness, but historians have shown that female committal rates to asylums, especially colonial asylums, were not always as high as men's.[34] This difference was true of St Giles, where women made up between 20 to 35 percent of admissions until 1948. In Fiji, the gender gap gradually closed after World War II when Fiji was still a colony. Equal gendered admission rates were almost reached by 1960 (see figure 4.3). After 1904, Indo-Fijian women made up a significantly higher percentage of total female admissions than female patients of other ethnicities, peaking during 1914 to 1923, when 68 percent of female admissions were Indo-Fijians (see table 4.1). During this period, many Indo-Fijians were admitted as destitutes (see chapter 2). Although twice as many Indo-Fijian men (140) than women (seventy) were admitted to the asylum, Indo-Fijian women made up a higher percentage of all female admissions than Indo-Fijian men did of male admissions.

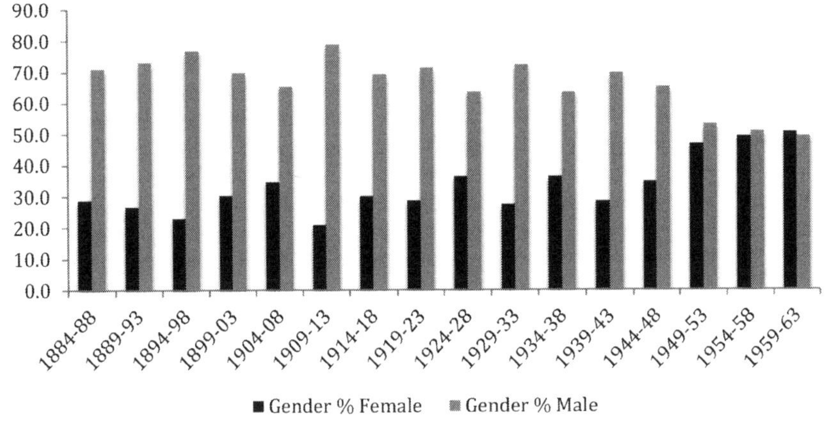

Figure 4.3. Gender as a percentage of total admissions to St Giles, 1884–1963. Patient data incomplete. Source: Author's database from patients' admission papers, St Giles Hospital, *Blue Book of Fiji,* Mental Hospital Register.

Table 4.1. Female admissions to St Giles

Years	Total					Percentage			
	Total	Fijian	Indian	European	Others	Fijian	Indian	European	Others
1884–1893	24	9	9	2	4	37.5	37.5	8.3	16.7
1894–1903	32	16	8	6	2	50.0	25.0	18.8	6.3
1904–1913	47	16	20	9	2	34.0	42.6	19.1	4.3
1914–1923	103	26	70	5	2	25.2	68.0	4.9	1.9
1924–1933	90	26	56	4	4	28.9	62.2	4.4	4.4
1934–1943	114	30	62	4	18	26.3	54.4	3.5	15.8
1944–1953	187	46	102	16	23	24.6	54.5	8.6	12.3
1954–1963	554	136	356	14	48	24.5	64.3	2.5	8.7

Source: Author's database from patients' admission papers, St Giles Hospital, *Blue Book of Fiji,* Mental Hospital Register.
Note: Patient data incomplete. These are repeat admissions.

Mortality patterns also indicate some gendered differences. As would be expected, when more men than women were admitted, they usually also made up a higher proportion of asylum deaths. With the exception of the years between 1909 and 1918, men were far more likely than women to die in the asylum than be discharged.[35] Some women may have suffered fewer terminal physical illnesses than men or have already received medical care if their insanity was linked with childbirth. Possibly most significant in explaining the higher mortality rate for men in the asylum was the tendency to discharge women earlier if they were wives and caregivers. Mrs. J.'s husband wrote a letter requesting her discharge two months after her admission in 1896. She was released the same day. When she was readmitted in 1905 as a widow, however, she remained there until her death in 1909.

Gendered and ethnic patterns also intersected with age. Older single women could spend much of their lives in the asylum. May, a European, and former nursemaid, was committed to the asylum in 1901 at the age of twenty-nine, ostensibly for "taking too many Williams Pink Pills."[36] These pills were unlikely to have caused her delusions, which included

> frequent conversations with the Prince of Wales, Duke of York & many others who tell her many obviously untrue stories; that all her relatives either shot or hung and that some have come to life again; that all the officers of the Royal Watch are all in Hell & looked after by her relatives who are also there . . . hears voices from monsters telling her that she is poisoned; says Governor Sir William Allardyce says she is to receive 6 years imprisonment or become the slave of a master; voices have told her that the Officers of the ______ and the Duke of York have ordered all the people in the town to be murdered, especially her mother and sister.

May's mother, a "needlewoman," signed her daughter's admission form. May remained at the asylum for thirty-five years, during which time her family never visited.

By World War II, St Giles had an increasing number of young patients. Before then, in 1928, a ten-year-old Indian child was admitted to the asylum as a congenital idiot. Five years later, Salefai, the night wardress, found the child dead in a cell.[37] The autopsy revealed that she had died from congenital heart disease. After the war, the increase in the number of young patients being admitted was notable, at least twenty-five, mostly Indo-Fijian females, age sixteen and younger, between 1947 and 1962. Their conditions included paranoia, schizophrenia, idiocy, and hysteria.[38] The average age of these patients was thirteen, possibly indicative of puberty. A doctor suggested that the cause of a fifteen-year-old Indo-Fijian's "imbecilic" and "childish" behavior and her attempts to assault other village children was "probably only a temporary puberty mental upset" that "would improve with proper care in an institution."[39] Attempts to treat her with electroconvulsive therapy failed and she lay in a fetal position for many years, recorded as being difficult to bathe and feed. In 2001, forty-eight years after being admitted, she died.

Parents may have worried that mentally subnormal girls were vulnerable to sexual abuse and could become pregnant. Amelia's mother had her thirteen-year-old daughter admitted to the asylum in 1960 because she was "moronic, cannot answer simple questions, doesn't know her name or age."[40] Her mother reported, "she has been a backward child, now wanders at large, doesn't want to wear clothes, cannot feed herself." Young women with obvious mental disorders were unlikely to marry, and for Indo-Fijians this could have implications for their siblings who negotiated suitable marriages. Unmarried adult women were a burden to their families, especially if they were unable to contribute to family labor.

Gendering Madness Discourse

Lay and professional categorization and diagnoses of mental illness at St Giles were grounded in cultural perceptions of appropriate gender identity and behavior as well as "the perception of emotional distress."[41] When doctors and magistrates filled out admission certificates to the asylum, they relied on family and community members for observations indicative of insanity.[42] Classification as insane was reproduced at several levels in Fiji and was discursively and subjectively framed—gender and ethnicity being threaded throughout—in different locations. As Stephen Garton pointed out, transgressions of feminine norms did not alone lead to psychiatric certification but depended on the material and social context and the community, which would decide that such behaviors could no longer be contained or tolerated.[43]

Both experts and family tended to link women's insanity with their emotional or reproductive lives. Early colonial debates attributed the rates of suicide and violence among *girmitiyas* to sexual jealousy (see chapter 2). In St Giles's records, however, relationships and sexuality were only occasionally cited as leading to men's insanity. One exception was a Fiji-born Tongan schoolteacher from Lomaloma committed to the asylum in 1895. The onset of his madness was attributed to his wife's infidelity, although the medical superintendent informed Lau's stipendiary magistrate that a medical examination revealed that the patient suffered from a cerebral disease and not insanity.[44] An Indo-Fijian male in 1940 was another exception. His mania and religious delusions were said to be caused because his "wife ran away" with their four children to live with another man. He also attempted to burn their house and threatened his wife and children.[45]

Unlike women's sexuality, men's was rarely judged on a moral basis, with the exception of a few cases of "masturbatory insanity," such as the diagnosis of an incoherent and delusional European male admitted from Levuka Gaol in 1885.[46] In this case, an earlier suicide attempt indicated other stresses.[47] In contrast to women's madness, men's madness were much more likely to be attributed to money or employment problems, organic illness, accidents, and substance abuse. Although money troubles were recorded as the cause of an Indo-Fijian woman's mental illness in 1936, this anxiety was considered delusional, as were her claims that that she was being impoverished and starved by her children.[48] Common causes of insanity among men and women were old age and physical illness. Men were far more likely than women to suffer from general paralysis of the insane (GPI): 84 percent of GPI sufferers between 1884 and 1940 were male. This gendered pattern reflected global epidemiology.[49]

Love, infidelity, jealousy, "matrimonial unhappiness," or "domestic troubles" apparently drove women (more than men) insane—not just metaphorically but for some into the asylum.[50] In 1928, Asenaca's "derangement of mind" was attributed to her stepmother's persistence in arranging a marriage for the eighteen-year-old with an "undesired suitor."[51] Being abandoned by a partner was much more likely to be cited as causal in women's insanity than men's. It is probable that illness contributed to the decision by one partner to leave, but records suggest that a husband was more likely to desert his mentally ill wife than vice versa. A few ex-indentured Indians returned to India, leaving behind their mentally ill wives. This happened to one patient in 1929, and her delusions, suicidal ideation, violence toward others, and lack of personal care were said to be due to being deserted.[52] Yet men of all ethnicities permanently distanced themselves from their wives—whether by emigration, divorce, or physically and emotionally removing themselves—and this abandonment was cited as the cause of the women's illnesses. The melancholia of Ro, a woman of Fijian chiefly status, was linked to her husband's leaving her eighteen months prior to her admission to the asylum in 1892.[53] The district constable reported that she had become severely withdrawn, "when she speaks it is only with impressions spontaneously developed in her mind and not from any resulting out of the remarks of other persons." The doctor observed,

> Persistent silence when addressed in ordinary conversation, whether by myself, or by her friend or by other natives. Neglect of her person and clothing. Frequent changes of expression of countenance as if in obedience to alternating trains of thought but yet no speech accompanying them. Quasi cataleptic attitudes.

The constable revealed the reason for her husband's leaving her. Ro was said to have drowned her child, though her admission papers do not mention infanticide. This case shows the complexities of attributing desertion as a cause or an outcome of mental illness, but the more frequent citing of desertion on women's, rather than men's, certification papers indicates how etiology could be gendered.

In other cases, domestic issues were given as the cause of a woman's mental distress, but such reasons often masked complex stresses in women's lives in the colonial Pacific. One of the few indentured women laborers from Ulawa in the Solomon Islands was committed as a lunatic in 1901 due to "jealousy and domestic troubles." To escape these pressures and her employer, she stowed away on a boat sailing from Levuka to Suva. On arrival in Suva, she was confined in the immigration depot but managed to escape. Her anguish was such that she claimed people were trying to hang her, and she threatened to hang herself.[54] Later, in 1956, a twenty-six-year-old woman was admitted to St Giles because of the break-up of a domestic relationship. Diagnoses of catatonic schizophrenia to manic depression show that her mental disorder was severe. She attempted suicide several times during her admissions to St Giles between 1956 and 1987.

Relatives noted changes in behavior and the transgression of cultural, class, and gendered norms as evidence of mental instability.[55] This could include that of personal appearance. Among the evidence of a European male patient's bizarre behavior was neglecting to wear a hat when wandering "aimlessly about . . . addressing people familiarly with whom he should have no business or social connections."[56] In 1943, a European woman admitted her husband, an accountant, to the asylum, saying that he "went to work without shaving for the first time."[57] More extreme in transgressing masculine norms was a twenty-year-old male Indo-Fijian cultivator admitted by his brother in 1948; he dressed in tattered clothes and emulated a female by applying lipstick and rouge.[58] Despite these cases and relative to women's, men's embodied gendered norms were rarely mentioned.

Mad women in Fiji disrupted civilized behavior and, possibly more so, feminine norms in all cultures. Dishevelment, lack of control, sexuality, excessive mobility, and violence were all signs of madness, but appearance and comportment especially embodied it for women. Nudity in public spaces was an extreme form of madness. When a female Indo-Fijian was committed to the asylum from a copra estate in Taveuni in 1925, evidence provided of her insanity included her disruption of feminine norms and nudity. She was

> restless, loquacious, continual gesticulation; continuously in an insane manner; apparently no regard for her femininity; general demeanour

> that of a lunatic . . . runs about without clothes; throws away husband's food; burns her husband's clothes; fights with other women in the lines; has attacked another woman with a knife.[59]

Madness was defined in relation not only to gender but also to ethnic stereotypes and transgressions, and such evidence was primarily cast as observations about embodied appearance and behavior. In 1920, an admission certificate for an Indian woman cited as evidence of her melancholia and insanity that she was clothed "not in accordance with the custom of Indian women."[60] Several observations confirming the insanity of indigenous Fijian women stressed transgressions of the norms of gendered and ethnic appearance and behavior (*vakamarama,* "to behave like a lady at all times"), as in 1915, when a Fijian woman was considered by a doctor to have dirty habits in a way "unusual among Fijians."[61] His assessment was based on evidence supplied by a native medical practitioner and a police officer: "for a long time in her village she has been filthy in her habits, has been stealing trifles from numerous houses, and at times goes about naked."[62] When Dr. Harper was medical officer of the Lau Islands in 1917, he observed that the "general behaviour, especially head gestures," of a Fijian woman "express a boldness or sometimes lustfulness not usual in Fijians." The woman's initial conversation with the doctor concerned "her monthly periods . . . no normal Fijian woman mentions these unless asked or there is some corresponding disease." The Buli Lakeba had seen her attending church "with her clothes obviously soiled by her menstrual discharge." She had previously been briefly admitted to the asylum in 1911 after attempting to kill her child and trying to provoke a fight with another woman during a church service.[63]

Neglected Work

The neglect of work was a dominant trope in lay perceptions of insanity in colonial Fiji, especially when paid and unpaid roles were not fulfilled. Expectations of work roles were framed along gendered, ethnic, and class lines. The resumption of appropriate occupational activities—according to gender, ethnicity, and class—indicated recovery.

Assumptions about masculine work expectations were problematic in regard to indigenous Fijian men. Most were not waged workers, so their insanity could not simply be equated to the transgression of Eurocentric masculine notions of paid work. As discussed, Fijian villagers could still be chastised for being idle, and *girmitiyas* who refused to work were accused of "malingering." Yet European men who stopped working were clearly of "unsound mind," such as a plantation manager who bathed his head in a creek and prayed all day instead of working.

Women's aversion to domestic work and childcare dominates perceptions of their insanity, though work-role expectations were framed not only by gender but also by ethnicity. When Emily was admitted to the asylum for a second time in 1904, she had, her daughter stated, neglected domestic work for six months.[64] Emily, a European, was expected to care for her large family, including her sister Anne, who had been discharged from the asylum in 1901.[65] Both sisters were re-admitted several times and eventually died in the asylum. After her husband died, Emily remained in the hospital from 1905 until 1935; Anne's final period was from 1911 to 1924.

Indo-Fijian men also complained about women neglecting their housework, and dereliction remained a prominent indicator of mental disorder. In Manibai's admission papers in 1943, her husband observed that "[she does] not attend to the house but stays outside under the trees or goes out shouting on the road."[66] In 1964, Nalini was admitted to St Giles during her sixth pregnancy. According to her husband, her illness began seven years earlier when she was also pregnant and refused to complete domestic chores. She threw her gold bangles into cow dung—a possible repudiation of her identity as a wife.[67]

Even when women engaged in serious acts of violence, their transgressions in everyday domestic duties still substantiated their insanity. When a Fijian missionary's wife returned from New Guinea in 1893, she was "frequently violent with peculiar animosity against her husband. Threw her child down some time ago and thereby has injured its spine . . . Took a quantity of cooked and prepared food and threw it out to the fowls."[68] Myesha, diagnosed as a schizophrenic in 1950, also exhibited bizarre cooking habits. She had "killed her poultry without reason" then cooked it with the feathers still on; in another basin, she mixed together unpeeled potatoes, rice, unshelled eggs, and oil. When her family objected to this, Myesha chased them with a knife and tried to set the house on fire.[69]

Immorality

When a twenty-five-year-old Fijian woman from Bau was admitted to the asylum in 1896 she was judged by villagers as having led "a loose and immoral life to excess lately," exhibiting "indecent behaviour, frequently exposing herself and using indecent language in her *mekes*."[70] Several texts incorporate other villagers' complaints of mad women behaving "extravagantly" and "indecently" and "desiring connection" with men. Women's virtue and controlled sexuality was central to Hindu and Muslim discourses and Indo-Fijian identities. Lay discourse on sexuality and immorality cut through all ethnicities and community assessments of women's insanity in Fiji. When a ten-year-old Indian child was admitted to the asylum as a congenital idiot, her irrational behavior included her "sexual actions."[71]

Sexuality was a powerful marker of colonized subject locations and the colonial hierarchy.[72] Mad Europeans, especially women, disrupted this order, especially when they flagrantly violated sexual and other norms. Descriptions of their sexual delusions or fantasies were abundant. The content of delusions, whether "rational" or not, deserves attention because this may open a window into past events, such as sexual abuse (see chapter 5). Notes concerning fifty-five-year-old Mrs. J. were preoccupied with her sexuality:

> obscene delusions—her language being incessantly filthy and unrestrained and always on the subject of sex and sexuality . . . said Governor asked to have her killed, that last night several lights turned on her, fired at with electricity by several people whom she had previously seen cutting out a girl's womb.

These graphic descriptions of Mrs. J.'s sexuality may have reflected the positioning of racialized and gendered sexualities: European doctors were shocked by the intensity of a European woman's embodied sexuality and sexual delusions, but often stereotyped Fijian and Indian women as sexually promiscuous. Details of the sexuality of European women were more likely to be recorded because the patients, doctors, and family all spoke English as a first language and thus did not need an interpreter (who were usually male). It is possible that an interpreter may have censored content and language they considered obscene when passing on information to European doctors.

The records of sisters Anne and Emily include examples of European women's obscenities. Emily had "delusions of a sexual behaviour, erotic statements. A man has gone to the colonies & a subscription should be raised to bring him to her." She claimed that she was totally mad because of this other man.[73] She later reiterated that two years previously she had

> coitus with a man who has since left Fiji, act was not properly consummated, led to flow of blood which has led to continuous distress; firmly believes that can't be cured except by completion of coitus with the man.

The doctor assessed this story as a sexual delusion, noting that Emily "is ready to tell it to whoever would listen."[74] Her sister Anne's admission notes in 1906 recorded that "nearly all her conversation is directed to such matters as rape, prostitution, adultery etc." By 1908, Anne was a resident of Cottage House, but the matron complained of Anne's violence. When Anne was readmitted to the asylum in 1909, the matron also reported that Anne "frequently talked erotically using foul language."[75]

Legal and medical authorities correlated the insanity of some women with prostitution. The term "prostitute" was ambiguous and could refer to "fallen," "stroppy," or assertive women as well as those with more than one sexual partner.[76] This chapter opened with references to some female *girmitiyas* who turned to prostitution as a livelihood. Complex circumstances were behind this change: some women may have found that sex work offered more autonomy and a better income than plantation work; others may have been pressured into sex work by violence and abusive relationships. The marital status of Indian women is indeterminate on medical records because many women were recorded as single even though they were in a de facto marriage. Jashomati was age sixteen and pregnant when she arrived in Fiji as a laborer on the *Hereford* in 1888. For many years, she cared for her son. She assumed another name and at various times was apprehended by the police. In 1902, she was admitted to the asylum, "constantly guilty of acts of shameless prostitution indiscriminately." She declared with "extreme volubility" that people wanted to kill her and her son.[77] She had been admitted as unmarried but she was discharged into her husband's care and was readmitted as married in 1905, still claiming that a man was trying to find and murder her; the doctor, though, dismissed this as "delusions of persecution."[78] She died five years later in the asylum.

In 1889, a seventeen-year-old Fijian was admitted from Naitasiri District with severe mental distress having attempted to kill her child. Found sitting in the doorway of her house "dirty, emaciated and apparently indifferent to all going on around her," she was taken from her village to Nadurulolo, where Dr. Joseph Barnes observed her

> lying prone on the ground, knees doubled under her and the child underneath her chest in imminent danger of suffocation, showed great resistance to being raised & with "greatest difficulty" child taken; her privates were exposed, "thrust high in the air and covered with excrement"; when child removed threw herself on ground with hardly any covering & "exposed her person to the numerous spectators with the utmost unconcern", made a "dogged and sullen resistance" to anything done for her & remained squatting in mud and rain performing a series of "pantomime" gestures—no sound—until "forcibly" removed to female lockup.

Despite this extreme mental distress and illness, her mental disorder was simply listed as "remorse for leading life of abandoned prostitute." After six months in the asylum, she was discharged and married the child's father, considered "generally decent" in personal habits, but, suffering from "mania of pregnancy," was later readmitted to the asylum. Her child remained with her there until almost a year later, when she was discharged into the care of her father on Kadavu.[79]

Wandering Women

In 1898, the native commissioner signed the admission certificate for Saini, age twenty-two. Her insanity was attributed to seduction. She had the

> habit of smiling inanely, sprawling on floor in unseemly way on public verandah, not seeming to know "other than seemly"; sings at inopportune times . . . wanders at night in and out of people's houses without purpose when she ought "by the customs of native propriety" be at home with parents; easily excited and angered; came over to Suva without leave and fell into the hands of the Police as being insane.[80]

These notes tell us more about Saini's movements than her seduction, but the focus is on her embodied madness, uncontrollable, unpredictable movements, and violation of cultural and physical boundaries. Gender is inflected within many reports of wanderers, in which women's mobility was linked more with their sexuality.

As in other colonies, the mobility of non-European subjects was regulated in Fiji, and this regulation applied more to women than men. Saini's case highlights how these colonial restrictions applied to indigenous Fijians, particularly women. Women were required to live in their *koro* (village), a restriction enshrined not only in colonial but also in native regulations. During the 1920s, the Great Council of Chiefs stipulated that Fijian women needed the *buli*'s consent if they were away from their villages for more than twenty-eight days.[81] Similarly, penal sanctions bound Indo-Fijian women and men to their workplaces. As we saw in chapter 2, colonial authorities considered former *girmitiyas* who became vagrants and unable to care for themselves as problems. In 1897, Chotki wandered around Ba province and was found lying on the ground in a filthy condition, refusing to eat and unable to "give an intelligible account of herself." She had been an indentured laborer but had no family in Fiji. Chotki was admitted to the asylum for seven days, but the superintendent was unable to certify her insanity.[82]

Cultural and religious values further restricted women's mobility.[83] The spatial movements and appropriate gendered activities of indigenous Fijian women were demarcated by customary authority of males over females, Christianity, and chiefly authority over commoners.[84] The sanctity of the family was strengthened with the reconstitution of Indo-Fijian identity during post-indenture years. Instead of Indian women being constructed as "whores," the colonial imagination now constructed them as the "world's best mothers."[85] Female virtue was pivotal, and family honor was linked with *purdah* (seclusion and modesty) and women's fulfilling their *dharma* (duty and roles).[86] These restrictions militated against women's participation in public activities and their mobility outside the home. Anthropologist Sue Carswell observed that Indo-Fijian women in a rural cane-farming community in Vanua Levu during the 1990s still needed their husband's consent to leave the home and that gossip censured a woman who was seen "rushing here and there."[87] Myesha's bizarre cooking habits have already been outlined, but she was also considered "unbalanced" because her husband said she was "wandering around house and town without any purpose," activity that included climbing trees.

Indigenous and Indo-Fijian women who transgressed spatial boundaries threatened moral as well as colonial order. Women's spatial and social restrictions changed during Fiji's colonial period, especially as women negotiated these restrictions. Other mediating factors may have been class and rural or urban locations. Women who crossed formal or informal spatial boundaries could be arrested, and if they exhibited other bizarre behavior, then such vagrancy rendered them liable to having their sanity reviewed by legal and medical authorities. Despite the weight of colonial strictures, the most frequent complaints came from husbands and families when women absented themselves from their domestic spaces. In 1940, nineteen-year-old Indrani was admitted from Nasinu near Suva. She was pregnant, and it was said "that she is constantly running away from her home and children neglecting her duties." She was discharged after seven months but readmitted three years later from the Women's Hospital in Toorak in a very weak condition. When she died two months after that, no relatives were known and two asylum warders were the only witnesses at her burial.[88]

Violent Women and Troubled Lives

Imaginaries of madness have evoked the violent subject, although many people designated insane have not displayed violence. The tragedy of madness and violence is that they provoke questions of why and when society decrees certain types of violence as not only criminal but also irrational or mad. The St Giles archive indicates that though communities and the law set boundaries concerning violence, the boundaries included gendered differences, which had implications for evidence of madness. Very little testimony commented on men swearing or using violent language, but when women were designated insane, their abusive language was recorded. This gendered difference crossed all classes and ethnicities and is constant throughout St Giles's records. In 1919, the superintendent of a plantation hospital observed a female *girmitiya* "talking loudly and foolishly and suddenly using foul & abusive language without cause . . . uses obscene expressions. Wild, rambling, incoherent statements."[89] Similarly, in 1953, an Indo-Fijian woman from a middle-class background was admitted who used "vile and filthy language."[90]

The ultimate rejection of feminine roles was a mother's violent repudiation of her children. In 1886, while her husband was at work at Rarawai Mill in Ba, Eliza attempted to cut off the head of her infant with a dinner knife. The following night she left the house and was found by her husband in the early morning standing at the river's edge with the child in her arms. Eliza had also tried to burn down their house and attack her husband with a knife. Her husband said that he sometimes had to prevent her physically from leaving the house. Eliza was discharged two and a half months after her admission to the asylum. Such relatively short admissions were common among mothers of young children. Eliza had formerly been a patient at Auckland Mental Hospital and was readmitted there in 1900.[91]

Emily also knocked her children about, "caressing them over roughly and squeezing throats so that they cried out," and threatened to cut herself with a knife. Her delusions of violence were caught up in her domestic world; she believed that she had poisoned herself by mistakenly consuming some unidentified powder instead of baking powder and then taking boracic acid to counter the effects of this poison. She also thought her husband and children had swallowed the poison. Her sister Anne threatened their mother, Emily's family, other family members, and residents at Cottage House with axes, knives, and stones. Anne accused her mother of murdering her children, a Mr. Singh of shooting her brother, a brother-in-law of killing her other brother and her sister's child, and a Fijian of poisoning her niece. She claimed to have killed and buried the wife of the police superintendent. Anne and Emily were members of a large European family in Fiji and kin tried to care for them, despite their imagined, threatened, and actual violence. The family was not wealthy, and a brother who was diagnosed as mentally ill compounded family tensions.

As noted earlier in Lani's story at the beginning of this chapter, women's madness was infused with sexuality, work, wandering, and their violence—and the violence and stress women endured in Fiji. Lynette Jackson's study of patients at Ingutsheni Mental Hospital in colonial Zimbabwe suggested that many African women who came to the attention of state authorities were "women interrupted" who had probable reasons for leaving their homes, including fleeing victimization.[92] In Fiji, women's delusions were recorded as indications of their madness, and, as Emily's and Anne's records depict, these were replete with delusions of violence. Little veracity is attached to Anne's accusations, but other women's narratives at St Giles are suggestive of the violent and troubled lives many women in Fiji endured.

The violence of indenture for female *girmitiyas* was compounded by lower pay rates than men and abuse from male workers and Indian and European overseers. When some women reported violence or economic deprivation, their complaints could be dismissed as delusional on the basis of their manic behavior. Deeti was admitted to the asylum in 1905 from Nausori Hospital. She was extremely physically and verbally violent, filthy, destroyed her clothes, and left the hospital to return to the plantation "lines," where she threatened to burn down her house and kill her infant child by placing it under a moving cane truck. Deeti said that "someone was hiding her money," but the hospital superintendent dismissed this report as delusional. Her accusation was plausible given the economic hardship most *girmitiyas* faced.[93] Similarly, in 1912, another female *girmitiya* admitted to the asylum counted sticks and said they were money. When she sobbed "that her *sahib* and *sirdar* beat her and get angry with her," the doctor rejected her accusations as delusions of persecution.[94] Totaram Sanadhya reported how Narayani's insanity was caused by an overseer who beat her horrifically. "This poor woman was beaten so much that her mind went bad, and until now she has stayed crazy." Her illness may also have been caused by the death of her newborn baby. The overseer had ordered her to resume work, but she had refused because regulations stipulated that a mother should not return to work until three months after the birth. The overseer was still found not guilty of any offense.[95]

Dukhni's case in 1921 indicates the violence and stress Indo-Fijian women experienced outside the plantation system. On admission to the asylum, she put her age at sixty though she was only thirty-three. She had suffered from mania "since meeting her husband 18 years ago . . . Imagines her husband continually wishing to assault her." A police officer stated that Dukhni had made several false reports of assaults. Immediately prior to her committal to the asylum, she went to "the police station with a knife saying if police couldn't find her somewhere to stay away from home she would chop up her husband." Her only record of actual violence is when she attempted to hang herself.[96]

Later records reiterate probable tensions behind mad women's violence, though the veracity of their claims was often doubted and their accusations considered delusional. By World War II, an increasing number of women were admitted as private patients; their violence and madness were attributed to "delusional jealousy." In 1941, a police officer's wife tried to choke her husband and son. She accused her husband of infidelity, and, though this claim was considered delusional, her insanity was attributed to "mental derangement following domestic troubles."[97]

Women in Fiji, as elsewhere, experienced stress that exacerbated mental illness and increased the possibility of their inflicting violence on family. Some of these women were abused by their partners, kin, or employers, but as Stephen Garton found in colonial Australia, when mad women accused their husbands of abuse, doctors questioned the reality of the claims.[98] Abuse was not just physical. During the early 1960s, an Indo-Fijian woman was admitted to St Giles by her father. She had been depressed, unkind to her baby, and violent toward her two other sons. Behind this behavior lay considerable physical and psychological stress. The woman had no formal education and had married at the age of twenty. Two years later, she had given birth to a baby that died. After three years and without warning, her husband deserted her and their children to emigrate. She was diagnosed with general paralysis of the insane, indicative of tertiary-stage syphilis.[99]

Self-Harm

Women's violence could be self-directed, but during the indenture years the high suicide rate of Indo-Fijian men raised the most concern in Fiji. As emphasized in chapter 2, prominent factors involved in suicide were gender disparity and women's sexuality and the impact these had on men. Suicide and attempted suicide may have been precipitated by more generalized mental distress and mental illness, factors that tended to be overlooked or subsumed into references to melancholia.

Chapter 3 also revealed gendered assumptions about suicide among Fijians in colonial Fiji, sexual jealousy and women's disobedience being implicated in the causes of men's suicide. Acting Resident Commissioner J. K. M. Ross pronounced certainty over Jone's suicide in 1882: "Cause seems quite clear—Luisa sits in the house of one fisherman . . . she refuses to help her 'Wati' (Fijian husband) in cleaning his garden—whereon the latter shoots himself." Ostensibly the suicide was due to Jone's jealousy and Luisa's neglect of her wifely obligations.[100] A death inquiry a decade later was more explicit in attributing suicide to sexual jealousy:

> The reason for the suicide was the "jealousy" of the deceased on account of his wife running about with the other women, neglecting her household duties and also begging tobacco from various men.[101]

The stipendiary magistrate ruled that Mere's death in Nalawa District in Ra in 1894 was suicide and attributed this to an impulsive act rather than as a response to her husband, Tokalau, or the situation she found herself in as a new bride. He claimed that "the suicide can only be attributed to one of those extraordinary freaks that Fiji females occasionally indulge in." According to villagers' testimony, after the Turaga ni Mataqali (chief) ordered Mere to go to Tokalau's home to consummate the marriage, she hanged herself from a tree with a vine.[102] Are such reports of women committing or threatening suicide because they refused to live with their husbands "freakish" gestures or an expression of agency? We need to be cautious against exaggerating such agency but still recognize self-harm and suicide as "the desperate communication of the powerless."[103] Katrina Jaworski argues that such actions have tended to be dismissed or "articulated through the feminine character of emotional turmoil."[104]

On May 5, 1890, a female Fijian prisoner facing a death sentence stood on her slop bucket, tied her *sulu* to the cell's window bars, and hanged herself.[105] Yet, as explained, suicides were rare in the asylum, and no instances of women doing so are recorded. Attempted suicides were far more common, in both the asylum and the community. Many attempts were undocumented. Those that were received scant attention compared with suicides, which is in line with other findings about the invisibility of women and attempted suicide.[106] A few records indicate the connections between suicide, mental illness, and possibly physical illness. Amriti, a female *girmitiya,* was admitted to the asylum in 1890. She had been transferred from another hospital where she had attempted to hang herself with a lamp cord and to drown herself and had attacked a mother and infant as well. Amriti was seriously ill, "crouching on the ground, senseless chattering, agitation of the head and limbs, and muscular tremor."[107]

Outside the hospital, concern about women and underreported or "invisible" suicides began to be raised only during Fiji's postcolonial years, although evidence of a rising incidence of suicide among young Indo-Fijian women dates from at least the 1960s.[108] Suicides were underreported among invisible groups, such as rural Indo-Fijian women and elderly Indo-Fijian men.[109] When Issac Karim and John Price surveyed reported suicides in medical records between 1965 and 1972, they found an alarming suicide rate among Indo-Fijian women.[110] Suicide was associated with rural residence and being a young female with low status in the family. Many such vulnerable women were isolated from community and family support, and often married at a young age. In Macuata, between 1962 and 1968, nineteen of twenty-eight married women who killed themselves had married before the age of seventeen.[111] Suicide and attempted suicide among women was an embodied act that could be an extreme response to the particular social and structural oppression that women in Fiji might face. It could be associated with diagnosed mental illness, but, in many instances of suicide, such a connection was not reported. Suicide was also linked to women's bodies, such as when a female *girmitiya* killed herself at Lautoka Hospital in 1909:

> A few days prior to her death when in hospital her menstrual period came on, and this the Hospital Superintendent informed me often causes a depressed state of mind which might account in her case for her action in taking her own life.[112]

Reproduction and Madness

Medical records at St Giles frequently linked women's, but not men's, reproductive bodies with disordered minds. In psychiatry, the causation and treatment of madness has been associated with menstruation, pregnancy, childbirth, miscarriage, and menopause.[113] Henry Maudsley stated in 1873,

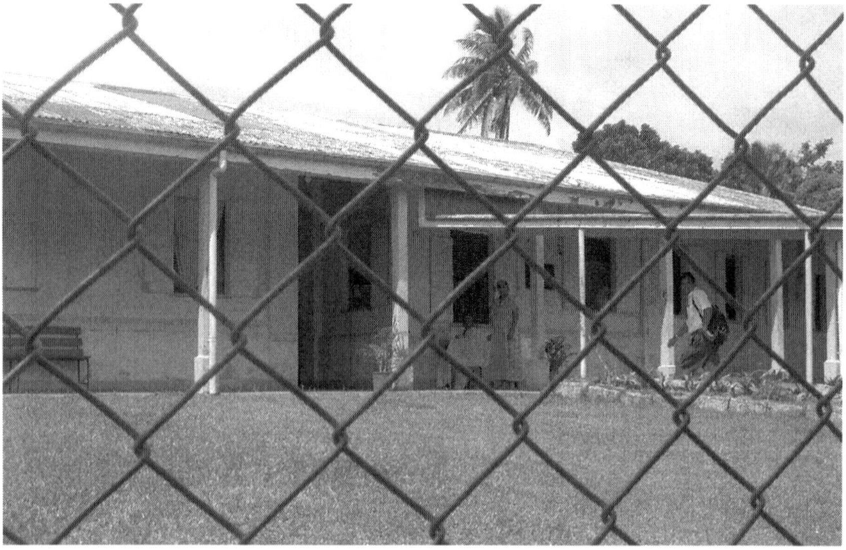

Figure 4.4. Women's ward, St Giles Hospital, 2002. Source: Author.

> The monthly activity of the ovaries which marks the advent of puberty in women has a notable effect upon the mind and body; wherefore it may become an important cause of mental and physical derangement. . . . .A sudden suppression of the menses has produced a direct explosion of insanity, or occurring some time before an outbreak it may be an important link in its causation.[114]

Maudsley's discourse on the female body was rejected.[115] The actual impact this had on medical practitioners is questionable.[116] Medical discourse and practice in colonial Fiji correlated women's biology with insanity. Women's menstrual patterns were scrutinized in the asylum, such as in these notes from 1914: "23 Sept S. (Indian female) very melancholic (menstruating) . . . 20 Oct S. very violent (menstruating)."[117] The outbreak of hysteria among schoolgirls at Qawa (discussed in chapter 2), was linked to women's reproduction and emotionality. Dr. Sell had never come across hysteria in boys and, like many doctors, believed that "the menarchal girl exposed to emotional tension is particularly at risk."[118]

Menopause was not considered an illness in indigenous and Indo-Fijian communities in Fiji.[119] This, though, did not inhibit doctors from attributing the onset of women's insanity to the "climacteric." Such assessments included a thirty-eight-year-old Indo-Fijian mother of nine, who was admitted in 1935 with manic-depressive insanity caused by the "change of life and cruelty," and a forty-five-year-old single Fijian villager from Lomaloma in Lau in 1921.[120] The older woman had attempted suicide, destroyed the walls of a house, thrown stones, stolen a canoe, and wandered around the island of Vanua Balavu.[121] Another Fijian villager with insanity ostensibly caused by the "climacteric" was a widow, diagnosed as an imbecile with manic depression.[122] In 1948, an affluent European woman was said to have manic depression caused by the "change of life." She was readmitted six times in the following decade.[123]

Although women's reproductive lives might have been considered causative of insanity, doctors usually diagnosed a gender-neutral condition, such as mania or manic depression. The exception to this rule was mental illness surrounding childbirth, categorized during the hospital's early years as mania of pregnancy, then for several decades as puerperal insanity, and later as postpartum psychosis or postpartum depression. Fijians regarded such illness as a form of *cavuka* (speaking nonsense or craziness); *na tadoka ni vasucu* (the flu of childbirth), associated with somatic symptoms of weakness and severe headaches, was usually less severe.[124] Sometimes women with puerperal mania might be delirious while running a puerperal fever.[125] Diagnoses of mental distress linked to the puerperium could be uncertain diagnoses, as shown in Devi's case history of throwing herself into a well in 1944. Both the cause of this action and the diagnosis were attributed to childbirth. She was later diagnosed with manic depression but in 1950 was readmitted with puerperal insanity. In 1954, she was again diagnosed with manic depression, a diagnosis that in 1963 was changed to paranoid schizophrenia.[126] The duration of the puerperal period was vague, usually lasting for six weeks after childbirth, but puerperal insanity could be linked to pregnancy, miscarriage, or lactation. Doctors sometimes applied this "convenient label" to mental disorders several years after the birth.[127] In 1882, a doctor suggested that Sukudaia's mania may have been linked to "extensive inflammation of the womb" and that "she may gradually improve, if not recover her reason."[128]

St Giles's early records replicate the reality of postpartum depression and psychosis common to psychiatric institutions worldwide. Between 1884 and 1936, approximately twenty-five admissions or twenty-one women had conditions attributed to puerperal insanity. This figure was around 10 percent of female patients, equivalent to comparable classifications in asylums elsewhere.[129] Outside Suva's asylum, many women were treated for postpartum complications, including depression and violent behavior, in their homes and communities. Indigenous Fijians and Indo-Fijians might follow a traditional healing approach. The wealthy hired private nurses or had mentally disturbed mothers treated outside Fiji. These were hardly options for poor women, including some European women in Fiji. One of the asylum's first patients, Annie, a European waitress from Nausori, admitted by her husband, was suffering from puerperal insanity. She was only twenty-one, but Dr. Patullo, the medical superintendent, reported that she had suffered two attacks of chorea and generally had had a hard life. She was suicidal, described as paranoid that violence was being inflicted upon her, and threatened violence against her husband. Annie spent a relatively short period of six weeks in the asylum, indicative of how doctors in the Victorian era optimistically expected that women with puerperal insanity could quickly recover.[130]

Women diagnosed with puerperal insanity in Fiji, as elsewhere, did not always have a "perfect recovery."[131] Two months after the birth of her child in 1898, Veniana, a twenty-two-year-old Fijian, was admitted to the asylum in a weak and emaciated condition; she was diagnosed with puerperal melancholia. Her husband reported that she "wanders; discards clothes; melancholy; refused to talk to anyone; complained devils after her; since birth refused to suckle child; won't have child near her and lost all interest in her; recently filthy habits in house." Veniana had been declared insane by a native medical practitioner and, on admission to the asylum, was noted as "melancholy, fixed fawnlike gaze, no particular purpose to it; stoops and bends incessantly and evinces tendency to remain in any position to which guided; won't speak . . . exhausted and drowsy." Veniana died forty-nine days later at the Colonial Hospital following emergency gynecological treatment and septicemia.[132] Physical recovery from childbirth was undoubtedly hindered by the asylum's inadequate sanitation, which sometimes resulted in septicemia, even death (see chapter 6).

Veniana's case reflects the precarious correlations between women's madness, their bodies, and surgical intervention. Women's biology was often considered causative of madness, so treatment could include gynecological surgery. Mrs. J. was admitted in 1896 suffering from "puerperal melancholia, with homicidal impulses." The chief medical officer later conducted a "special gynecological examination . . . as a knowledge of the sexual apparatus is essential to a proper radical treatment." He "found a condition which could be advantageously healed at the Colonial Hospital with a fair hope of success and of permanent cure of her mental irritability."[133] This treatment may have been a hysterectomy, indicating that surgery was considered a possible cure for puerperal insanity.

Doctors in Fiji advocated such surgery for some mentally ill women, to treat madness, to prevent further pregnancies, and to rectify painful and possibly life-threatening gynecological conditions. This intervention was not always followed through because of objections from patients or their husbands. In 1967, Dr. Macgregor urged the termination of a patient's pregnancy along with sterilization. If she refused, he recommended that her physician proceed with a D&C (a uterine scraping that would have precipitated an abortion) followed by the insertion of an intrauterine device for contraception. Macgregor feared "that she is in grave danger of a major schizophrenic breakdown," which she had earlier experienced after giving birth. He thought that this woman "minimizes her complaints because of morbid preoccupation with fear of having to have an operation."[134]

Conclusion

Gender is central to understanding mental disorders as well as to constructions, classifications, patterns, and treatments of madness. Gender underlies patterns of admission, discharge, and the care of insane patients in Fiji. Contrary to earlier feminist literature on women and madness, women did not have higher rates of admission to the asylum than men in Fiji, and neither was madness represented as a female malady there. Lay people and doctors located evidence of madness within a gendered framework, but in Fiji this reading intersected with ethnicity and, to a lesser extent, class and indigenous status. Among all ethnicities, gendered role expectations especially linked women's insanity to domestic life and work, and gendered assumptions were made about sexuality, violence, and spatial mobility.

This chapter has also focused on the pressures mentally ill women faced. Their underreported suicides and attempted suicides were further outcomes of this stress. Gender was prominent in the discursive framing and management of madness in colonial Fiji. But St Giles's records go beyond this. Sukudaia's and Lani's sketchy narratives reflect how women in Fiji from different ethnicities and living a century apart experienced similar poverty, physical and mental illness, violence, and opportunities for work and survival.

Mad women were often rejected or ignored by their partners and families once they were confined in the asylum. Although some became resigned to being abandoned, others were anxious about the families, especially the young children, they were forced to leave behind. As a mother wrote in a letter to the doctor in 1963, "Please I want to go home this week. My children need me and I need them too."[135] Usually, the lunacy archives reveal little of mothers' anguish—less so, the fate of their children. In 1914, a destitute Muslim woman was admitted to the asylum.[136] Who cared for her four children while she was there and after she died from anemia and nephritis in 1919? A Hindu mother of two children became a patient in 1920, and while there she gave birth to another baby. She remained in the hospital until her death from dysentery and "dementia praecox exhaustion" in 1939. Her children were put under the care of the Catholic Mission at Savusavu.[137] Sala had puerperal sepsis and a diagnosis of puerperal insanity a month after giving birth in 1943. She was unable to feed or care for her baby, who initially remained at Colonial War Hospital. Sala's husband stopped visiting his wife, and so the child probably had no contact with its birth mother. Sala's health deteriorated. She developed prominent abdominal swelling (ascites) and edema as well as shortness of breath, indicative of congestive heart disease, and died in the asylum at the age of twenty-seven.[138]

It appears that kin and the community cared for the dependents of women confined to the asylum. This love extended to the patients. This chapter ends with a plea from an Indo-Fijian man in 1941 for his wife to be discharged. His request to the medical superintendent was made in a letter that the head attendant had written in English; when the letter was interpreted to the husband, he signed it with a thumb mark. He had visited his wife five times during the previous month and stated that

> when I visited her, she talked to me in the proper manner as she used to talk some years ago when she was healthy and of sound mind. When I visited her yesterday she begged me to take her home. She

> asked how the young son of my brother Pardessi was, whom she was very fond of. She appears to be homesick and very anxious to see the home people.

She was released a month later. There are no records of her returning to the hospital.[139]

CHAPTER 5

Diagnoses and Discourse of Mental Disorders

Assessments of madness by the community in Fiji could be both certain—"he is a *pagali,*" "she is *lialia*"—and ambiguous. The interface between lay and medical jurisdiction over the mentally ill was equally slippery, partly because of the costs involved in hospitalization, partly because of the legal ramifications and stigma of being declared insane. As stressed in previous chapters, the medical and legal authorities who signed committal papers attached considerable importance to evidence provided by kin, community leaders, employers, and police. This testimony could be thick with accurate description or based on hearsay. Doctors also relied on observations from other health professionals. As Akihito Suzuki explains, historiography has established that, by the late nineteenth century, professional and scientific authority was firmly discrediting "the lay etiology and illness narrative."[1] Until after World War II, most European doctors in colonial Fiji had minimal or no training and experience in psychiatry, but they would have been convinced of the superiority of medical over lay knowledge and assessments of madness. Alienists in Europe usually had vastly different backgrounds to their patients; in Fiji, doctors faced far greater cultural gulfs and complexities. Even when biomedical discourse became pervasive in global psychiatry after World War II, doctors in Fiji had to remain cognizant of community and traditional understandings of madness. This insight could be overruled given that medical practitioners increasingly relied on powerful new drug and shock therapies as well as biomedical tests. The new interventions gave doctors greater confidence in controlling and treating mental illness, which in turn offered hope to affected families, but patients challenged these therapies (as we will see in chapter 6).

Discourse from various sources about a patient's madness constructed the mental patient—at which point a person assumed a file number in the St Giles archives. This framing was based on lay, medical, and legal discourse and occasionally that of the patient, as reported through "facts," causes (etiology), diagnosis, and classification (nosology). Facts and causes were subjectively based on the kind of lay assessments discussed in previous chapters and on doctors' clinical examinations. Sometimes patients' opinions were considered, but more often they were overlooked because they were not fully understood, whether due to the patient's mental condition or to language barriers between patient and doctor. The content of patients' delusions and hallucinations were usually dismissed, though doctors might regard it as significant in offering explanations of what caused the disorder. This disregard of patients' opinions was common in psychiatric assessments, as Sadowsky found in colonial Nigeria, where "most reductive biopsychiatry, holds what the lunatics *said* is not so important as what they *had*."[2] Doctors in Fiji examined the content of patients' delusions if it were evidence of the nature of the disease. For example, delusions of grandeur were a recognized stage in the prognosis of general paralysis of the insane (GPI); hearing voices or having religious visions was often implicated in schizophrenia. Doctors might interpret fears of being penetrated by radio waves or electricity as paranoia. Although doctors recorded the verbal content of raving, they did so usually to verify a disease and only occasionally to offer insight into the causes. Patient introspection was generally absent in an institution where medical staff were not trained in psychoanalysis or talking therapies. Facts and causes of insanity formed the basis of medical diagnoses and allocation into the disease classifications that separated the insane from normal and healthy people.

Classification as "mad" operated at several levels in Fiji and was discursively framed in different social contexts. Only a tiny minority of those considered mad by their communities were or became legally insane. Previous chapters have revealed how communities long accorded madness to those displaying repeatedly aberrant behavior, outside localized norms of rationality. The community or the lunatic's family often provided the impetus to hand over the care of such individuals to the state. As anthropologist Mary Douglas observed, although communities could tolerate peculiar behavior, the same behavior became intolerable once people were formally classified as abnormal; "a threshold of tolerance [was] marked by entry to a mental hospital."[3] Admission certificates to St Giles were replete with evidence of eccentric behavior that, taken individually, could hardly have constituted either a danger to self or others, or evidence of insanity. The dangerous and insane individual was often constructed through the accumulation of "facts" in a retrospective inventory provided by lay people to medical authorities, and these observations reveal how madness was identified in the community.[4] Ultimately, the observations of the (usually) European doctor determined the clinical diagnosis, and the doctor's observations, along with their medical knowledge designated a patient's madness as a recognized disorder or disease.

Even so, the meaning behind these disorders was not fixed. As psychiatric nosology changed elsewhere, classificatory systems in Fiji were revised. The meanings of melancholia, mania, and dementia were very different in early colonial Fiji than they were later. GPI was a standard disease category during the late nineteenth century, but by the 1960s it rarely featured in St Giles's reports.

Much of this chapter is based on my database of 3,866 admissions to St Giles between 1884 and 1964 derived from admission papers, the Mental Hospital Register, and the *Blue Books*. Data on the admission certificates and in the register was often incomplete and sometimes contradictory. It also conflated cause, facts, diagnosis, and the final disorder assigned to a patient; for example, GPI might be listed as a cause, symptom, and diagnosis as well as a cause of death. This chapter analyzes selected symptoms, causes, and classifications to consider how universal biomedical discourse was transferred to Fiji. The local became entangled with Western biomedical frameworks, unfolding as the colonization of madness. Cultural and historic causes of mental illness for indigenous Fijians and Indo-Fijians have been explored in previous chapters; this chapter also identifies substance abuse, loneliness, disasters, disease, and war in Fiji's context. Although universal psychiatric nosology is addressed, the chapter examines several patterns in Fiji, such as with GPI. Culture and ethnicity are crucial factors in understanding psychiatric etiology and nosology in Fiji.

Facts Indicating Insanity

The diagnosis of mental illness began with the details entered on the admission certificate. The diagnosis could become fixed, or it might be revised by the same or a different doctor, because of shifts in medical knowledge and nosology, or due to changes in the patient's behavior and mental state. To arrive at a disease classification, doctors itemized "the facts indicating insanity," although ultimately they used their judgment to assign a classification and to record the cause of the disorder.[5] Stipendiary magistrates usually lacked medical expertise, but they still had to record and decide on the validity of what became medical facts. These facts point to the subjective nature of assessments of madness, dependent on observation as well as assumptions of rationality, morality, and normality. These assessments were finally produced through Eurocentric eyes, and, even if these viewers were cognizant of local customs, the scope for misunderstanding within the cultural complexity of Fiji was enormous.

Madness came to the fore when humans appeared to behave as animals, when they were not just devoid of rationality but also embodied animalistic qualities. Bizarre behavior and attributions of animality might be linked to race.[6] Yet only a few references to animality, across ethnicities, were found within admission certificates between 1884 and 1964. In 1925 and 1948, two Indo-Fijian patients with mania were described as monkeys: one patient had "monkey-like antics and capers . . . animal like howls"; the other "jumped around the floor like a monkey; squatting down and pawing the floor."[7] In 1899, a Fijian male "opens mouth & gapes & groans like an animal," and in 1931 an Indo-Fijian female "jabbers, acts the animal by going on all fours, eats excreta."[8] In 1899, a European patient "devours food like an animal," and in 1927 an Indo-Fijian patient jabbers & slavers "like an animal."[9] These latter two probably had GPI. Not all those likened to animals were diagnosed with mania, such as a European patient with melancholia, who "rolled eyes, ground teeth & hissed like an animal."[10] In 1955, a doctor used a variation on the madman as animal when describing a nineteen-year-old Fijian male who was diagnosed as a schizophrenic catatonic, saying that he "stands with a sly animal look of cunning."[11] In Fiji as it had globally, sound, such as howling, was one aspect of the animalistic representation of madness.[12]

The universality of sound within madness discourse is striking, and sound and language feature throughout observations of lunacy.[13] In Fiji, madness texts were similar to those produced in other contexts. In 1909, a doctor observed a patient "raving at times to herself or others, and talking nonsense."[14] Sounds and speech might be unintelligible, out of place, or inappropriate, such as "hysterical crying & laughing" in court.[15] Smith, the chief warder, reported that Taniela was "always awake when visit him—not sleeping; hear him mekeing through the night."[16] Signs of madness included unrelenting noise, screaming, chattering or singing or the absence of sound or refusal to answer. Noise or silence could indicate patient agency within the asylum. Piercing screams and painful moans can still be heard from within St Giles today—echoes from a soundscape that conjures up a world of madness to those outside.[17]

In the past, both indigenous and European authorities listed sound and language as one of the facts indicating insanity. Until the mid-twentieth century, Europeans issued all certificates of insanity; some understood vernacular languages, but most relied on interpreters—if available. It is difficult to understand whether comments such as "incoherent speech" or "rambling talk" reflect the communicative limitations of the subject or the observer.[18] The comment that a Fijian patient "imagines & is quite satisfied that he can speak English; when incited to do so talks utter gibberish" might imply that the patient had limited ability in English or that the doctor could not understand Fiji English; in fact, this patient also talked nonsense to the Fijian police.[19] Observations about incoherent speech were less likely to be made about Europeans: between 1884 and 1936, 218 out of 1,141 admission certificates recorded that the patient was incoherent, but only eighteen of these recorded notes refer to thirteen Europeans.

Speech as well as flows of ideas might be incomprehensible to members of the same ethnic group. Taituse's speech was "at times very thick, & at times unintelligible to other Fijians."[20] In 1956, a Fijian senior nurse reported to doctors that a patient from Lau "cannot understand or speak Fijian (he being a Fijian) sensibly to convey meaning to others."[21]

The sudden switching of Fijian dialects or languages was also considered a sign of mental abnormality. In 1905, staff observed a female who "changes dialect without cause" and spoke "incoherent prattle."[22] Shifting between dialects or distinct languages for no apparent reason was taken as a sign of abnormal behavior and thought processing. Mohamed was incoherent when he talked, "wildly mixing English, Fijian, Hindustani and Malayalam languages."[23] An Indian sent from the leprosarium on Makogai Island confounded Dr. Bridgeman and the district commissioner in Levuka because she had a Fijian name and talked "incoherently & increasingly in English, Fijian & Hindi" and spent "hours doing native dances" as well as conversing with imaginary people and hearing voices.[24] Teiphal, also an Indian, spoke Fijian at Waiyevo Hospital on Taveuni in 1943; native medical practitioner Elikini Lauroutu, however, could not understand him and concluded that he was a lunatic who was deficient in mind.[25] Isoa engaged in long conversations with his Fijian friends and Europeans, though they did not always understand what he called "Vosa Peritania" (language of Britain).[26]

"General Appearance under Attack"

Appearance was also considered potentially indicative of madness. Vague and subjective assessments of appearance were common, such as the comments in these notes: "General appearance that of an insane person" or "facial expression indicative of insanity."[27] Embodied madness was linked with diagnoses. Mania might be exhibited through a "wild look in eyes" when under attack.[28] Dr. Duncan Macpherson diagnosed a woman with manic depression in 1937, noting that she "presents an appearance of abject misery. She is unkempt and dishevelled in her appearance, is gesticulative and has the general demeanour of a melancholic subject."[29]

Doctors recorded the physical details of patients who were severely mentally impaired. Vitendra rolled his eyes and head, was "drooling," and looked "obviously mentally deficient."[30] Occasionally, doctors took head measurements or noted the shape; for example, a doctor noted that Teiphal had a "Head badly shaped, physically wasted."[31] Doctors' observations of the body reflected cultural expectations of the normal body and behavior as well as scientific measurements.

During the twentieth century, they increasingly ran biomedical tests to assess intellectual abilities, to identify neurological disorders, and to verify the presence of physical disease that could indicate mental deterioration, notably GPI.

Dress and how it was worn was also noted as evidence of insanity. A sixty-nine-year-old male villager "dresses in extraordinary manner" and a police constable sported a "beard and moustache and peculiarity of coiffure."[32] As discussed in previous chapters, appearance was judged according to ethnic, gender, and class norms. Although in 1886 Graham's other bizarre conduct caused more concern, it was noted that he, as a European, failed to wear a hat in public.[33] In 1943, a European woman found her husband's behavior unusual because he went to work without shaving for the first time.[34] Emori had an "attitude & demeanour totally different from those of a Fijian of normal mental condition." Meanwhile, Ganesh's "manner, appearance & style of speech" was "not that of a normal Indian."[35]

Of concern were those whose appearance and behavior endangered their health. One woman was "careless of her person, soiling clothes, allowing her finger to become stinking & almost gangrenous from constriction by 5 rings."[36] Some people were preoccupied with rubbish—considered evidence of insanity—indicative of human and cultural norms to categorize and separate that which is dirty and clean. This distinction between clean and dirty can be interpreted according to cultural boundaries of purity and danger.[37] In Fiji, however, markers of cleanliness and sanitation were also part of the colonial order.[38] Some patients of all ethnicities and occupations collected or wore rubbish; for instance, a male teacher dressed with flowers and rubbish.[39] A *girmitiya,* pursued by "ghosts" from Calcutta, started covering himself with rubbish and eating it when he arrived at the hospital.[40] Collecting and hoarding items considered useless or dirty in the community could assume different meanings. Tekuka, an indentured Tokelauan admitted in 1890, "collects in a box all kinds of rubbish, sticks, stones, pieces of cloth, leave, which she says the devils have put in her way on purpose to annoy her."[41] An indentured Solomon Islander tried to "make himself [into] a white man" by taking dirty zinc coated dressings from a rubbish tin and smearing himself with them.[42]

"Strange and Unwarrantable Behaviour"

Among the reasons for Graham's five admissions to the asylum was his "purposeless," "strange and unwarrantable behaviour," which included painting small pieces of rope, an "undue fondness for dabbing in water," "asking for articles of diet in a public house & mixing them foolishly together with water," and repeatedly washing the same article of clothing in a public place.[43] This preoccupation with water and paint possibly arose from his former occupations as a waterman and as a painter. Although Graham was a European, he transgressed class boundaries by "addressing people familiarly with whom he should have no business or social connections." He was also a nuisance when he threw paint on buildings, an action referred to as "endangering the integrity of buildings."

Some Fijian patients broke class and ethnic boundaries. One patient "tries to grasp people . . . when ordinarily a Fijian would never touch, and turns his back upon his superiors." Another assumed a "listless, lounging attitude and totally different from that of a 'normal Fijian native.'"[44] Samu dared to smoke while talking to the doctor, exhibiting an "Attitude & manners [that] are not such as befit a Fijian of his standing."[45] In 1901, a nineteen-year-old private serving in the Fiji Armed Constabulary showed "unnecessary & unusual saluting & formality" to his superiors and assaulted and terrorized others.[46] In 1929, an Indo-Fijian car driver made "frequent references to matters considered indecent and unmentionable by persons of his race and class, eg passing water, defecating, etc."[47]

Communities might tolerate strange behavior for years, but a sudden departure from daily patterns, especially with regard to work, raised concern. In 1945, an employer was "amazed" when an employee suddenly refused to work although he had always been known as a very industrious and regular workman.[48] This thirty-one-year-old laborer was diagnosed with "typical acute mania" and died in the asylum two years later. As noted in chapter 4, work roles were gendered, and a woman's neglect of domestic work and family was often a sign of mental instability.

"His Mind and Reason Are Imperfect"

This phrase appears in Dr. Alfred Munckton's notes about Bhagal, the first patient admitted to St Giles. It shows how medical expertise had the final word in assessing whether a patient's mind was unsound or insane. Munckton appears to reproduce universal psychiatric discourse of his time, yet it remains unclear how such discourse was transmitted between the metropole and colonies and between colonies during the early years of Fiji's asylum. Only some doctors in Fiji had experience working in asylums elsewhere and access to texts on mental disease. Munckton based his assessment on Bhagal's answers to questions, but we have no record of this exchange and how the meaning and understanding of the conversation might have been lost in translation. During subsequent decades at St Giles, global psychiatric discourse continued to be inscribed on admission certificates even though its content changed. Doctors typically recorded a patient's flow of ideas and reasoning and whether the patient's answers were relevant to the conversation. In 1928, a doctor noted a Hindu priest's "inability to fix attention; rapid flow of disconnected ideas expressed with considerable incoherence."[49] "Insight" (or the lack of it)—that is, self-awareness of one's mental illness—is a common concept in modern psychiatry, and it was in use at St Giles by the late 1930s. A *yagona* addict diagnosed as manic depressive had "clear insight."[50] This was unlike an epileptic patient prone to several fits daily, who had "no insight . . . subject to outbursts of erratic behaviour leading to conflict with the law."[51]

Delusions—true beliefs for the patient but false for others—offered flamboyant evidence of an "imperfect mind."[52] So, too, did hallucinations or imaginary sounds, smells or visions. Dr. Philip Harper recorded these observations of an Indian storekeeper on July 9, 1938:

> 1. Facts indicating insanity observed by myself.
> (a) Hallucinations. He states that he sees persons in Nadi stores who as a matter of actual fact are known to be in Labasa.
> (b) Delusions of persecution. He states that persons of Labasa & Nadi are defrauding him but can give no rational account of the fraud.[53]

Some cases discussed in previous chapters suggest that delusions might reflect real situations the patients faced, such as gendered oppression, violence, or economic troubles, even if the detail was exaggerated. Religious delusions could be prophetic and shared by followers or those with similar beliefs. Women's sexual delusions feature more than those of men in the asylum records. Does this mean that women were more likely than men to express sexual delusions or that doctors were more likely to note what they judged as heightened sexuality in women? As several cases show, delusions were colored by the cultural and historical context and what counted as wealth or power. Chaju, who was a planter in 1918, believed that he owned the sugar mill. His hallucinations of seeing a boiler coming toward him nearly resulted in a fatality when he climbed onto a cane carrier. The mill had to be stopped to remove him. He also stated, "I am Ram," and said that the sun and moon were his sons.[54] For Fijians, pigs could signify status and wealth, which may have been why one patient claimed that he owned a thousand pigs as well as a thousand pounds.[55]

Delusions often mirrored the colonial world of which patients were a part. Several patients believed that they were kings, whether of Fiji or Britain, or perhaps a rajah in India. One Indo-Fijian, who worked for the Penang sugar company in 1917, believed that he was the king of a large kingdom with power over many ships and Europeans.[56] In 1929, a *ratu* was convinced that a "man of war" was coming to take him to see the king of England. He wanted to see paramount chief Sir Lala Sukuna to obtain one thousand pounds rent money to purchase ceremonial gifts of *tabua* (whales' teeth) and mats for this impending visit. The *ratu* also possessed fifty million pounds.[57] In 1958, a sixteen-year-old Fijian woman believed that she was Sukuna. She said she was God and the devil.[58] Sukuna featured in the delusions of some Indo-Fijians, such as a retired civil servant in 1951 who said he had purchased a house from Sukuna for two shillings and sixpence. He also declared that "King George V is his adopted grandfather and that Mrs King George VI is his adopted mother."[59] Two other Indo-Fijian patients claimed Gandhi as their grandfather or father.[60] Others believed that they were connected through marriage to prominent local Europeans, such as Sir Henry Marks in 1925.[61] Some delusions featured racial hatred and fears. A Fijian in 1917 believed that he had the "power of life and death over all Indians with whom he came in contact."[62] In 1921, an Indo-Fijian mother reported four times to police that Fijians had murdered her children.[63] In 1924, a Chinese carpenter stole and burned a roll of cloth from a Japanese store in Levuka; he had an "exceptional hatred of Japanese & 'much silly talk' about their killing of children & men generally," including an "irrational description of the Japanese war & actions of various Japanese officials & others."[64] Delusional insanity was a major classification from around 1900 until the 1930s (see table 5.1); more men were diagnosed with it than women. Not all patients with delusions were diagnosed with delusional insanity, however.

As these examples indicate, the "facts indicating insanity" were often subjective lay and medical observations embedded in the cultural, religious, and historical context. However, as this chapter shows, medical views exerted authority, ostensibly supported by scientific evidence. The rare instances in the St Giles archive when degeneration was recorded reveal the ambiguity amidst scientific dis-

Table 5.1. Percentage of major mental disorders, St Giles

	1884–1889	1890–1899	1900–1909	1910–1919	1920–1929	1930–1939	1940–1949	1950–1959	1960–196
Mania	19.6	15.6	13.2	43.1	40.1	24.6	1.9	13.3	9.3
Manic depression	0.0	0.0	0.0	0.0	0.6	10.3	33.6	21.1	13.1
Melancholia	0.0	5.2	5.3	8.7	6.3	4.4	0.8	0.6	1.0
Delusional insanity	0.0	0.0	4.0	2.9	9.5	16.2	0.0	1.5	0.0
Schizophrenia	0.0	0.0	0.0	0.0	0.0	1.6	1.9	31.1	58.1

Source: Author's database from patients' admission papers, St Giles Hospital, *Blue Book of Fiji*, Mental Hospital Registe
Note: Patient data incomplete and numbers indicative only.

course. Unlike many other colonies, the term appears much later in Fiji and not explicitly for Europeans.[65] During the late 1930s, Macpherson listed bearing a "distinct stigmata of degeneration" among the facts confirming the insanity of Indo-Fijian, Kalidas, and i-Taukei, Joape.[66] Degeneration theory, favored by many doctors during the nineteenth century, accounted for a supposed racial weakening from behavior such as alcoholism or masturbation.[67] It was believed that such weakening could lead to hereditary mental illness, linked to physical and intellectual disabilities. These illnesses could be exhibited through physical stigmata, though stigmata were also a euphemism for a mark of moral decay. Although degeneration theory continued to have popular currency until World War II, very few traces of this theory exist in the St Giles archive. "Hereditary" was given as a cause and diagnosis of illness for only a few patients, and not usually equated with moral degeneration. Macpherson's descriptors were therefore unusual. In Joape's and Kalidas's cases, it appears that the doctor could actually see embodied signs (stigmata) of degeneration, though it is ambiguous whether this was a moral judgment or a medical assessment based on pseudo-scientific theories. Other facts from these patients' histories appeared to confirm moral "degeneration." Joape had attacked two women; Kalidas had a previous prison sentence for rape. The night before his admission, Kalidas had assaulted an Indo-Fijian woman. Both men believed that their madness was caused by supernatural causes. Kalidas had been diagnosed with epilepsy; Joape was later diagnosed with paranoia.

Supposed Cause of Insanity

Certification papers required that a "supposed cause of lunacy" be stipulated.[68] This section was often left blank, possibly because those filling out the paperwork were ignorant of the patient's medical and personal history, the committal process was often done under urgency, and because medical knowledge of the etiology of mental disorders was (and still is) limited and contested. Information listed under cause and disorder was sometimes repeated or interchanged—alcohol, for example, might be recorded as both the cause and the condition.

Social and economic pressures and the occasional moral failing were more commonly listed on earlier admission papers than on those in later decades. Sometimes a specific cause was given, such as "internal troubles with his Mataqali" or "talks of Native Lands Commission."[69] Most causes, however, reflected the approach of British psychiatry by the 1880s, identifying somatic-pathological or organic origins rather than moral or psychological origins of mental disorder.[70] Doctors in Fiji were unable to unravel the complexities behind their patients' mental illnesses, not only because of the cultural divide but also because of their medical backgrounds. The understanding of mental illness etiology in global psychiatry further unfolded during the twentieth century with debates over the role of functional and psychodynamic etiologies or organic and biochemical etiologies in individuals and in specific diseases.[71] Medical personnel in Fiji likely found it more challenging than doctors in more developed countries to construct a patient's history or access resources for biomedical tests.

Other chapters have examined the context of mental disorders within Fiji's communities. Chapter 2 focused on Indian migrants and highlighted the role played by displacement, loneliness, violence, physical disease, and destitution in mental disorders. Chapter 3 discussed how many of these causes affected indigenous Fijians. Religious insanity was cited as the cause and diagnosis of madness for some prominent Fijian patients. Patients of other ethnicities had "religious insanity," but this condition was far less likely to be associated with women. Gendered roles and norms predominated among the causes given for women's mental illness. Women's insanity was mostly linked to their emotional or reproductive lives, in contrast to men's illness being caused by financial or employment issues.

Chapter 2 showed how work and money were key causes of mental breakdown among Indo-Fijians. Employment and business was frequently associated with the mental troubles of European men. Arthur Carr was admitted to St Giles five times from 1897 until his death there in 1907. His manic and depressive outbreaks were linked to his failure as a banana and plantation farmer, and to his worry about land transactions.[72] Carr had earlier been treated for mental illness in Sydney and then emigrated to Fiji with his family to join his brothers, who were sugar planters. Carr's story shows how European ambitions in Fiji could be shattered by many factors, such as the environment, economic slumps, and colonial restrictions on access to land and labor.[73] Economic failure, often combined with loneliness, could affect Europeans who were mentally fragile and could result in bizarre, aggressive, compulsive, or addictive behavior.

Before World War II, alcoholism was mainly a white man's burden. It ravaged Michael, a European civil servant, as did his profound guilt over his masturbation.[74] Yet "masturbatory insanity," another common cause and classification of mental disorders during the Victorian period, was rarely noted in Fiji.[75] Masturbation and alcoholism were considered moral failings and causative of pathological disease. So, too, were forms of substance abuse more specific to Fiji.

Kava and Opium Abuse

Yagona or kava abuse was the distinct cause of four cases of mental illness in Fiji between 1884 and 1964.[76] The linking of madness to *yagona* probably had more to do with who these patients were than to the mildly psychoactive plant. None of these patients were indigenous Fijian men, for whom kava consumption and the rituals surrounding it had been the norm for centuries. Indo-Fijians did socially use kava. Women rarely drank kava, so it is surprising that in 1888 villager Mele's excessive *yagona* drinking, replaced her food and was listed as causing various behaviors, including

> ridiculous appearances when under attack . . . Rapid alternations of temper, changing from manual violence to servile politeness. Aimless wandering at large both by day and by night. Neglect of person, which was not formerly her habit . . . Undue familiarity toward strangers her superior in station, without any reason. Wanton destruction of property . . . Abusive to former friend and a near relative who has continued to treat her well.[77]

Another female patient, diagnosed with manic depression, was said to have drunk *yagona* "all day."[78] One Indo-Fijian male with manic depression was labeled a "yagona addict"; another with schizophrenia was described as a heavy *yagona* user.[79]

Although opium was probably introduced in Fiji by Indians, it was not mentioned in their mental illness records. It was, however, implicated in the madness of a few Europeans and part-Europeans. An elderly sailor and trader was committed in 1895 after he sought medicine from a doctor because he was ill and craved opium.[80] In 1903, opium and alcohol were given as the roots of a planter's paranoid delusions and violence.[81] The final reference to opium in the hospital archives is in 1918, when "opium smoking" was entered as a disorder.[82] Alcohol is discussed later in this chapter.

Loneliness, Disaster, and Disease

For those unaccustomed or without community support, Fiji's environment could be challenging and induce mental distress. Environmental causes and loneliness mainly featured on Europeans' admission papers, which resonates with nineteenth-century views that Europeans were unsuited to settle in the tropics because of their predisposition to undergo physical and mental breakdown there.[83] This assumption was underpinned by the concept of racial degeneration from the admixture of moral and physical decay. Yet some Indian and Pacific Islander laborers—"naturally" suited to working and living in the tropics—were also prone to loneliness and mental breakdown, partly from the effects of a different, hostile, or isolated social and physical environment.

Selina, age forty-five, was admitted to the asylum in 1918 from one of the most isolated locales in Fiji: the small island of Wailagilala, in the far north of the

Lau Islands. The cause of her "religious mania" was listed as "solitude, over 20 years at Wailagilala," yet she had refused to leave the island, asserting that she had a divine order to be there. Selina also said that God had told her to leave her husband. Selina probably sailed to Wailagilala with her husband soon after her marriage in 1897.[84] He was possibly the keeper of the lighthouse, which was strategically located to direct shipping through the dangerous Nanuku Passage. It is not known who else lived on the island besides the couple or how frequently Selina had contact with others during the decades she lived in this remote region. In 1935, loneliness was given as the cause of another patient's mania, religious obsessions, and depression. She was from Fiji and had been living in the Gilbert and Ellice Islands, where her husband was an engineer on a cable ship.[85]

Climatic extremes were implicated in causing a few cases of madness in Fiji but not to the extent as at a Melbourne asylum in the 1870s, when sixteen males were admitted following sunstroke.[86] As Coleborne explains, sunstroke was as revealing about white men's vulnerability in the tropics as it was caused by the environment. In Fiji, although Graham was likely accustomed to the harsh sun when he was a waterman and lived on Nukulau Island, his insanity was initially attributed to sunstroke. Carr's lunacy in 1897 was first attributed to "sun." But not all patients with sunstroke were white men. Heat stroke was given as the cause of an Indo-Fijian poultry farmer's sudden violence and brief admissions to the hospital in 1939.[87] A severe hurricane and flood in 1931, which led to the death of at least 225 people, were thought to have caused two European women to have mental breakdowns. One of these women suffered from melancholia, and, although the other had an attack in 1931, she was not admitted to the hospital until 1939, when she was diagnosed with psychoneurosis caused by worry and shock. These women may have been closely involved with the disaster, which was intense when it hit Ba, where one of the women was a teacher and the other was married to a road overseer.[88]

Disease was noted as the cause of some mental illnesses. In 1886, disease as well as climate ("dengue fever with sunstroke") were given as the causes of the delusions, hallucinations, sleeplessness, and incoherence experienced by a European storekeeper from Savusavu.[89] Measles, typhoid, and influenza, among other diseases—which were linked to high fever as well as febrile convulsions, exhaustion, or depression—were all said to have occasionally caused madness in Fiji.[90] Influenza was sometimes implicated in causing or being a form of mental illness, as documented with Sailosi Ratu's first admission in 1899, although he had been reported as having religious mania for several years.[91]

Seven asylum patients had mania linked to the influenza pandemic that arrived in Fiji between November 1918 and April 1919.[92] The pandemic's impact in

St Giles was tiny relative to the nine thousand deaths across the colony.[93] In very rare cases. influenza could have neurological effects, but the pandemic more generally fomented anxiety and despondency in a population that faced so much debilitation and mortality.[94] A destitute patient was wrongly admitted to the asylum: although he was acutely delirious and diagnosed with mania caused by influenza, he was not considered mentally ill.[95]

Another wrongful admission involved a Tahitian patient with leprosy in 1897. The patient was assessed by the medical superintendent as "not apparently insane in a serious degree." The patient was transferred to a leprosy hamlet adjoining the main hospital.[96] A patient died in the asylum in 1919, the cause of death listed as leprosy and dysentery.[97] The admission records indicate that at least eight other asylum patients with leprosy were admitted from or discharged to the leprosarium on Makogai Island in the years after it opened in 1911. The fear and stigma of leprosy featured in some patients' delusions: another Chinese patient in 1929 dreaded leprosy and syphilis, was constantly worried "about his genital organs," and desired "to make an end to his existence."[98]

Organic Causes

Mental conditions were therefore linked to organic causes, including infectious diseases such as influenza; yet other diseases were considered to be a direct pathway to neurological pathology. GPI was linked with syphilis but, as discussed shortly, doctors in Fiji also linked yaws (*framboesia,* known as *coko* in Fiji) with GPI and mental illness. GPI was understood to be a progressive disease leading to profound mental and physical deterioration. Although GPI could cause dementia, and not all dementia was caused by GPI, both were in keeping with late Victorian understandings of mental disease as a teleological progression toward "the common form of insanity" and the "common goal of dementia."[99]

Dementia as a cause and as a classification embraced a wide range of conditions associated with mental deterioration.[100] For example, in 1916, a thirty-year-old Fijian male was diagnosed with dementia apparently caused by a headache.[101] He had previously been admitted to the asylum when he was seventeen after threatening violence and experiencing delusions. On his third admission in 1924, he was diagnosed with delusional insanity. The neurological disorder chorea was given as the cause of dementia in a thirty-five-year-old female laborer in 1935.[102] Usually, dementia and senility were associated with elderly patients, but the mental illness of some young people was classified as secondary dementia.

Age categories and concepts are culturally and historically constructed and could be associated with forms of mental illness.[103] A diagnosis of senile dementia caused by age was not unusual in an eighty-six-year-old European woman whose behavior had severely deteriorated. She was a former schoolteacher who could no longer recall either recent events or who her children were. She also threatened violence against others and herself and to burn down her house, imagined seeing people in her bedroom, talked to inanimate objects, and was not "properly dressed" for public outings.[104] Yet age could be relative, such as when "old age" was provided as the reason for admitting an Indian aged fifty in 1957.[105] Age-specific causes and diagnoses were also given for young people. Adolescent insanity was the cause given for seventeen-year-old Nand's manic depression.[106] In 1897, adolescence itself was listed as the form of mental disorder for an eighteen-year-old Fijian from Ovalau.[107]

Insanity was sometimes linked to accidents. In 1940, a sixty-year-old retired Wesleyan minister was admitted and diagnosed with senile dementia, attributed to a fall from his horse some years earlier. By the time of his admission, his destructive and frightening behavior was no longer tolerated by villagers, behavior that had led his wife to flee. He appeared much older than his age, was feeble and blind, and died in the asylum ten days after admission.[108] It is not clear whether there was a direct link between the cause and his diagnosis because sometimes, when behavior became intolerable, the community might search for a vivid past event, such as an accident, to explain subsequent strange actions. Patients whose insanity was linked to an accident, usually to the head, were all men.

War Trauma

Some mental illness was linked to war. Although some traces of World War I were found, World War II featured more prominently in the archive. The war had a huge impact on Fiji, which was a crucial base for the South Pacific Area Command.[109] The effects of military command, the presence of thousands of foreign troops, and the threat of Japanese invasion were entangled in the fears of many Fijians, so it is hardly surprising that war was implicated in the mental conditions and delusions of some patients, especially their "paranoia." In 1944, sixteen patients (approximately 15 percent) were recorded as being paranoid.[110] "War" was given as the cause of a Samoan's mental illness: he had had attacks since the outbreak of World War II. He said that he had caused this war and burned his military uniform because God had directed him to do so.[111] "Religious worries and war" were the causes provided for the admission of a Fijian patient in 1941. He had been in trouble with the police and military for breaking military curfew and for attempting to board the USS *Monterey* so that he could win the war.[112] A Kailoma patient was diagnosed with hereditary mental instability, along with a raft of other disorders, including possible epilepsy, "great depression," and "suicidal intent"—all supposedly caused by "conditions of military life and discipline affecting psychopathic mentality." He was discharged from the Fiji Defence Force.[113] "Stress of service" was the cause given for a Rotuman patient's manic depression and "sense of persecution" in 1945.[114]

The horrific impact of combat—once referred to as shellshock, combat or war neurosis, and now combat stress reaction—was cited as the cause of mental breakdown.[115] A few patients were briefly admitted with mental disorders caused by the ongoing effects of shellshock from World War I; one was an Australian fireman on a cargo ship in 1925; another was a British clerk in 1933.[116] When Kameli was escorted back to Fiji from the Solomon Islands in 1943, shellshock was given as the cause. He had been violent toward his comrades, was subject to depression and memory loss, had dreams and olfactory hallucinations of a dead man, devils, snakes, and dogs, and was "full of fear and self defacement." The medical superintendent assessed Kameli's condition as "anxiety neurosis," but the acting director of medical services suggested that it was dementia praecox.[117] Three New Zealand soldiers stationed on Fiji during World War II were admitted to the mental hospital.[118] When two American servicemen were transferred from the 71st Station Hospital in Tamavua to the mental hospital in November 1942, they were never officially recorded on the register.[119] War-related trauma continued to be associated with mental distress after World War II. In 1953, a twenty-two-year-old Fijian soldier was repatriated from Singapore; originally treated at the British Military Hospital in Kluang, Malaya, where Fijian troops had been serving with the British Army during the Malayan Emergency, he was diagnosed with paranoid schizophrenia but died in the mental hospital in 1957.[120]

Form of Mental Disorder

Madness assumed a legitimacy and historical permanence in colonial Fiji once the "form of mental disorder," derived from diagnoses made on admission and recorded in the hospital register, was officially recorded. A large variety of disorders was squeezed into broader published classifications. This tidiness followed bureaucratic categories applied in Britain and other British colonies, as one scholar noted, "for all doctors in the colonies, using statistical tables was a concrete expression of connectedness to British standards of expertise."[121] The list of mental disorders offered a nosology of mental disease in Fiji, which gradually shifted with changing conceptualizations in British and global psychiatric nosology.[122] International experts fiercely debated classifications that would lead to the International Classification of Diseases, Injuries and Causes of Death (ICD) adopted by the World Health Organization in 1948. The nomenclature, classification, and causes of morbidity became a foundation of Western biomedicine, but no single universal classification of mental illnesses existed.[123]

In colonial Fiji, classifications of mental diseases varied between admission papers, the asylum register, annual reports, and the *Blue Book of Fiji*. From 1884 to 1922, the *Blue Book* standardized mental illness into categories based on the patients' behavior or potential risk: maniacal and dangerous; quiet chronic; melancholy and suicidal; and idiotic, paralytic, or epileptic. From 1923 forward, the patients' outcome was filed, being assessed as idiots and imbecile (including epileptics); presumably recoverable; chronic and presumably irrecoverable. Chronic patients were further classified into being turbulent and dangerous, suicidal, sick and infirm, general paralytics, epileptics, senile dements, or able bodied.[124] From 1909, published annual reports categorized patients into broad categories of mental disease: mania, melancholia, dementia, delusional insanity, and GPI.[125] These categories were not mutually exclusive and embraced a wide range of behaviors and symptoms. The unpublished annual reports, register, *Blue Book*, and admission papers broke down the general categories into more specific disorders, such as the types of mania, psychosis or dementia, epilepsy, idiocy, alcoholic insanity, puerperal insanity, hysteria, neurosis, or paranoia.[126]

All Embracing: Mania, Melancholia, and Manic Depression

According to published records, mania was diagnosed for the largest group of asylum patients in Fiji until the early 1940s (see table 5.1), similar to findings in asylums elsewhere.[127] Mania was both an all-embracing and an ambiguous category. Mania was also more precisely labeled as acute, subacute, chronic, intermittent, simple, incendiary, incipient, transient, hysterical, religious, alcoholic, puerperal, or megalomania, or linked to other conditions, such as epilepsy, GPI, dementia, and melancholia.

Table 5.2. Percentage of selected mental disorders of St Giles' patients, 1884–1964

	Total	Female	Male	Fijian	Indian	European	Others
Mania	17.6	18.6	16.9	18.7	18.0	8.7	17.0
Melancholia	2.8	2.6	2.9	1.6	3.2	3.8	3.5
Schizophrenia	22.5	28.0	18.8	20.5	24.8	7.7	24.2
Manic depression	13.3	16.1	11.5	14.4	13.8	7.7	10.7
Dementia	7.3	5.1	8.8	6.3	7.6	12.6	5.2
Delusional insanity	3.5	2.0	4.4	2.9	3.0	12.6	2.1
Depression	0.6	0.9	0.4	0.2	0.9	0.0	0.3

Source: Author's database from patients' admission papers, St Giles Hospital, *Blue Book of Fiji*, Mental Hospital Register.

Note: Patient data incomplete and numbers indicative only.

Table 5.2 presents a more detailed breakdown of the gender and ethnicity for patients whose diagnosis was mania or manic depression. These figures are approximate because many patients who presented with manic symptoms could have been classified as melancholic or with other conditions and much data was incomplete. When data was available, between 1884 and 1964, mania was recorded for 18.8 percent of women and 17 percent of men, with similar percentages (17 to 18 percent) for Fijians, Indians, and Others. Europeans had mania noted as a diagnosis on 8.7 percent of admissions. The classifications used before the 1930s cannot be equated with later nosology (notably manic depression or bipolar disorder), which makes it impossible to determine clear epidemiological patterns over time. Ali, discussed in chapter 2, was diagnosed with mania in 1915, dementia in 1922, but—on his final admission between 1930 and 1943—with manic depression.[128] Table 5.1 reveals that manic depression became more commonly recorded by the 1940s, although many patients continued to be diagnosed with mania. Henry had eleven admissions between 1923 and 1945, during which time he married and worked as a carpenter. He could be "violently insane" and "intensely melancholic," and in 1924 was restrained in leg irons and handcuffs "for his own safety."[129] Dr. Thomas Clunie diagnosed him with manic depressive insanity in 1926: "Has intervals of lucidity but always reverts to mania followed by melancholia." Subsequent records, however, list mania as his disorder.[130]

Melancholia embraced mania as well as a wide range of conditions, including psychosis, mania, anxiety, irrationality, delusions, nostalgia, suicidal attempts and ideation, and acute and chronic depression.[131] Western psychiatric concepts of depression were also problematic to apply in a cross-cultural context.[132] Although doctors in some African colonies underdiagnosed melancholia or considered that depression was rare among indigenous patients, both diagnoses featured in Fiji.[133] Until 1922 "melancholy and suicidal" was a category in the *Blue Book,* though admission papers and suicide reports used the term melancholic or similar terms. As outlined in chapter 2, melancholia and depression were prevalent among Indian migrants in Fiji. In addition, more Indians than Fijians were diagnosed with melancholia, 3.2 and 1.6 percent respectively (see table 5.2). Melancholia was diagnosed in 3.8 percent of Europeans and in 3.5 percent of others. Depression emerges as a standalone diagnosis only from the 1950s and is featured on only 0.6 percent of admissions between then and the 1960s.

In 1938, a "modern classification" of mental illnesses was introduced into the mental hospital's annual reports.[134] These new categories indicated how changing theoretical concepts and debates within psychiatry reformulated mental disease classifications. Changes in knowledge and nosology were usually transmitted to Fiji when doctors trained overseas were appointed in Fiji or when local medical personnel participated in international conferences and visited hospitals elsewhere. It is perhaps no coincidence that Fiji's new mental illness classifications were instigated by the medical superintendent, Dr. David Hoodless, who was also the principal of the Central Medical School. He had returned to Fiji in 1935 after training at Charing Cross Hospital in London.[135]

The 1938 classification of mental diseases in Fiji resulted in a prominence of manic depressive insanity, seventy-seven cases of 121 being classified as such. In 1935, only two of 124 had been. Theories underpinning manic depression and schizophrenia (formerly known as dementia praecox) had been established by Emil Kraepelin, Eugen Bleuler, and other psychiatrists by the early twentieth century, but doctors in Fiji did not apply these terms until later.[136] The 1938 classification only reported two cases of schizophrenia but identified twenty-two cases of reactive and toxic insanities (which could include psychosis induced from alcohol or drugs, tuberculosis, influenza, fevers, puerperal sepsis, or syphilis). Hoodless remained dubious about the new classifications and suggested that they might need periodic reexamination. Reactive and toxic insanities did not persist as significant categories in subsequent annual reports.

Dementia: "Wires Inside My Head Pull It About"

Clara, a seventy-eight-year-old European, explained herself in 1922 as "wires inside my head pull it about." These words convey the confusion and cognitive impairment that many patients at St Giles diagnosed with dementia experienced. Clara was disorientated, could not recall familiar things or places, and was "impossible to converse with." A nursing sister from the Colonial War Memorial Hospital described Clara as sleepless, restless, wandering, noisy, quarrelsome, sometimes violent, and prone to disrobe in public. Clara's symptoms were associated with "senile decay" (possibly Alzheimer's disease).[137] Other patients with dementia did not have all of her symptoms but might have others. A forty-year-old Indo-Fijian in 1924, for example, had lost control of his arms and legs and was diagnosed with dementia paraplegia.[138] In the early asylum records, dementia sometimes was interchanged with other disorders, such as GPI or melancholia.[139] Sukudaia was classified as having dementia, but it remains unclear what this implied.[140] The Board of Visitors was uncertain about the form of dementia a twenty-five-year-old Fijian male had in 1892.[141]

Clinicians' understanding of dementia has greatly changed since the nineteenth century, yet the diagnosis is still sweeping.[142] Dr. Jude Ohaeri's description in 1997 makes this clear: "a chronic condition, characterized by insidious onset (months to year), marked memory loss, disorientation in spite of a fair degree of clarity of consciousness and deterioration of personal habits, judgment, intellectual and social functioning."[143] Patients of widely varying ages and abilities came under the category of dementia, such as Miss G. M. and Karuna, both patients during the early 1960s. Miss G. M., an eighty-four-year-old part-European, was admitted to St Giles from the Home of Compassion in Suva with senile dementia.[144] Karuna was age seven when diagnosed with post-encephalitic dementia (probably caused by an infection).[145]

Dementia as a general category declined as new diagnoses were introduced, especially manic depression and schizophrenia, but by the 1930s senile dementia occurred more often in the records. In the 1920s, dementia was the diagnosis in 12.6 percent of known admissions, versus 4 percent from 1960 to 1964. Mr. F. K., a thirty-year-old Chinese market gardener, had been classified with senile dementia in 1912. He was admitted a month after he received news from China that one of his children was ill. This news probably sparked F. K. to search for his wife and family in Fiji even though they were in China. He believed that they were living in the home of another Chinese resident in Fiji. There, F. K. tried to abduct a child and threatened the father with a knife. F. K. died in the asylum in 1938.[146] During the 1920s, the number of patients with senile dementia gradually increased, and the diagnosis was linked more with older patients on first admission. The hospital's oldest recorded patient, a Gujarati male, was one hundred years old in 1948.[147] Remarkably, he was discharged to the care of his sons after ten months. Despite the advanced years of several patients with senile dementia, many were discharged. Table 5.2 shows that dementia featured more frequently as a diagnosis for Europeans (12.6 percent of admissions) than for other ethnic groups. The elderly had a valued and active role within Pacific and Asian that may have protected against dementia. Elderly Europeans in Fiji were more likely to lack family support than other ethnic groups, especially once Indian communities were formed.

GPI: Certain Diagnosis, Uncertain Causes

GPI, also known as general paresis or dementia paralytica, is the disease classification that is perhaps the most confounding in the St Giles archives. This disease no longer appears in contemporary psychiatric discourse, but, during the nineteenth and early twentieth centuries, a large proportion of patients throughout the world were diagnosed with it.[148] Estimates in Fiji suggest that until 1940 about 10 percent of patients were diagnosed with either GPI or neurosyphilis. In some years, such as 1910, as many as 25 percent of patients were treated for GPI.[149] The first record of GPI was in 1890 on the death of a laborer from Vanuatu.[150] The last reference in my database concerned a twenty-nine-year-old Fijian woman admitted in 1962 who was also diagnosed with schizophrenia.[151]

Due to the terrifying physical and mental impact, GPI evoked such fear in asylums worldwide that it was known as "the most deadly disease of asylumdom."[152] Taniela of Nanukuloa village in Ra was diagnosed with it, and the course of his illness was recounted by Harper and conformed to the stages outlined by Thomas Smith Clouston (superintendent of the Royal Edinburgh Asylum from 1873 to 1908).[153] Taniela's illness probably first manifested in 1906, when he was hospitalized for several months for backache. Severe bodily pains are listed as part of the disease's preliminary, along with other symptoms, such as tiredness, slight depression, and changes in disposition. By 1916, Taniela's relatives were concerned about the dramatic change in his personality and behavior, as he went from being an upstanding community member—"exceptionally trustworthy, well-behaved, government official of a very religious turn of mind"—to someone who behaved indecently and was explosive. Taniela showed signs of Clouston's first stage of GPI, typified by slight speech defects, slurring, eye symptoms, facial muscular incoordination, morbid elevation, and grandiose delusions. Taniela first consulted Harper in 1915 because, for the previous three months, he had been tremulous, especially in his fingers, and was becoming inarticulate. His relatives reported that he had become thin and weak, whereas he had formerly been an "unusually powerful man." Taniela claimed that he was a harbormaster and that he owned vast and valuable land. He offered to give some of this land to Harper, when in fact the land belonged to Europeans. Harper treated Taniela for three months, but Taniela's mental condition rapidly deteriorated until he was committed to the asylum in January 1916. At this point, Taniela was in the second stage of GPI, which Clouston identified as characterized by "mental confusion, apathy, silliness, and further loss of face expression and speech," widespread muscular incoordination, and paralysis. Taniela reached Clouston's fatal third stage when he died of exhaustion in the asylum nine months after his admission. By that stage, patients were often bedridden, inarticulate, and paralyzed.

Delusions of grandeur often reflected real—albeit exaggerated—aspirations in the patient's world. Men with GPI in Fiji often desired wealth, power, or high status, which in reality was beyond their reach because of their ethnicity or class. Land was highly valued in Fiji for both cultural and economic reasons, so it was not surprising that it featured in delusions, as seen with Taniela. Autiko, admitted in 1906 with GPI claimed to possess a large cutter and a steamer, which were very desirable in a maritime environment but impossible for ordinary Fijians to own.[154] He also said that he had one thousand wives.

GPI evoked alarm in Western Europe because it had once been a disease that linked morality to madness.[155] During the nineteenth century, some European alienists believed that GPI was hereditary, but greater medical opinion linked it to moral failings, such as alcoholism or debauchery, and considered it a "disease of civilization."[156] From at least the 1860s, links were made between syphilis and GPI and, during the late nineteenth century, heated debate emerged within European medical centers over whether syphilis caused GPI.[157] By 1906, the Wassermann test enabled doctors to identify the presence of the syphilitic spirochaete within the bloodstream of patients with GPI.

Meanwhile, in Fiji, doctors were recording GPI among the symptoms and classifications of madness. They based this on their observation of patient behavior, speech, delusions, and physical symptoms, as in a Fijian's notes in 1912:

> Tremor of tongue, mouth, lips, hands & feet; incoherence & difficulty of articulation, perception. Condition of legs indicating early GPI . . . Noisy, incoherent & difficult to control. Speech uncontrolled, very difficult to understand.[158]

"Weak and tremulous" was a common descriptor of GPI patients on admission to the asylum, but it was also used for patients with other mental and physical disorders, such as epilepsy. An eye condition known as an Argyll Robertson pupil was associated with neurosyphilis. Harper provided a description of this condition in Taniela's friend Tiacoro, who had GPI: "the pupils were small, equal, and sluggish in their reaction to accommodation and there was absolutely no reaction to light. The sight was not affected." This condition is noted in a few asylum records in patients with GPI or syphilis, although the physical evidence of GPI may have been underreported. Harper suggested that it was difficult to examine many Fijians for neurological disease because it was masked by other physical conditions.[159]

In 1927, the Wassermann test became available in Fiji.[160] It tested blood or cerebrospinal fluid for the presence of spirochaetes, but it was not conclusive in identifying the presence of syphilis or yaws. The test was only used sparingly in Fiji and, by the 1940s, was superseded by the Kahn test. Although the Kahn test was also not always reliable in determining the underlying disease, it was routinely administered to patients diagnosed with GPI or possibly syphilis.

One hundred and four patients diagnosed with GPI or syphilis died in the asylum between 1884 and 1940. Only eight patients with GPI were discharged before 1940. GPI was often listed with other causes of death—such as aneurysm, cardiac failure, and exhaustion—consistent with the end-stage of the disease.

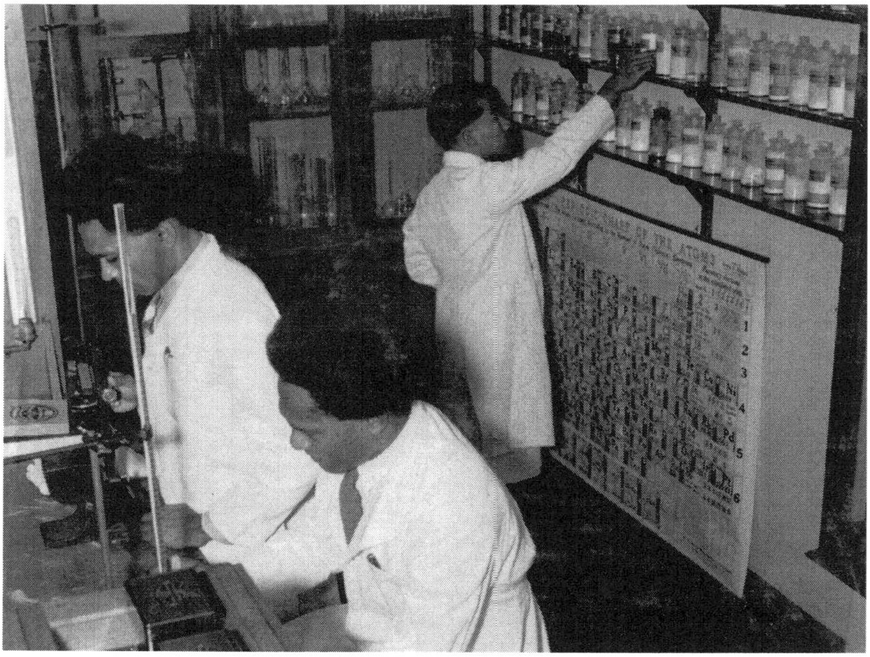

Figure 5.1. Native medical practitioners in the pathology laboratory, Colonial War Memorial Hospital, Suva, 1945. Source: Neg. no. 1126, NAF.

The impact of, or even causative agents of, aortic disease and aneurism—diseases common among Fijians—were not addressed in understandings of GPI.[161] Instead, during this era, medical doctors and psychiatrists worldwide were confident in diagnosing GPI and assigning it as a cause of death.[162] An autopsy could confirm pathological changes in the brain.[163]

The epidemiology of GPI in Fiji confounds comparisons with the history of psychiatry elsewhere. This is because the majority of those diagnosed with GPI were indigenous Fijians. Table 5.3 presents the ethnicity of those patients with GPI (or paralytica insanity) mentioned in their records, either as a symptom or a cause of illness or death, between 1884 and 1940: sixty Fijians, thirty Indo-Fijians, ten other Pacific Islanders, two Europeans, one Indo-European, and one Fijian-European. If patients with syphilis but not GPI mentioned in their records are included, the number of non-Fijians affected slightly increases. Dr. Sylvester Lambert reported that an analysis of death records between 1909 and 1929 showed that forty-two of 182 "Fijian natives, Melanesian and Polynesian," admitted to the asylum died from GPI but did not have syphilis.[164] This finding verified

Table 5.3. Asylum patients with general paralysis of the insane, 1884–1940

	GPI	GPI with Syphilis	Syphilis	Total
Fijian	60			60
Indian	21	9	3	33
Other Pacific	10			10
Fijian European		1	1	2
European	2	1	3	6
Indian European	1			1

Source: *Blue Book of Fiji* and patients' admission papers, St Giles Hospital.
Note: The ethnicity of two patient deaths during this period is unknown. These categories refer to whether syphilis was mentioned with GPI as a symptom, disorder, or cause.

earlier medical assessments that syphilis was absent among Fijians.[165] The common wisdom was that yaws offered immunity to syphilis.[166]

Some doctors did report that yaws, like syphilis, could produce severe neurological effects. During the early twentieth century, these doctors pointed out that tertiary stage yaws produced GPI symptoms.[167] By 1911, the arsenical compound salvarsan, an anti-syphilitic treatment, was successfully being administered in Fiji for tertiary stage yaws, but Dr. Montague did not administer the drug for GPI, "so common among Fijians." It was unlikely that salvarsan would have offered any relief.[168]

William Chapple, a New Zealand surgeon, and Harper reported on the similar effects of yaws to syphilis. Chapple wrote,

> This peculiar disease is Fijian "syphilis," and is not contracted venereally. It has a similar germ to syphilis, produces the same symptoms and signs all through the life of its victim, has the primary, secondary and tertiary manifestations, produces locomotor ataxia and general paralysis of the insane, and can scarcely be distinguished from the European disease.[169]

Harper reported in *The Lancet,* "Locomotor ataxy, general paralysis of the insane, and aneurysm, well recognised as sequelm of syphilis, seem to have been generally overlooked as remote results of framboesia."[170] He ruled out syphilis as the cause of such effects in Fijians and stressed the link to yaws. Harper published three case studies of Fijians who had tabes or GPI but who did not have syphilis.[171] He had seen several other similar but less clear cases in his medical district of six thousand Fijians, where

> there is a very high rate of such nervous disease amongst the Fijians, but it must be remembered that the whole Fijian population has been

> infected with yaws, and probably the case-rate following yaws might not greatly differ from the case-rate following syphilis.

Chief Medical Officer Dr. Lynch reported to the Australasian Medical Congress in 1913 that GPI was common among Fijians because of framboesia, not syphilis.[172] Maciu, diagnosed with GPI in 1922, had apparently had "framboesial insanity" as an infant, although he had no other tertiary lesions. His "lunatic behaviour" resurfaced at the age of twenty-eight, when he became "morose & sullen" and, subsequently, increasingly violent.[173] Some Fijian patients had yaws noted as a cause of their insanity, GPI being recorded only after their deaths; a few of the patients with yaws noted as a cause never had GPI mentioned in their records. however.[174]

Although some doctors in Fiji linked yaws (and not syphilis) to the extreme mental anguish of indigenous Fijians with GPI, their clinical observations had little traction within esteemed medical circles in Europe.[175] It was only much later that some researchers reviewed Fijian and comparable global literature on yaws and concluded "that congenital, visceral, ocular, and neurologic involvement can indeed occur in yaws."[176]

The accounts of GPI in Fijian villages take us back to chapter 3, where it was stressed that madness was not just about disease but that it was also a social outcome. Villagers did not associate yaws with shame and usually cared for those affected with tertiary stage yaws and what doctors labeled GPI. They did so for Taniela, for example, until his increasing physical incapacity and violent and immoral behavior became unacceptable after he exposed himself to a NMP's wife and made indecent suggestions to her; Harper then had him committed to the asylum.

In contrast to yaws, syphilis invoked moral alarm in Fiji and was especially linked with the sexual immorality of Indians. Only a small percentage of those who contracted syphilis also contracted GPI (neurosyphilis). Once penicillin was available from the 1940s, GPI dramatically disappeared as a mental disease globally and locally. Simultaneously, GPI also declined in Fiji once yaws was controlled and then eradicated in the late 1950s Although syphilis started to emerge among indigenous Fijians, GPI did not reappear because both it and syphilis could be treated with antibiotics.[177] GPI was a significant mental disease category in colonial Fiji, reflecting actual organic and mental conditions, but it was also a disease constructed by contested discourse. In 1939, Hoodless reported, "9 out of the 21 deaths at the Asylum were indicative of spirochaetal infection," but it was not possible to "evaluate the part played by syphilis or yaws in the incidence of mental disease in Fiji."[178] That mystery remains.

Alcoholic Insanity

Another mental disorder that warrants discussion is alcoholic insanity, because alcohol and substance abuse figured far less in the etiology and classification of insanity in colonial Fiji than elsewhere.[179] Alcoholism was a predominantly male European disorder in Fiji before World War II, and alcohol abuse by Europeans was probably more widespread than the asylum records indicate.[180] Before 1964, only two females were admitted to St Giles with alcohol listed as a problem. Alcohol-related admissions tended to be brief, the asylum offering a space for short-term detoxification. Among such acute cases were travelers and sailors, such as a fireman on the SS *Atua* in 1911 who was only admitted for two days after throwing himself overboard and attempting to assault officers and crew.[181] Alcohol abuse was a problem for crew on Pacific steamships, the problem partly exacerbated by working conditions, boredom, and depression.[182]

Alcoholism could lead to much longer stays in the asylum. In 1924, for example, a European shipping clerk was admitted with delusional insanity; he died in the asylum in 1932, age thirty-nine, from phthisis, with toxemia and exhaustion.[183] In 1902, a European patient admitted with "alcoholic insanity" died four years later from thrombosis in the brain, dementia, and exhaustion, thought to be directly related to his alcohol abuse. A former baker, he continued in the asylum to believe he was still baking loaves every morning. He was also convinced that people were trying to cut off his head.[184] Other alcoholic patients were admitted several times: Mani, an Indian storekeeper, had six admissions between 1934 and 1962.[185] He was diagnosed initially with dementia, then with mania, and only on his fourth admission with alcoholic psychosis.

As Mani's history revealed, alcoholism could present with other mental disorders. Michael, a European civil servant, was admitted to the asylum as an "alcoholic maniac" after attempting suicide by drinking perchloride of mercury. Consuming this compound could be lethal, and it is unclear how much he ingested or what the long-term repercussions were. He endured severe and complicated mental distress while in the asylum from September 7, 1910, to January 17, 1911, which was longer than an initial period of detoxification; this distress included delusions, violence, anorexia, depression, and additional suicide attempts. Michael saw his madness as a moral struggle with the devil that had driven him to drink and chronic masturbation. Two days after his admission, he saw a conflict between God and the devil; the devil won, and Michael's presence on earth thereby damned a million people a day. He had slept and talked with the devil and proclaimed that, against his wishes, he had to accompany the devil to hell or else "all mankind will be damned." Michael had asked the police to lock him up because he was directed by voices to commit murder, including that of a Fijian policeman's child. Once in the asylum, he claimed that he had only feigned madness so that he could be committed. He urged the medical superintendent to cut out or open his genitalia, presumably to stop him from masturbating. Two weeks after his admission, Michael appeared more cheerful but continued to insist that he had been anointed by the devil, given that his violence, manic behavior, and anorexia resurfaced episodically.[186]

One reason alcohol abuse was predominantly a white man's disorder was its availability to Europeans. In Fiji, non-European access to liquor was either prohibited or limited through permits. Restrictions on access to alcohol were not removed for men until 1962 and for women until 1969. Alcohol was banned in most indigenous Fijian villages, and many Hindus and Muslims abstained. Alcohol was illegally available from the informal economy and bootlegging, thanks to the presence of thousands of Allied troops during World War II. Patterns in alcohol abuse in Fiji changed after the war, alcohol being noted slightly more often on admission certificates. Indo-Fijians rather than Europeans now made up the majority of these cases, which may have reflected more non-Europeans being allowed to purchase alcohol along with more disposable income and changing attitudes in some Indian communities about alcohol. The majority of Indo-Fijians admitted with alcoholism were storekeepers (seven), who would have had easier access to alcohol. Contrary to stereotypes in Western countries of the alcoholic as homeless, no destitutes admitted to St Giles during the colonial period appear to have had serious alcohol problems.

Some doctors, notably Lambert, believed that alcohol had a toxic effect on Pacific Islanders, given that they supposedly lacked Europeans' "acquired immunity," though, as historian Annie Stuart points out, "the Pacific abounded in examples of non-immune whites."[187] Only two indigenous Fijians were admitted to St Giles before 1964 with alcohol as a cause of illness.[188] One of the two was a young NMP who had drunk methylated spirits and, after being disciplined for doing so, became acutely depressed and refused to work. He did not resume practicing medicine and was diagnosed with manic depression.[189] The tragic death of Mesulame Taveta in 1935 highlighted the effects of mental stress, isolation, and alcohol abuse. He was another Fijian NMP, posted to the island of Malakula in the New Hebrides. T. Clunie, the Central Medical School head tutor, had warned about the impact of overseas postings on the mental and physical health of NMPs, saying, "few natives lifted out of their natural sphere escape death from alcoholic poisoning."[190] Taveta was treated with disdain by the French doctors and the British administrators in the New Hebrides and began drinking heavily. He was forbidden to consume alcohol further but continued to binge drink. He then contracted malaria and blackwater fever while attending a European patient in a remote part of Malakula, but was refused admission to the hospital because the doctor thought he was drunk. He died soon after.

Intellectual Disabilities

Several patients were classified with disorders that identified them as idiots, imbeciles, retards, mental defectives, feeble minded, or spastics. This discourse was commonly used in medical and lay circles during the colonial period. The disorder "idiot" often had no explanation, or doctors simply stated either "idiot since birth" or congenital idiocy. Patients with cerebral palsy were called spastics. The terms used in one category on admission papers did not always equate to the legal certification.[191] A patient classified with idiocy might be admitted with unsound mind or as a lunatic rather than as an idiot, or someone certified as an idiot might show symptoms of what doctors diagnosed as manic depression.[192]

Between 1911 and 1946, the general census in Fiji gathered information on people with mental disabilities. It asked respondents to "State the name of any person in this dwelling or establishment who is . . . 'Lunatic, imbecile, or feebleminded.'"[193] It is not clear how respondents understood this question because the terms were also derogatory, abusive, or shameful. It alludes to the colloquial use and the cultural context and translation of such discourse—terms discussed in earlier chapters, such as *pagla, buddhuu, lialia,* or *jaurara,* and the Fijian term *gone gogo,* which could refer to a "dull child, undeveloped mentally."[194] The census was not an accurate way to gauge the extent of mental disabilities in Fiji, and numbers were clearly underreported.[195]

Even in the 1970s, a more scientific survey in Fiji suggested that the number of children with intellectual disabilities was underreported, including in the number of females attending schools for the intellectually impaired.[196] John Price, medical superintendent at St Giles between 1970 and 1972, put this down to families' keeping daughters with disabilities at home because of shame and worry about their marriage prospects or those of their siblings. They were also protecting their vulnerable children from public abuse. Only a few intellectually disabled people were admitted to the hospital. According to Hoodless in 1939, the "number of mental certified mental defectives in Fiji up to the present is too small to warrant the erection of a separate institution."[197] Some of these patients died soon after admission, and, at a young age, from physical illness: a twelve-year-old admitted in 1934 died a year later from pneumonia as well as "congenital idiocy."[198] Severely mentally and physically disabled patients often required intensive care, which was the case with twenty-five-year-old Magan in 1948. Until that year, he had been cared for by his family but had never learned to speak, could not hear, and had frequent epileptic fits. Magan was admitted to St Giles after he started wandering and attacking adults and children. He required an attendant to feed and bathe him until his death eleven months later.[199]

Other patients with mental disabilities, known as chronics, remained in the hospital, because families were either unwilling or unable to offer care and because of the lack of suitable alternative institutions. Patients with widely differing intellectual and physical abilities shared the same space at St Giles. In 1967, the medical superintendent highlighted that "the mixing of disturbed patients and defectives with other patients continues to present problems." He recommended that an outpatients' block and reception ward be established near the hospital's entrance to allow "defectives" to be segregated in the main wards.[200] This structure would reduce overcrowding and disruption but was also probably suggested to shield patients with obvious impairment from public view. Although most of those born with intellectual and physical disabilities continued to be cared for by their families, after World War II, the number of young people, several of whom were classified as "idiots," admitted to St Giles increased. These youths had epilepsy, schizophrenia, manic depression, and other affective disorders.

Epilepsy

Those with epilepsy, especially children, were often relegated as "mental defectives." The 1938 classification listed epilepsy as a mental disease though today it is referred to as a neurological and seizure disorder.[201] Between 1936 and 1964, epilepsy, epileptic seizures, or epileptic fits are mentioned in approximately 6 percent of admission records, but in all the admission records I consulted going back to 1884, epilepsy is noted in only 3 percent. As in global patterns of the illness, most patients were male. Only a small proportion of those having epileptic seizures received medical attention in colonial Fiji, and only those with frequent and severe seizures, other coexisting mental disorders, or whose families could not care for them were committed to the asylum. In Fiji, some tolerance toward people with epilepsy was typical, but, as elsewhere, they might be called mad, subjected to stigma or ridicule, or assumed to be possessed by a spirit. Patients with epilepsy often had repeat admissions. Epileptic seizures were linked with other mental disorders, and epilepsy was listed as a cause of death. An eighteen-year-old male who had frequent epileptic seizures and was described as a "poor weak patient [who] could not help himself in any way" died a month after he was admitted to the hospital in 1942.[202]

Delusions of Persecution

Paranoia also appeared in the new mental disease classifications in Fiji in 1938, though the term had first appeared in Pita's admission records in 1913.[203] Pita was one of the controversial Fijian leaders discussed in chapter 3, as was Penioni Ravoka, who was diagnosed with paranoia in 1935 and called a paranoic. After Pita, paranoia did not feature on admission papers until 1932, though other terms, such as "delusions of persecution," were used. In 1920, a European planter was convinced that he had to be "on the alert" because a group of men was "after him" and that they had fired electric shocks at him.[204] Many doctors believed that paranoia, unlike schizophrenia, did not exhibit marked thought disorder and that delusions were "well organized, coherent and systematized," often reflecting the actual world, such as being talked about, under surveillance, or affected by war.[205] Paranoia was mostly diagnosed during the 1930s and 1940s (3 to 4 percent of admissions). Beginning in the 1950s, more patients were diagnosed with paranoid schizophrenia.

Schizophrenia on the Rise

Hoodless thought it necessary to reexamine patient classifications periodically; a pattern borne out by the dramatic post–World War II rise in those classified with schizophrenia in Fiji. This rise in diagnoses replicated a global shift within nosology from manic depression to schizophrenia although the diagnostic criteria in the United Kingdom and the United States diverged for several decades.[206]

Dementia praecox was first recorded in Fiji in 1924 on Deeti's admission papers. Deeti had emigrated to Fiji in 1908 when she was sixteen. Her husband said that she was "apparently normal" for a year but had since been insane. The doctor observed that Deeti was "totally incapable of coherent speech; untidy & dirty in habits; facial appearance, gestures, attitude, etc suggests a mental condition advanced to dementia." Dementia praecox was given as the cause, but her disorder was still recorded under the classification of mania, and her postmortem established GPI and heart disease as the cause of death in 1938.[207] This case indicates that, though some doctors may have acquired modern psychiatric terminology, confusion and ambiguity remained about etiology and diagnosis. In contrast, in 1936 Macpherson offered an almost textbook diagnosis of dementia praecox:

> He [the patient] is dishevelled in his appearance non cooperative in his attitude, and apparently disorientated to some extent in regard to time and place. He is noisy, showing little ability to answer direct

> questions and no logical flight of ideas. His behaviour would appear to indicate a . . . form of dementia praecox.[208]

Schizophrenia first appears on a St Giles record as the diagnosis given to an Indo-Fijian patient admitted in 1931. He would spend most of his life in the institution and was not discharged until 1971.[209] Twenty-one-year-old Cathy was also admitted by her mother in 1931, when she was diagnosed with dementia praecox, attributed to overstudy. Cathy said that worms were crawling out of her mouth and snakes were under the bed clothes and that, when she walked in her sleep, men tried to seduce her. She was violent and used obscene language. In 1948, her diagnosis was redesignated as schizophrenia.[210] By 1956, ninety-six patients were listed in the mental hospital's annual report with schizophrenia to seventy-eight with manic depressive psychosis.[211] The number of patients diagnosed with manic depression declined, and, as table 5.1 shows, the number with schizophrenia increased dramatically during the 1950s and 1960s (31 percent and of 58 percent as the final diagnosis respectively). Among 322 patients in 1963, 187 were diagnosed with schizophrenia, compared with forty-four with mania and only three with depression.

It could be suggested that this changing nosology reflected shifts in the kind of patients being admitted to the hospital rather than changes in medical knowledge and nosology. More women were admitted to the hospital in the decades after World War II, and a high percentage were diagnosed with schizophrenia (28 percent to 19 percent of men). Indians and Others were slightly more likely than Fijians to be classified with schizophrenia, but only 8 percent of European admissions were. Because schizophrenia was more commonly diagnosed in Indo-Fijians than in indigenous Fijians, an increase in the number of Indo-Fijian patients admitted to the hospital was matched by an increase in the hospital rates for schizophrenia.[212] The tendency was to diagnose disproportionately certain groups with particular psychoses, as Jackson found for Africans, especially women, in colonial Zimbabwe.[213] Fiji's clinic was not immune from racial and gender stereotyping, but, as discussed at the end of this chapter, doctors had doubts about equating race with the form of mental disorder. Price and Issac Karim suggested that the higher number of Indo-Fijian patients with schizophrenia may have been because schizophrenia was tolerated better within Melanesian extended families and that those admitted were very disturbed.[214]

Closer reading of the archive suggests that categorizations were often only vaguely indicative of a patient's condition. The frequent blank spaces under "disorder" suggest that doctors often did not know how to complete the section. As explained, a patient might have their disorder changed from manic depression to schizophrenia or another category. Such shifting classifications could reflect changes in a patient's symptoms, in nosology and medical knowledge, or in the turnover of medical personnel.

Mental illness classifications were revised again in 1965 soon after Duncan Macgregor was appointed as the first psychiatrist to head St Giles. Macgregor conducted a local study to assess whether the United Kingdom's diagnostic criteria were applicable in Fiji. The largest group of 29 percent of discharged patients in 1965 was diagnosed with schizophrenia. Manic depression may have been subsumed under the old category of mania (26 percent) or depressive disorders (10 percent).[215] Macgregor's classifications were revised by Dr. David Sell a few years later to provide more simplified disease classifications under the broad categories of psychoses, neuroses, personality disorders, drug dependence, epilepsy and allied disorders, and mental retardation. These revisions brought classification more in line with the Eighth Revision of the ICD.[216] Sell did not include symptoms that Macgregor had listed, such as tantrums, frenzies, epileptic furies and confusions, and outbursts in mental defectives.

Heightened and Altered Reality: Hysteria, Neuroses, and Anxiety

Hysteria, neuroses, and anxiety disorders encompassed a variety of symptoms and meanings and were not significant among diagnoses for hospitalized mental disorders in Fiji. Nineteenth-century discourses of hysteria embraced nervousness, neurasthenia, nerve prostration, and hysterical insanity that were interpreted as a form of degeneration and "out and out madness."[217] On November 14, 1906, Cutt Schroeter, the paymaster on the German warship *Condor*, was admitted to the Colonial Hospital suffering from neurasthenia. He had "heart affections," difficulty breathing, insomnia, and was depressed; after learning that there would be a delay in his being sent to Sydney, he hanged himself in a bathroom.[218] Another seaman with the British Royal Navy was admitted to the Colonial Hospital in 1922; Dr. Mildred Staley diagnosed him with neurasthenia. He began to hear voices and could taste a nasty smell of smoke emanating from his heart. He believed that he had religious mania and needed to confess his crimes. After he was transferred to the mental hospital, his diagnosis shifted to mania.[219] Busfield summed up twentieth-century clinical assessments of neuroses as an exaggerated response to reality rather than a loss of contact with reality.[220] The understanding and treatment of hysteria and neuroses shifted over time, and, possibly because of the psychological basis to these conditions, European doctors in Fiji were less likely to apply such terms cross-culturally. The notable exception (as outlined in chapter 2) was in 1968, when doctors identified spirit possession among schoolgirls at Qawa as mass hysteria. Only the "trigger girl" was administered antipsychotic medication and psychological tests.

Hysteria was more likely to be the diagnosis on first admission, but this diagnosis often changed once doctors had observed patients or when patients were readmitted. Sodhi was twelve when she was admitted to St Giles in 1957 with hysteria, following a nightmare after a religious ceremony. She continually gesticulated, talked, shouted, threw herself about, and refused to eat. After a second admission the following year, Sodhi's diagnosis changed to schizophrenia. By 1964, she was diagnosed with cyclic manic depression and having "a moderate degree of intellectual retardation."[221]

Hysteria has long been considered a woman's disease and a metaphor of feminine stereotypes throughout modern Western history. The Fiji records show that the label of hysteria was applied to other cultures.[222] In 1949, Rukhmini's husband's employer sent her to Lomaloma Hospital after she had a long argument with her sister, threw most of the furniture and glassware outside, tore her clothes, and sat alone, talking aimlessly. She did not sleep for six days. Rukhmini was nineteen years old, newly married, and living with her husband on an island in Lau. She wished to return to her parents in Navua, an unsurprising desire for a young bride living on a remote island far away from her natal home. The assistant medical practitioner assessed that she was not "seriously ill mentally" but "more a case of hysteria rather than lunacy." Nonetheless he sent Rukhmini to Suva for further examination for mental illness where her condition worsened and she attempted to hang herself. Dr. Oldmeadow and Dr. Doran diagnosed her with manic depression; she spent seven months in the mental hospital. She was readmitted in 1960 for nearly five years.[223] Yet in the fourteen patients diagnosed with hysteria in the St Giles records from 1884 to 1964, the gender breakdown was equally split, and ethnicity may have been of more significance. Nine of these patients were Indo-Fijians; three were Europeans. Georgina, a fifty-eight-year-old single European from Levuka, was the only patient diagnosed with hysteria before the late 1930s. She was admitted in 1910 with a profound conviction that she was dying. She did die three months after being admitted to the asylum, though her postmortem stated that she had suffered from acute mania rather than hysteria and that she had died from exhaustion.[224]

Only eight patients were diagnosed with nervous conditions between 1884 and 1964, among whom were four Europeans and two part-Europeans. Six of these patients were males. Most of the admissions were very brief. In 1936, an elderly Indo-Fijian woman spent three weeks in the hospital as a "victim of an anxiety neurosis," though the recorded disorder was delusional insanity.[225] More undisclosed people likely suffered from anxiety neurosis outside the hospital.

Many were treated through the outpatient services that started during the 1960s. Sell predicted that the number of outpatients with stress neuroses would increase as Fiji developed.[226]

Conclusion: Fiji as an Ideal Natural Laboratory

Neuroses may not have been commonly reported or as alarming in Fiji as symptoms linked with mania, depression, schizophrenia, or GPI, but an occurrence, such as the Qawa hysteria incident, raised questions about the boundaries of normality or abnormality within cultures and the universality of biomedical discourse. The meanings attached to the symptoms and classification of madness changed over time and were mediated by culture, gender, and status. This was one reason psychologist and sociologist Glenn Wilson described Fiji as an ideal natural laboratory.[227] The cultural and religious diversity in both Fiji's asylum and community offered rich potential for the growing interest in cross-cultural psychiatry after World War II.

Cross-cultural psychiatry, comparative psychiatry, and ethnopsychology are also concerned with identifying culture-specific mental disorders.[228] Fiji's ethnic complexity raised tantalizing questions over the universality of psychiatric disorders, although these questions did not address how Western biomedicine and psychiatry were culturally constructed or grounded in modern capitalist society.[229] Canadian psychiatrist Eric Berne, who established the transactional analysis school in psychotherapy, studied psychiatric epidemiology and some patients in Fiji and Papeete during the late 1950s. This research confirmed his view that there is no causative link between culture, history, or geography and mental illness, and that etiology, symptomatology, diagnosis, and therapy could be transferred between cultures.[230] Berne's conviction as to the universality of mental disorders was verified by his assessment that rates of psychiatric disorders in Fiji's two main ethnic groups were probably similar.[231]

Duncan Macgregor introduced a local concept into psychiatric nosology. He identified the Fiji Syndrome, which was reported in 14 percent of discharged patients in 1965 and about half the patients admitted with acute excitement "on the borderline of clinical acute mania."[232] Macgregor modified the Fiji Syndrome to refer to a form of transient mania or hysteria common throughout the South Pacific and seen in Malaysia that was rarely caused by major mental illness or required specialist treatment.[233] *Matiruku* went further and was identified as a culturally bound mental syndrome.[234] *Matiruku* could be a colloquial term for madness, but a study by Price and Karim suggests that it was a form of hypomania, which manifested in Fiji with a short duration, frequent recurrence, and intensified symptoms in the morning.[235] It was likely to affect people when the tide was very low or possibly very high. Karim was later uncertain as to how much *matiruku* could be applied to psychiatric diagnosis.[236] The Fiji Syndrome was discounted.

Other researchers investigated patterns in ethnicity, symptoms, and mental disorders.[237] Transcultural psychiatrist H. B. M. Murphy, from McGill University, teamed up with St Giles Medical Superintendent Ram Narayan to study mental hospitalization between 1972 and 1975. They found that Fijians were more likely to exhibit mania, while Indo-Fijians were more prone to depression,

> It is commonly recognized that Fijians, as well as being the more robust, are the more likely to act out under stress, and this can give their mental disorder a manic character. The slighter Indians, in contrast, are more likely to withdraw into themselves under stress, and any turning of anger in on the self, as can easily happen during such withdrawal, is likely to show itself as depression or, in the extreme, as suicide, a condition which occurs much more often in the Indians than in the Fijians. The "Other" ethnic group category does not show any special diagnostic features.[238]

Later Karim remarked to me that, although the mental symptoms might present differently between different cultures, the condition was the same. He qualified any correlation between ethnicity and psychiatric nosology: "that was just impression, later on when we started looking at the figures and so forth it doesn't hold up."[239] Macgregor was also careful to emphasize the difference between outward presentation and psychiatric diagnoses along ethnic lines:

> I have found that depressive illness is very liable to present as something else: the Fijians start off with a fighting frenzy, the Indians with a paranoid reaction and the Europeans with a severe anxiety.[240]

His comments could be regarded as racial stereotyping but also point to how culture could impinge on symptomology and potential diagnoses. Community assessment was significant in providing the "facts" of mental illness but doctors were also swayed by their training, knowledge, and cultural preconceptions. In practice at St Giles, medical opinions about symptoms, etiology, or nosology had limited relevance to treatment or management. The demarcation between Europeans and natives was maintained in the asylum, as it was in the community, during the colonial period. Even these boundaries could be porous. Within the asylum, patients with widely varying conditions, from severe mental and physical disabilities from birth to sudden, acute psychosis, shared the same wards and often the same treatments, which is the focus of the next chapter.

CHAPTER 6

Struggling with Madness

Control, Treatments, and Resistance

Testimony about the asylum's diet is buried within the Fiji National Archives as part of a series of letters that patient Martin Syljeseth wrote in 1923 to J. S. Neill, head of the asylum's Board of Visitors.[1]

> It is only fair to state that the food, bar the bread, is generally good, but it is now a fairly well known fact that science condemns white, or hulled rice, because of its lack of an all important vitamin and that lack of course makes it undesirable as a food for anyone let alone one whose brain tissues have weakened to a point where he is classed as insane.[2]

Such remnants of patient voices are rare because "most senseless letters from patients" were usually destroyed.[3]

Syljeseth was among the minority of patients who were literate in English. Colonial authorities sometimes procured translations of Fijian and Hindi testimonies for persons of high status or when a serious legal matter was under consideration. In the asylum, only selected (usually European or "mixed-race") patients had access to pen and paper; this lack of writing paper may have been the reason that Grace, a patient between 1958 and 1965, wrote scrawled messages on clean toilet paper.[4] During the asylum's early years, even if staff were willing to assist patients, warders had limited English literacy. Status and power hierarchies, overlaid by ethnicity, gender, and class, meant that asylum patients were unlikely to approach higher-level hospital officials. The divides of mental ability and disability and sanity and insanity also determined noncommunication. When patients did resist, it was often in nonverbal or nonliterate ways. This situation makes it even more remarkable that evidence remains of Syljeseth's exercising his legal rights of patient advocacy. Patients were permitted to write confidentially to the Board of Visitors and communicate with them during the board's visits to the hospital. Such provisions were rarely exercised, which is not surprising given the severe intellectual disorders of many patients.

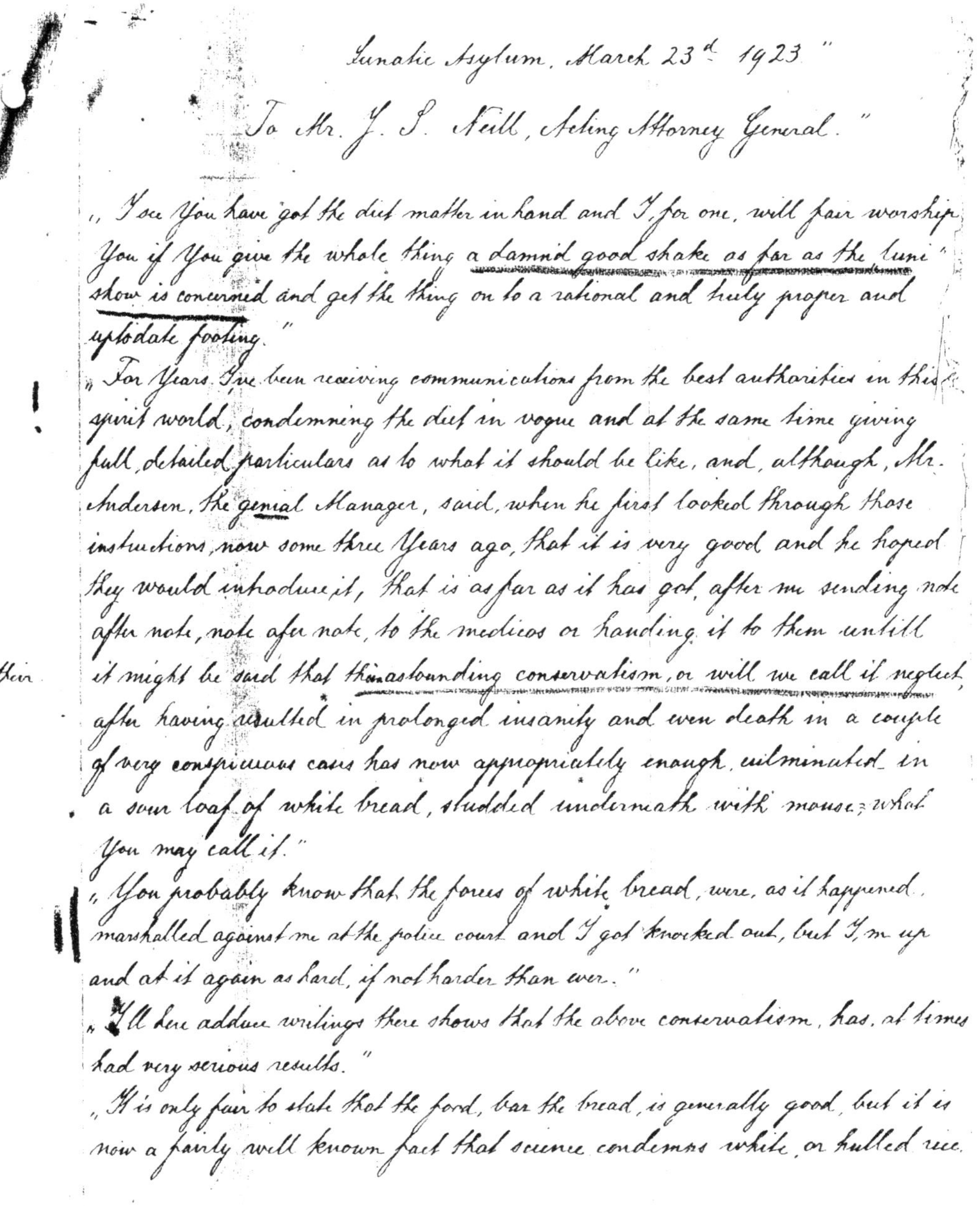

Lunatic Asylum, March 23rd 1923."

To Mr. J. S. Neill, Acting Attorney General."

" I see You have got the diet matter in hand and I, for one, will fair worship You if You give the whole thing a damnd good shake as far as the luni" show is concerned and get the thing on to a rational and truly proper and uptodate footing."

" For Years I've been receiving communications from the best authorities in the spirit world, condemning the diet in vogue and at the same time giving full, detailed particulars as to what it should be like, and, although, Mr. Andersen, the genial Manager, said, when he first looked through those instructions, now some three Years ago, that it is very good and he hoped they would introduce it, that is as far as it has got, after me sending note after note, note afer note, to the medicos or handing it to them untill it might be said that their astounding conservatism, or will we call it neglect, after having resulted in prolonged insanity and even death in a couple of very conspicuous cases has now appropriately enough, culminated in a sour loaf of white bread, studded underneath with mouse= what You may call it."

" You probably know that the forces of white bread, were, as it happened, marshalled against me at the police court and I got knocked out, but I,m up and at it again as hard, if not harder than ever."

" I'll here adduce writings there shows that the above conservatism, has, at times had very serious results."

" It is only fair to state that the food, bar the bread, is generally good, but it is now a fairly well known fact that science condemns white, or hulled rice.

Figure 6.1. Letter (detail) by patient Martin Syljeseth to J. S. Neill, March 23, 1923. Source: CSO MP 23/1111, NAF.

Syljeseth was a tailor from Norway who had probably spent several years in New Zealand before sailing to Fiji.[5] He was first admitted to the asylum in 1918 as a fifty-four-year-old destitute.[6] In December 1922, he was discharged but three months later was readmitted; he remained in the asylum until his death in 1933.[7] His only property was a "useless sewing machine." Syljeseth often wrote his beautifully neat and articulate letters as Dr. Jenner, the pioneer of the smallpox vaccine, whom Syljeseth regarded as a "leading medical authority in this spirit world."[8]

Syljeseth advocated "rational" and "truly proper and up to date" dietary changes in the hospital. He was cognizant of the diversity of patients' cultural dietary preferences but insisted on similar dietary principles for all:

> it is to be exactly the same for every one in the asylum never mind what race, creed or colour he or she happens to belong to, but out of the asylum we expect the European will swear by his bread, the Asiatic by his rice and the Fijian by his taro, yam etc for his staple food, and glorious stuff those Fijian root crops are, but Dr Jenner insists that after being thoroughly scrubbed and washed they must, one and all, be boiled in their skins, for otherwise an invaluable element is lost.[9]

Syljeseth was deeply concerned about other patients and closely watched their diets as well as how they were treated. He claimed that a European patient "would, without any operation, have become quite contented after one week in the asylum if he had got one or other of those diets so strongly insisted on."[10] As Dr. Jenner, Syljeseth was not happy that the family of "the big Indian" could bring him "the most refined food possible," as this "keeps his digestive apparatus constantly disturbed."

Syljeseth also wrote about "the Chinaman," but it was with "the Honolulu man, Kepah" that he took on the most visible role of patient advocate. He wrote in the third person, as Dr. Jenner observing Syljeseth's interactions with Kepah: "As Martin was just passing, he [Kepah] spoke to him and begged him to speak for him so that he might be allowed out in the sun and not be kept without any clothes and without any bucket in the cold cement room." Syljeseth documented Kepah's physical and mental deterioration following his admission to the asylum.

> When the Hawaiian first arrived at the asylum he was by no means very bad and I thought he would be out again in a few weeks for he looked a splendid stamp of a fellow. Presently I got information from

> the spirit world as to the real cause of his insanity and insisting on a change in the unfortunate chaps diet, but as per usual the doctor took not the slightest notice of the carefully detailed note I handed him and the poor man went from bad to worse.[11]

Syljeseth reported how representatives of the spirit world found Kepah lying on the floor and presumed him dead. Realizing that he was only asleep, "providence then enlightened us that the real thing will happen in from three to five weeks, unless that man's diet is altered." Syljeseth had informed an attendant and the chief medical officer how to prepare wholemeal rice, but they ignored the instructions. Kepah died about six weeks later.

Syljeseth's documentation was accurate. Kepah was John Kepper, a Polynesian, who was either a Tongan or Hawaiian. He had been sentenced to two years hard labor for larceny in Tonga and was committed to prison in Suva before being transferred to the asylum on 21 July 1922.[12] He was probably placed in solitary confinement because during his manic periods he would break plates and buckets with "no sense of wrongdoing for this." His death was attributed to exhaustion and chronic sepsis. Syljeseth was dismayed by the "medicos," through

> their astounding conservatism, or will we call it neglect, after having resulted in prolonged insanity and even death in a couple of very conspicuous cases has now appropriately accumulated in a sour loaf of white bread. . . . Just think of it. People loosing their health, and, in some instances their very reason and ending in lamentable tragedies simply through lack of a little bran.

The colonial secretary dismissed Syljeseth's letters despite the serious issues he raised, writing, "The ravings of this lunatic, need not have been officially registered. My experience of Martin is that he never expects a reply to his scintillating effusions, but derives mental peace from writing them to all & sundry!"[13]

Syljeseth's letters articulated the signs, behind the walls of the asylum and within the archive, of overt and hidden struggles among patients and staff. Patients struggled against institutionalization, the asylum, community, family, and living with madness. They most openly used violence, escape, and suicide to repudiate confinement and the daily regimes it entailed, but other expressions of patients' agency can be traced in the archive. Their letters represented internal worlds, mostly incomprehensible to others. Although such voices may appear bizarre, they are indicative of patients constructing individual worlds of rationality. In putting words on paper, through letters or other media, patients were inscribing their identity, as literate human beings attempting to communicate outside themselves. Talking to oneself could be an expression of sanity in the insane world of the asylum. In 1961, "one of the old chronics," who had been in the hospital for twenty-two years, said he "talked to the air," because he must practice talking or he might forget how to do it.[14] Similarly, Syljeseth's letter writing represented a rich internal world that reflected his mental condition but also showed how he resisted and coped with the biopolitics of care in the asylum.

Staff were also engaged in a struggle against madness, whether with compassion and moral management or by control. The biopolitics of care ranged from the most intimate aspects of daily regimens to revolutionary and experimental technologies and therapies. Such care equally could punish patients who did not accept the rules of confinement.

Previous chapters trace the link between care and control for those deemed mad, long before they were legally certified as insane. Some patients had been constrained, sometimes for many years, by family or in police custody, before admission to the asylum. Others had been relatively unfettered and cared for in homes and villages. Some had led transient lives, wandering between villages or around towns. This mobility abruptly stopped once they entered the asylum, where all patients encountered embodied, spatial, and therapeutic constraints, ostensibly as part of their care and asylum management.

Fragments of testimony reflect patient voice and their limited agency. Doctors either ignored or heard this perspective to a limited degree. In colonial Nigeria, Jonathan Sadowsky found that patient voice was generally not seriously scrutinized; content was attributed to psychosis, or the individual voice became literally or metaphorically subsumed within the general cacophony of the psychiatric ward.[15] Catharine Coleborne suggests that female patients in Australian colonial asylums in Victoria internalized institutional aims to accommodate the realities of institutional hegemony, possibly so that they could be discharged.[16] Compliance with hospital rules and routines, and the inculcation of this as personal regime were considered therapeutic and a sign of recovery and normalcy that might eventuate in release. Sadly, many patients were abandoned at St Giles and became long-term patients. Those who were permanently confined, such as Syljeseth, often accommodated the most to the institution.[17] This acceptance could be disrupted by cyclical changes in their mental state and was constantly tested by the hospital's conditions and tensions with other patients and staff.

Yet, despite the grim realities of institutional life, patients and staff also expressed humor, so important in Pacific cultures.[18] Humor is difficult to trace in the archive, but its subversive, equalizing, and "normalizing" roles were evident to me when I was researching at St Giles. Snippets of humor and irony as a form of agency include the patient who talked to the air, Syljeseth's reference to the chief medical officer as "the same old sinner," or, as discussed later in this chapter, when patients reprimanded staff for not performing their duties. Silly or disrespectful behavior could verge on mimicry or parody, as when Bagnath displayed "unnecessary and absurd servility of behaviour" to the doctor in 1885.[19]

Resistance and agency not only were a response to the immediate conditions in the asylum but also indicated how the external world was transmitted through patients' internal worlds. For Roy Porter, the content of patient discourse matters: the mad person's "immediate oppressors mainly existed only in their heads . . . they were commonly the analogues of ogres out there in society, in the culture."[20] Previous chapters emphasize community influences on patients' mental states. Women's responses and resistance show how gendered and ethnicized role expectations could be entwined with the path into madness. Women's crazy embodiment, violence, or sexuality was construed as evidence of madness, but it could show agency to gendered oppression.[21]

The extent to which struggles within the asylum reflected a broader struggle against biopower and political hegemony is contentious. For Michel Foucault, the biopolitics of care reproduced external hierarchies of power and the exercise of state and class hegemony, and for Frantz Fanon, also colonial control.[22] Richard Keller's study of colonial psychiatry in French North Africa connected broader political tensions with those in the asylum: "Psychiatric diagnosis exposed a deep rift between colonizer and colonized, and the doctor-patient relationship in this setting often took shape as a contest for hegemony."[23] James Mills similarly highlighted the link between confinement in colonial India and patient resistance: "These inmates may have lost their freedom as they were incarcerated in a colonial institution but they were determined to resist the imposition of an alien order on their bodies."[24]

Having started with Syljeseth's polite criticisms of diet and care, this chapter follows patient experience within the asylum, especially the daily regimens of meals, bathing, hygiene, dress, work, and other activities. These aspects were integral to patient care and treatment, as well as asylum management and the control of unruly bodies and disordered minds. After World War II, the rapid introduction of modern radical pharmacological and shock treatments became part of the hospital's daily patterns and would alter not only patients' minds but also patient-staff dynamics. The asylum was a space where the goals and realities of control and confinement, care and cure, constituted the exercise of biopower and delineated structures within which patient agency and resistance operated. This agency was sometimes overt and demonstrated through channels that authorities understood (even if they dismissed the content), such as formal or verbal complaints. Patients were more likely to be agentive in embodied and often oblique or covert ways. Such expressions could be incomprehensible or consigned by staff to madness. This chapter traces agency and patient voice in the archive against the structural context of institutional control, care, and treatments.

Patient resistance and agency to institutionalization and biopower at St Giles was expressed in various ways, from formal letters to violence and the extremes of silence and suicide. Agency might sometimes be written or spoken, but more often it was embodied. The body and the mind were key sites of control and agency, and this struggle often manifested over daily activities, such as bathing, eating, or working, as well as invasive treatments involving medication or shock. Patients were concerned about common issues, ranging from diet to wrongful committal or the behavior of staff and other patients. Resistance could be voiced through what doctors regarded as delusions, such as Syljeseth's imaginary identity, Dr. Jenner. Delusions like this might also be a way of highlighting material deprivation and mistreatment in the asylum.

Controlling the Body to Tame the Mind

Resistance to confinement often began prior to a patient's arrival at the asylum. In 1910, Michael, under the sway of "alcoholic mania," attempted to jump off a cliff during his transfer from the general hospital to the asylum. Staff were instructed to constantly watch him and, if necessary, constrain him with a straitjacket.[25] Violent, manic, and suicidal patients were often heavily constrained on arrival. Even if patients were not violent, institutional control over their bodies began immediately. All patients were stripped, searched, and washed, and those with *kutu* (lice) had their head shaved or hair cut very short. Personal belongings were confiscated and might never be returned, such as seven gold bangles, tied with white and red striped cloth, and five silver bangles, wrapped in brown paper, marked "owners not known."[26] Personal intrusion, such as when clothing and jewelry was removed, could be culturally sensitive and traumatic for patients. A profoundly disturbed Indian woman might regard herself as a widow or divorced when her jewelry was confiscated, not only signifying her vulnerability as a woman without a husband but also divesting her of personal wealth.

The embodiment of institutionalization extended to a patient's clothing, which became another site of struggle and control between staff and patients. Patients were washed and then dressed in asylum clothing, which varied according to gender and ethnicity (see figure 4.2). Many mentally ill patients refused to wear any clothes. They destroyed clothing and bedding because these were two of the few items left to attack. In 1905, after Kauvuo ripped up his *sulu* and bedclothes, he was issued with a canvas *sulu*.[27] Compliant behavior might be rewarded with permission to wear personal clothing, as a patient in 1948 was allowed, with the proviso that "at the first sign of an attempt being made to escape he will go back to institutional clothing."[28]

Appropriate dress was considered important for female European patients. Soon after her admission in July 1896, Mrs. J. destroyed her dress, after which the chief medical officer requested reports on the progress of a new dress and her acquiescence to wearing it.[29] Her comportment was observed, and by the end of that month she was "in a fairly quiet and playful mood, her features relaxed, lost a good deal of that hard, set, look."[30] Wearing the new dress was an indication that she was "improving." After her second admission in 1905, Mrs. J. "exceeded herself in her violence, abuse and obscenity," again destroying her clothing and towels as well as assaulting a patient and a warder. When she tore up her mattress and dress on January 11, 1909, her bed was removed.[31]

Embodied resistance extended over other forms of personal hygiene, but asylum conditions tested the ability of patients and staff to maintain cleanliness. For many years, patients were locked in the wards and "left to themselves until morning."[32] The acting medical superintendent condemned this practice in 1914, although regulations still stipulated that wards were closed between 6 p.m. and 6 a.m. Attendants were supposed to check patients regularly during the night, and in 1914 a tell-tale clock was installed to watch the watchers.[33]

During the asylum's early decades, patients usually had their own rooms, but, in later years, when patient numbers were higher, several patients were confined together in two main wards segregated according to gender. European wards continued throughout the colonial years, but disruptive Europeans could be punished by being consigned to the native wards. On March 27, 1951, a European male who had voluntarily sought admission damaged his bed and room. He then jumped over the asylum's wall and was later apprehended by police on a launch in nearby Walu Bay. He was sent to the native ward until April 6, when he was "moved to European quarters as he ha[d] settled."[34] Permission to remain in a superior space ("quarters" as distinct from "cells") was not just an entitlement of race but also depended on acquiescence to institutional rules and appropriate behavior. Dr. Steenson put this another way when he decided to house Emosi Saurara in the European ward: "accommodation is arranged according to the natural customs of the person concerned, and his mental condition." Although the hospital operated racially labeled wards, Steenson provided assurance that "there is no discrimination between paying and non-paying patients of any race."[35]

The demarcation between European and native wards was especially ambiguous for patients of mixed ethnicity such as Molly. Here, too, a patient's behavior could determine which ward they were allocated to. On Molly's first admission in 1948, she was classified as part European and given a bed in the European women's ward. The next day, she was sent to the main women's ward after threatening to hang herself with clothing and being "uncontrollable." She resettled in the European ward but after a month attempted to escape and so was returned to the "native cells."[36] It is unlikely that she remained there, but on subsequent admissions her race was recorded as part-European.

During the 1920s, the average patient population increased to sixty-nine and by the 1930s had risen to eighty. An unpublished report stated that, in early 1955, 143 patients were resident in the hospital, despite there being only eighty official bed spaces: "sixty men and women must sleep on the exposed verandahs. In the cold weather or when the verandahs are wet with rain these patients lie huddled in their blankets on the cold wet cement."[37] This situation sparked complaints by the unofficial members of Fiji's Legislative Council.[38] A few years earlier, after a surprise hospital visit in 1951, the chair of the Board of Visitors, E. C. Woodward, remarked that such crowded and substandard conditions exacerbated tensions between patients, with overcrowding of dry spots causing "quarrelling and annoyance."[39] Officials also feared immorality, suggesting that overcrowding required constant supervision "if the perils of homosexuality are to be prevented."[40] Overcrowding continued to be a problem, the hospital accommodating around two hundred inpatients at a time during the 1960s.[41] The official bed capacity was half this, at ninety-eight, but the true occupancy was not revealed in annual reports.

An inadequate structural environment compounded violence among patients and between patients and staff, and also made it difficult to contain infectious disease, especially diarrhea and, more seriously, dysentery. Patients in single rooms usually had a bucket to urinate and defecate into during the night, but such provision was next to useless when several patients were confined in one ward. During the daytime, only a few latrines were available to a large number of patients. Following a 1927 inquiry, after Sarjudei had died from septicemia, the acting medical superintendent, Dr. Philip Harper, pointed out that sanitation was difficult to maintain in light of defective latrines, overcrowding, and overworked staff. He blamed these structural issues and the government's inadequate expenditure on the asylum for a high death rate due to dysentery: "the Asylum is in fact starved & we work against great difficulties until something goes wrong."[42] When Chief Medical Officer and Medical Superintendent Dr. Aubrey Montague returned from leave, he denied these assertions but did admit that he had "been willing to pinch, perhaps unduly, the expenditure on the asylum" because of other financial demands. Instead, Montague racialized the cause of dysentery:

> Lunatics, particularly native & Indian lunatics, are often so filthy in their habits, defecating promiscuously, that the provision of septic tanks will make very little if any difference in the incidence of dysentery.[43]

Despite the inadequate sanitary conditions, medical superintendents could become fixated on patients and their bowel "action."[44] Regular fecal evacuation was considered essential to health, and if occurring at a prescribed time and within a latrine, it aided in patient management. Mrs. J.'s bowel motions were closely monitored because of her tendency to constipation or defecating on the floor. On one occasion she refused to go to the closet (latrine) and instead defecated on the verandah, telling the warder that she had had a baby.[45] Patients who did not pass motions were prescribed laxatives or administered an enema. Some constipated patients, such as a European female in 1914, had their bowels left open with "slats."[46] Violent patients like her were often prescribed laxatives, indicative possibly of control, punishment, and biopower as Mills suggested in asylums in colonial India.[47] During the Victorian era, some doctors considered purging bowels as a way of expelling physical and mental disease from the body. Treatments advocating the curative properties of bowel regularity may have still been practiced in Fiji during the early twentieth century.

Bathing was a site of control and resistance over the body that frequently resulted in violence. Several attendants might be required to control and bathe a patient, which heightened violence between patients and staff.[48] In June 1905, Mrs. J.'s resistance to bathing resulted in a black eye, said to be caused by her striking her head against the bath. Six months later, her head was also wounded when she struggled with warders in the bathroom.[49] For several years, the bathroom was reserved for Europeans and a few others who were ordered to use it.[50] Native patients bathed outside, and truculent patients were doused with a hosepipe. Dr. Karim recalled that, during the 1960s, some wards were hosed to wash excrement into a central drain. The "hosepipe treatment" was also a way for staff to control and punish unruly or disobedient patients, such as to John, a soldier from the Fiji Military Forces admitted during World War II who had torn up his army uniform.[51] He refused to answer the doctor's questions, was described as stubborn, tense, and maniacal, and attacked an elderly Indian patient. He also spent time in a concrete cell.

Diet was central to mental health regimes and, as Syljeseth articulated so well, prompted complaints. Food is a highly contentious issue in institutions such as schools, workplaces, prisons, and hospitals, especially for long-term residents. Meal times commonly became occasions for resistance, when patients might refuse food, vomit, or throw food around. Michael's notes recorded that he "seems very determined to starve." He also resisted being fed liquids through a nasal tube.[52] When staff were able to force-feed him, he induced vomiting by forcing a finger down his throat.

Anorexia could reflect severe depression or be a slow suicide. Prolonged refusal to eat could suppress appetite. Anorexia can also be considered a form of embodied resistance, struggles over eating being a contest for power over the patient's body and life. In 1946, a newly admitted Indo-Fijian female refused to eat solids.[53] A week earlier, she had attempted suicide. She survived but was readmitted to the hospital in 1950 and again in 1963.

Vereniki, Singh, and Govind—three prisoners sentenced for murder and admitted to the asylum from jail—starved themselves, which probably caused Vereniki's death in 1947. On January 17, 1945, Vereniki was sentenced to penal servitude for the savage murder of his wife, but, on April 18, he was transferred to the mental hospital. His notes state that from the time he was admitted "He was a man who offered no help to try and get well just gave in."[54] Sentenced on December 5, 1916, to twenty years' imprisonment for murdering a woman, Singh was admitted to the asylum in the throes of severe depression on March 3, 1926. He threatened staff with violence, stripped himself naked, and played with his feces, but his refusal to eat—save for "fancy dishes" such as whiskey-egg flip—caused the most concern. His case notes suggest that he refused to eat because he was "endeavouring to kill himself." Singh claimed that a warder stole his food to give to his children and that staff wanted to kill him.[55] A year later, in a letter to the governor written on his behalf by a European patient who seemed to "write most inmates' letters" (possibly Syljeseth), Singh pleaded to be repatriated to India. He reported that he was eating and complying with the asylum's regime: "I was told to feed up and behave and I am doing so. I listen to what Dr Harper and Mr Anderson tells me to do. . . . I have behaved myself all along in the Asylum."[56]

Singh's reference to his compliance through eating, and his inclusion of this detail in a letter bargaining for his repatriation, indicates that food could be part of a complex negotiation between patients and authorities. Paranoia and psychosis convinced some patients that their food was being poisoned. Serving a life sentence for murder since December 1930, Govind was transferred to the mental hospital in 1941. He believed that he was being made to eat poisoned food, so Dr. Hoodless temporarily allowed him to cook his own food.[57] Staff used food as a form of punishment and reward. Daniel Bower, who began working at St Giles as an orderly in 1970, recalled how troublesome patients were confined in seclusion, and, if they continued to be noisy, they were given a "half serve of food."[58]

In 1970, a letter to the editor of *Pacific Review* reported that patients who refused to work were locked up in Bua Ward and kept on half rations.[59] In contrast, patients' relatives could bring in treats, such as special food on Indian festival days.[60]

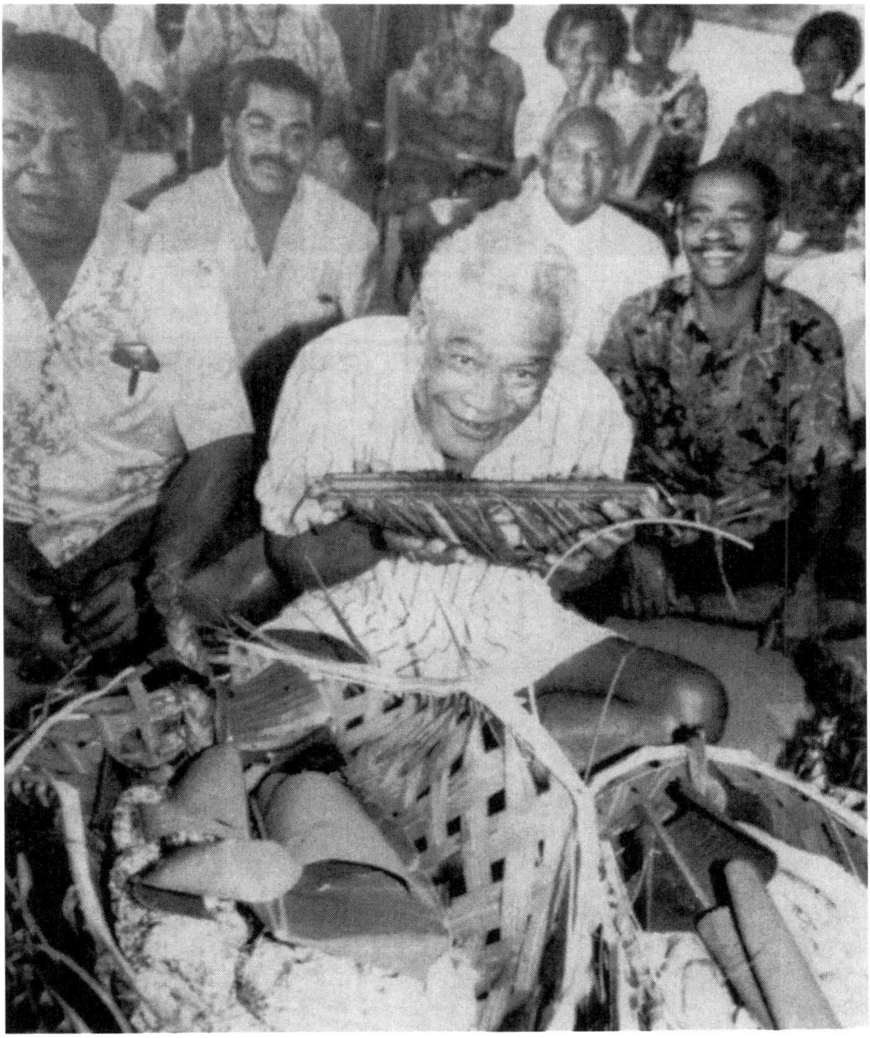

Figure 6.2. In 1996, members of the *tokatoka* Saganimara of Vatoa Island, Lau prepared *lovo* food for their relative, Suliasi Suka, and St Giles' patients and staff, to mark the end of Mental Health Week. Suka had been a patient at St Giles since 1976. Source: *Fiji Times*, October 14, 1996.

An important part of the daily routine, work could erupt into a contest between patients and staff. During the late nineteenth and twentieth centuries, psychiatric hospital staff believed that work was therapeutic and restored moral, mental, and physical normalcy.[61] The Board of Visitors treated this subject lightly in 1887, commenting on how some patients were being "permitted to amuse themselves in gardening close to the Asylum grounds, under the supervision of a warder."[62] Patients' labor and food production was needed to supplement the meager asylum budget. The asylum's chief warder was refused temporary prison labor in 1888 because "the work must be done, as opportunity occurs, by the patients who may be physically fit."[63] In 1916, a request from G. R. Anderson, the head attendant, for a gardener was declined because the colonial secretary hoped that the chief medical officer could "induce the chronic patients to cultivate the available land.—It is the practice at Lunatic Asylums in other Colonies."[64] Patients produced crops such as *dalo* (*taro*), cassava, yams, bananas, and pawpaw.[65] They maintained the asylum lawns and gardens and at times did heavier labor.[66] Many patients enjoyed participating in familiar routines, such as planting, weeding, and harvesting crops that were valued activities in Pacific cultures. Working alongside staff strengthened rapport and possibly contributed to healing.[67] Bower's recollections of St Giles during the 1960s were peppered with psychiatric "therapy-speak": patients were "well trained," "well occupied," "well activated," and "well organised." More warmly, he recalled patients "coming out to work in the garden right by the hillside there, mornings, it is quite fun. I can remember talking to patients, they have been gardening, gardening cassava and *taro* under the supervision of four orderlies."[68]

Those capable were expected to participate in cleaning the wards, and some patients were selected to clean the staff quarters.[69] Before World War II, some patients served as messengers for staff. In 1896, Mrs. J.'s progress was noted when, at her request, she was washing and ironing asylum clothes with the female attendants.[70] In 1914, regulations stipulated that the European female attendant was to "endeavour to find occupation for all the patients, such as reading, gardening, sewing clothes, washing, scrubbing, and other suitable occupation."[71] When Singh presented his case for repatriation to India, he mentioned that he had made envelopes for the government.[72] At various times, a few patients worked in painting, carpentry, the asylum's laundry, and other maintenance tasks.

By 1929, concern was raised in the Legislative Council over patients frequently carrying supplies and wood from the town and prison to the asylum. The official response reinforced the desirability of the work cure:

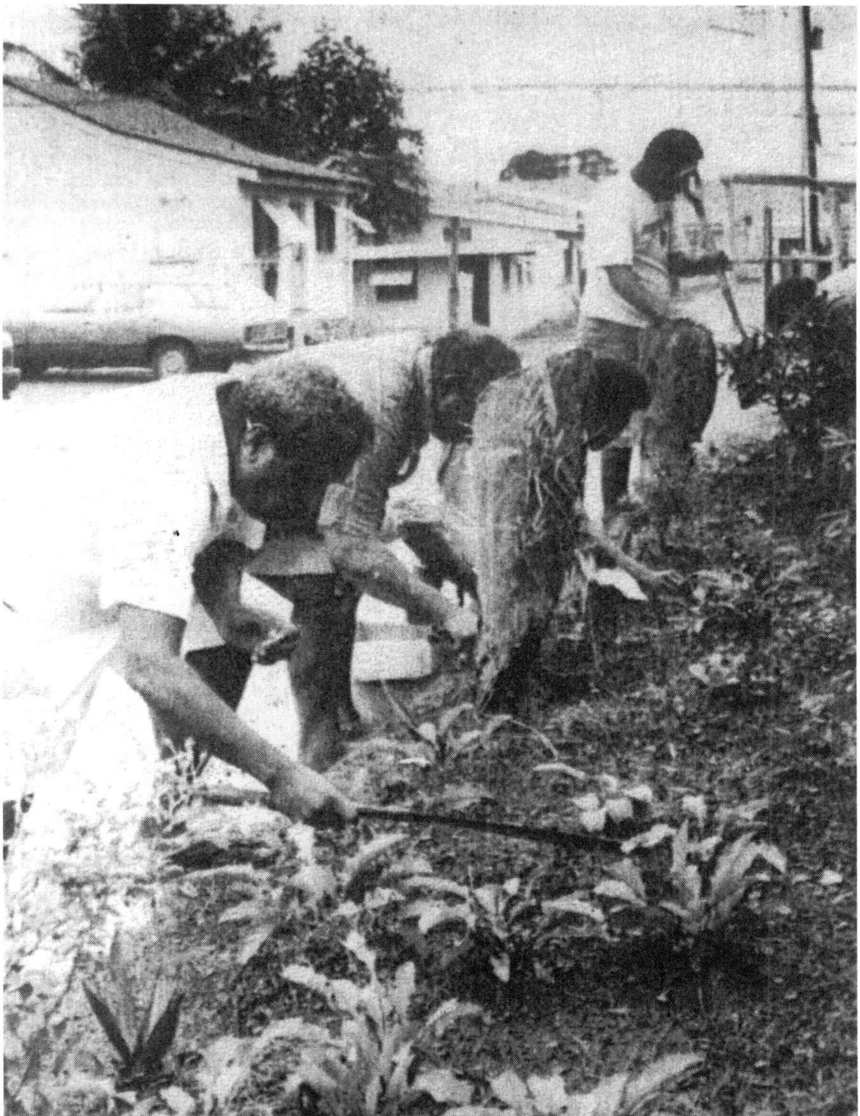

Figure 6.3. Patients gardening at St Giles Hospital. Source: *Fiji Times*, April 9, 1994.

> The Government is of the opinion that there is nothing degrading or menial in the performance of useful labour in public, by persons who while mentally unsound are capable of performing the service without hardship and whose bodily health in some cases is materially benefited thereby.[73]

In 1941, Dr. Macpherson, the director of medical services, suggested that the mental hospital could be developed like a farm colony, where the "more fit inmates" could undertake market gardening and milk production to supply government departments. But activities in spaces outside the hospital were also seen to offer opportunities to escape, or threaten the patient safety, as well as the sensibilities of the public:

> despite the utmost vigilance occasional escapes of mentally deranged persons is almost inevitable under the existing circumstances. The patients must be protected against themselves, as well as the general public and there is, moreover, the aesthetic aspect. A number of patients tend to divest themselves of clothing, etc., and accordingly public scandal may be provoked.[74]

Work and occupational therapy was not always possible at St Giles. Weather was a major constraint at this "fair weather hospital." Rain prohibited outside work and confined patients indoors or on verandahs, often in cramped conditions and with no activities. In 1966, Macgregor identified the lack of facilities for occupational rehabilitation as a major problem and suggested that this problem affected the speed of patient turnover.[75] Monetary and personnel constraints also determined the range of occupational activities on offer. It could be oppressive for patients to be forced to work or cajoled into occupational therapy when they were mentally confused, unwell, or unmotivated. Encounters like this contributed to tensions between patients and staff.

On March 1, 1924, Aiyaz wrote a letter to the "Protector of the poor," making serious allegations about forced labor and other conditions.[76] He stated that "we are treated as prisoners," male patients working between seven and nine hours a day, having to carry firewood and stones. Patients were beaten and held, he said, suffering "blows on our stomachs." He also complained about no food or just receiving one piece of bread and one plate of rice with a very small quantity of curry. However, even as he protested against the violence in the hospital—"we should not be beaten"—Aiyaz voiced concerns about the plight of the mentally ill in political terms as well: "the Government arrest us helpless

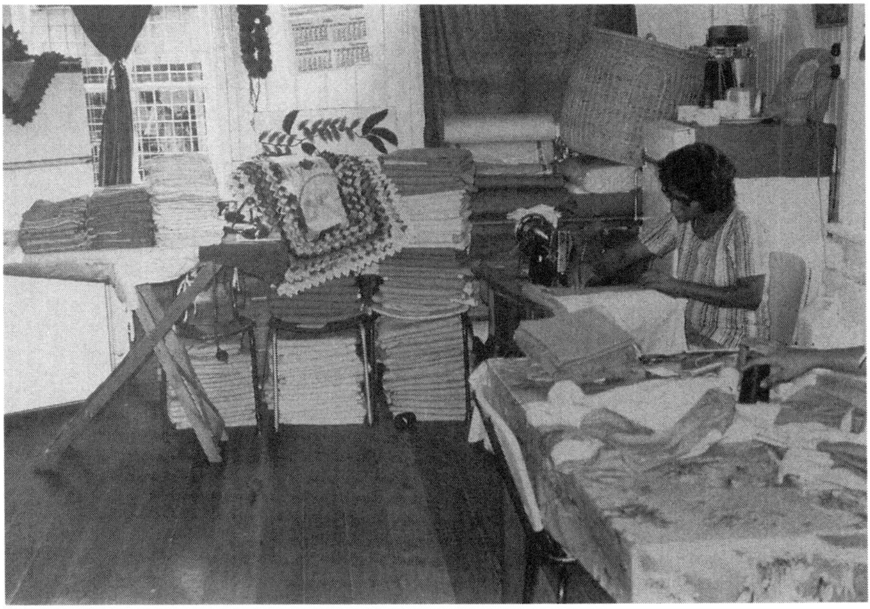

Figure 6.4. Work therapy at St Giles Hospital, probably early 1980s. Source: St Giles Hospital.

persons, lock us up and get Samoans and Fijians to give us trouble. The Government should be ashamed of themselves. Woe to their ruling us in this way."

A Site of Violence

Aiyaz was correct in describing the asylum as a site of violence. Ill, angry, and frustrated patients hurt themselves and lashed out at their immediate surroundings, other patients, and staff, as Dr. Halley noted of a thirty-two-year-old Fijian villager in 1904:

> Acute mania . . . Menacing behaviour on examination towards dr. & then the wall, needed restraint to prevent patient hurting himself. Attacked warders. Fought on being put back in cell. Stamping & beating cell walls. . . . Violent since admission to jail. Natural habits "perverted"—play with bucket or try & destroy, wallow in faeces.[77]

At times, staff were violent toward patients—whether to control them, protect themselves, or retaliate.[78] A Fijian patient in 1920 not only attacked others but also tried to drive the devil out of a patient.[79] Staff could become desensitized to violence. For example, they expected Ananaiasa to become manic and violent toward patients and staff every month. When, during the early hours of August 22, 1906, Ananaiasa and Autiko fought in their room and Autiko lost four upper incisors, was bitten, and suffered various abrasions, the chief warder described him as only "somewhat hurt."[80]

The habitual violence recorded in the hospital's case books seems a far way from the codes of moral management laid down in the asylum's 1887 regulations. These stipulated that close supervision should be given with a minimum of restraint and that "all officers of the Asylum must treat the patients with especial kindness and forbearance." The onus for moral management and treatment fell on asylum staff and the example they set. Warders were to refrain from "improper language and be strictly temperate in their way of living."[81] The 1887 report from the Board of Visitors suggests that moral management was followed:

> The chief warden is most attentive to his duties, and appears to have an aptitude for acquiring a kindly influence over the patients. The under-warders take an interest in their work, and are on good terms with the patients. The patients have as much freedom as is consistent with their safety. Those of them who can be trusted outside the bounds of the Asylum, are taken out for a walk every week by the Chief Warder.[82]

This account probably referred mostly to European patients. Later regulations, in 1914, continued to emphasize that the matron should "see that nurses and female attendants perform their duties with diligence, gentleness, and kindness" but also stipulated measures for staff to minimize violence towards and between patients.[83] Attendants were advised to sooth or control patients "by gentle means" or to be "put as quickly as possible into a room provided for the purpose which shall be safely guarded." Patients were not to be locked in the same room and the use of seclusion, violence, "harsh or intemperate language," or punishment against patients was prohibited. Despite these regulations, before the widespread use of psychotropic medication at St Giles after World War II, attendants restrained uncontrollable patients through seclusion or with mechanical devices. Although Mrs. J. was restrained with mufflers and knee and ankle straps during July 1896, warders still found it difficult to prevent her from injuring her head.[84] On May 26, 1905, she was put in a straitjacket for two hours, but, because she struck people when the opportunity arose, she was confined to her room. She had periods of comparative calm and engagement in work and social activities in the asylum. It is unlikely that restraints were therapeutic for her, but they offered respite for the staff from her violence, incontinence, and noisy "blasphemous obscenity." Restraints were also a form of punishment.

The Lunatic Asylum Return in the *Blue Book of Fiji* displayed the number of patients placed under restraint as well as the duration and the category of restraint. These statistics are questionable, not only because staff were unreliable in keeping records, but also because recording and timing the duration of every instance of a restraint was impractical. Possibly because of the small number of warders, solitary confinement and mechanical restraints were used more than personal force during the nineteenth century, compared with later years. Restraints included handcuffs, leather mufflers, leg irons, elbow, thigh, and ankle straps, or solitary confinement. During the asylum's early years, only a few patients were frequently restrained. The most extreme case was Qaqa, who was confined in irons for five months in 1884. In 1897, four patients were put in solitary confinement twenty times; one was placed in mechanical restraints ten times. The one part-time and four full-time warders recorded only fifteen incidents of restraint affecting three patients. By 1917, these proportions had greatly changed: thirty-eight patients were placed in seclusion under lock and key 1,089 times and sixty-eight patients were restrained by attendants in 1,250 incidents, though mechanical restraint was only used twice for the same patient. By then, twelve full-time and three part-time attendants, assisted by visiting nurses from the Colonial Hospital to care for female patients, oversaw a daily average of fifty-nine patients.

After 1922, only mechanical and seclusion were listed as categories of restraint in the statistics, so there is no way of ascertaining whether restraint was through being confined in a room or by an attendant. As early as 1887, the Board of Visitors recommended that a padded cell be constructed, the rationale being that this was more modern than physical restraints:

> At present there is no place in which a patient, who is violent, can be put and left to himself without fear of injuring himself. Violent patients have at present, when their paroxysms come on, to be confined in their movements by a careful system of strapping, which although perfectly humane and painless is hardly in accordance with modern ideas.[85]

Dr. William MacGregor objected to this recommendation because, when working in mental asylums outside Fiji, he had never used or seen such strapping or a padded cell.[86] Cloth, such as canvas, sheeting, or blankets, was used for strapping to tie or "bundle" a patient. This strapping inhibited a patient's movement and assisted attendants in lifting a patient who was struggling. Straitjackets allowed patients to walk and were probably in use until the 1960s at St Giles.[87] Strapping continued to be used occasionally as late as 1950, when a patient was diagnosed with puerperal insanity after the birth of her third child. She was kept in bed by bandaging her arms to the bed, but she refused fluids and food and died five days after admission to the hospital.[88]

The demand for a padded cell continued in the early years of the twentieth century, especially following the death of a twenty-three-year-old *girmitiya* in 1910, who had died from heart failure after he had severely battered himself while confined in a wooden cell with a cement floor.[89] Dr. Lynch had refused to use a straitjacket on the man because he considered this to be "weakening." The coroner concluded, "It is regrettable that no padded cell has yet been provided for the inmates of the asylum." Padded cells were installed at the asylum, but patients who destroyed the padding were confined in an unpadded concrete room; one such patient was John Kepper, about whom Syljeseth was so concerned. Suicidal patients were also put in padded cells. In 1922, a European patient was confined in this way but became very anxious and after a month asked to be released from the cell.[90]

Statistics suggest that the frequency of patients being put in seclusion increased from 1923; the record was 1,487 occasions in 1938. Again, this form of restraint affected a small proportion of male patients only.[91] Of approximately eighty-six patients that year, only seven were secluded, which equated to 212 seclusions each. These figures fail to reveal how many times each patient was secluded, and the returns on the duration of seclusion are meaningless. Ten hours seems to be the maximum ever recorded between 1884 and 1940, apart from Qaqa's confinement and the twelve hours a patient was secluded in 1887. Beyond the mental terror of confinement, patients would have found it stifling, especially during Suva's hot, humid months. The padded cells had concrete floors, and padding on the walls did not last. By 1946, plans to install new padded cells were shelved as the Board of Visitors recommended waiting to assess the impact of a new drug regime.[92] The introduction of potent antipsychotic and sedative medication after World War II provided staff with a new arsenal to control patients, even if these new treatments did not eradicate violence from the hospital.

Violence was embedded in the culture and management of the institution. Many of the warders or attendants were poorly trained or lacked the temperament to soothe or "talk down" a manic or violent patient. On February 28, 1940, Hoodless warned the Samoan warders that they must deal with violent patients in the "proper manner." This warning followed a complaint from the outspoken politician, Vishnu Deo, and a patient's father; the man's son had been ill-treated by a Samoan warder after the patient had struck the warder on the mouth. Similarly, in 1944, another visitor complained that a Samoan warder had "roughly handled" an elderly male European patient. The visitor's objections were as much about transgressions of race and status, as "colored hands" were placed on this retired military officer.[93] Hoodless defended the warder's actions, explaining that no force had been used and that the warder was doing his duty in restraining an overexcited patient who was trying to leave the hospital.[94] As a result of this complaint, Hoodless recommended that patients be allowed only two visitors and for twenty minutes per visit.

Some patients directly complained about violence in the asylum, although most were more likely to withdraw into themselves or retaliate with violence. Not so the one in 1967 who reported an attendant for applying a headlock, ostensibly to stop the patient fighting with another. The incident was not brushed aside, and the attendant was found guilty and severely reprimanded. This outcome did not satisfy Dr. Duncan Macgregor, who wrote a scathing memo titled "The Machinery of Discipline" to the director of medical services protesting about the decision not to dismiss the employee.[95] Standing orders for the hospital in 1964 stipulated that striking a patient was a criminal offense punishable by imprisonment. Because legislation had failed to prevent abuses, Macgregor intervened by speaking to staff, lecturing, and demonstrating nonviolent methods of handling patients, and promoting caring and sensitive nursing.

> I explain that this law is not enough: that absence of ill-treatment is not good nursing; that something positive is required. Namely a recognition of the fact that deprivation of liberty is a terrible blow to the self esteem of patients and that every step must be taken to restore their sense of personal dignity.[96]

Macgregor's efforts aside, the warder maintained, "I did not strangle the patient—I only put a headlock on him" and "I kicked the patient in the stomach in self defense."[97]

The inciting role that staff played in the escalation of violence was reported in a 1970 issue of the *Pacific Review*, in the article "Are Mental Patients at Suva Subjected to Cruelty?" The article was based on a patient's letter to the editor:

> Some orderlies excite other patients to violence and when the patients start fighting among themselves, the orderlies appear to derive sadistic

> pleasure out of it and simply stand and watch and actually kick some of the patients and provoke them to fight. This, of course, does not happen every day.[98]

This allegation was made at the close of the colonial era, and, although medical authorities challenged its veracity, it points to an institutional culture of violence.

Controlling the Mind to Tame the Body

Physical restraints were applied less frequently once staff could inject drugs to sedate acutely violent patients, especially after long-term drug therapy became the norm from the 1950s onward. The use of medication at St Giles followed global psychiatric trends, but in Fiji choice was restricted because of the availability of supplies, cost, and doctors' prescribing preferences and knowledge of new medications.[99] After World War II, a radical breakthrough in the regime at St Giles came with the introduction of psychotropic drugs and shock therapies. Although these new therapies were used to treat mental illness, it was no secret to staff that they were powerful forms of control and punishment, especially for violent or truculent patients.[100]

Before the 1950s, drugs were primarily administered for sedation and control or to alleviate mental and physical conditions.[101] Bromide and the foul-smelling paraldehyde were commonly used for sedation and as anticonvulsants, especially for epileptic seizures.[102] Phenobarbital (known as Luminal in Fiji) became available during the early twentieth century. By the 1950s, some patients received Dilantin (phenytoin sodium) for seizures. Arsenical drugs were the only treatments available for syphilis until antibiotics were introduced in the 1940s. Chloral hydrate, though sometimes available for sedation, was too expensive for general use at the asylum. From the 1940s to 1960, Nembutal tablets and gas were given to alleviate depression and insomnia, as were the long-standing remedies of morphine and sodium amytal. By the 1940s, "hyoscine cocktails" were served in Fiji, such as the mixture of hyoscine and morphine injected into a very excitable Fijian in 1947.[103] A belladonna mixture was prescribed in 1943 for an elderly female.[104]

A major breakthrough came when the "pharmacological revolution" of psychotropic drugs offered the possibility for seriously mentally ill patients to participate more in activities within and outside the hospital. Some new psychotropic drugs were dispensed in Fiji from the late 1940s, but 1955 heralded a significant shift with the introduction of Largactil (chlorpromazine), only a few years after its adoption in Western Europe and North America (where marketed as Thorazine).[105] Largactil was both a major sedative and an antipsychotic drug. The medical superintendent, Dr. Helen Rushton, outlined the promise the "therapeutic revolution of 1961" brought:

> The regime used was that of bringing patients rapidly under control with large doses of the appropriate drug, followed by a gradual reduction to the minimal dose compatible with social integration within the hospital environment. Provided that the patient remained reasonably well on this maintenance dosage, he was retained in hospital for as long as improvement of his condition continued and was then, wherever possible, released on trial to continue therapy on a domiciliary basis.[106]

This quotation indicates how curative drugs such as Largactil, also a new form of biopower, could be used to restrain patients in Fiji, as was the practice in hospitals elsewhere.[107] Rushton emphasized the positive results of the new medication: the considerable improvement in patient behavior and a fall in domiciliary patient numbers. Her optimism appeared vindicated in 1961 when eighteen patients were discharged completely and 208 patients were "on trial." This cautious approach was revised during the following decade when a large number of patients were readmitted to hospital.

During the early 1960s, a more peaceful atmosphere in the hospital allowed authorities to introduce into other wards some amenities previously limited to the European wards; curtains, mats, pictures, chairs, dining tables, and cutlery. More nursing care was required with Largactil and its possible severe side effects, which came under medical conditions termed anticholinergic, extrapyramidal, Parkinsonism, akathisia, and tardive dyskinesia. These bodily and mental changes could include dry mouth, blurred vision, jaundice, skin rashes, constipation, weight gain, edema, sun sensitivity, urinary hesitance, lowered libido, falls, bizarre muscle contractions, drowsiness, emotional blunting (or numbing), withdrawal, apathy, a shuffling gait, tremor, restlessness, involuntary grimacing, lip smacking, or tongue protrusion. The effects depended on the dosage and how long the patient had been medicated and whether anticholinergic counteractive medication, such as Lysivane, was prescribed or available in Fiji. A patient admitted in 1961 became partially blind by 1972 because her eyes were affected by Largactil toxicity.[108]

Given these possible severe effects, it is hardly surprising that noncompliance and rejection of psychotropic drugs became issues. This response was not new: patients at St Giles had often violently and covertly rejected medication. On

July 26, 1896, Norman Smith, the chief warder, observed that Mrs. J. probably kept a sedative in her mouth, rather than swallowing it, given that it had had no effect.[109] Some patients, such as Singh and Govind, refused medicine, claiming that staff were trying to poison them.[110] Following a course of modified insulin therapy in 1961, Mrs. S. B. was prescribed reserpine (an antipsychotic and antihypertensive medication) but after three weeks refused "point blank" to take it.[111] She was injected with reserpine two months later, but after another two months the Parkinsonism became so distressing that the drug was stopped.

Mrs. S. B.'s treatments indicate that some patients at St Giles were the subjects of drug trials, individually and not in a planned way, because of the expansion of the global pharmaceutical industry into developing countries. During 1962 and 1963, eight chronic patients who had shown little improvement with other treatments were trialed on Seranace (haloperidol), the "ultimate neuroleptic."[112] This trial was at the suggestion of Searle (Australia) Limited. The timing was significant in that Searle (United States) had refused to market haloperidol there, though it distributed Seranace elsewhere. Although the drug had limited effect in this Fiji trial, in 1964 Macgregor asked Searle to supply a free sample that he would report on. Five hundred and fifty ampoules for injection were provided. Macgregor was also in correspondence with Dr. A. J. E. Rowe at May and Baker in Dagenham regarding a possible comparative trial of Majeptil (thioproperazine methanesulphonate) and Neulactil (pericyazine).[113] Macgregor also wrote to Roche asking about the safe use of the sleeping medication Mogadon in children. He offered to conduct an "open uncontrolled trial" to assess its use locally.

Shock Therapy

On October 15, 1947, the brave new world of shock therapy came to Fiji when a woman in her late twenties suffering from postpuerperal manic depression was injected with Cardiozol (Metrazol).[114] This and other shock therapies, primarily electroconvulsive therapy (ECT), had a radical impact on mental health treatment in Fiji, as throughout the world.[115] Modified insulin coma therapy (ICT) was also trialed at St Giles but was soon abandoned along with Cardiozol therapy because of the cost and dangerous and severe side effects, a pattern found globally in many mental hospitals. Medical staff found ECT comparatively easier to administer and it was quickly adopted at St Giles. ECT could also be abused as a punishment and a form of control over patients.

Mrs. D. V. was an early experimental subject for shock therapies in Fiji. Age twenty-six, she was initially admitted and diagnosed with hysteria prior to the birth of her third baby in November 1947. Over a lifetime of convulsive and drug therapies, her diagnosis changed to schizophrenia and later to manic depression and paranoia. Sixteen days after the birth of her baby, Dr. Donald Oldmeadow began to administer her a course of twenty-two Cardiozol injections, the first producing a "satisfactory fit."[116] This therapy was traumatic, as documented by American psychiatrist Lothar Kalinowsky:

> the patient does not lose consciousness before the onset of the convulsion, which starts several seconds after the injection. During this interval he experiences a very unpleasant feeling of impending death and precordial sensations which are remembered as a frightening experience, and the fear derived therefrom is a severe setback for subsequent treatments. . . . Failure to obtain a convulsion makes the patient very apprehensive and uncomfortable.[117]

Mrs. D. V. undoubtedly would have undergone these terrifying experiences, especially because she did not always convulse after being injected. Her veins thrombosed, and as she regressed she strongly resisted injections toward the end of her Cardiozol therapy.[118] By February 25, 1948, she had "Completely regressed. Anointing herself with faeces, destruction & had to be confined to cell with nothing which she can destroy." Her recollections of injections at St Giles are suggestive of this trauma: "At times she said that the Dr was endeavouring to kill her and said that he only failed due to his inability to find her 'life-vein'. She cited the case of an Indian lady who had died after an injection."[119] Mrs. D. V. was discharged on March 11, 1948, conditional on her husband's admitting her two weeks later for a tubal ligation. Instead, her mental condition worsened, and she was readmitted. By September, she was on ECT.

ECT for humans had developed from experiments with pigs in a slaughterhouse in Rome. By the 1940s and 1950s, it was being extensively used in the United States and Europe in the treatment of schizophrenia and depression. Oldmeadow introduced ECT into Fiji in 1948 (complete with his own machine) amid acclaim from the Board of Visitors, who said, "this public-spirited service on the part of Dr. Oldmeadow deserves commendation."[120] He gave 558 ECT treatments, and in 1951 ninety-nine patients received 1,379 procedures.[121] Oldmeadow was so impressed with the results of ECT that it was a significant factor in spurring him on to specialize in psychiatry.[122]

Despite the internationally acclaimed therapeutic benefits of ECT, it raised widespread controversy and posed many problems. During the early years of its application in Fiji, electric currents were difficult to control, and anesthetics and muscle relaxants were not used. Some patients sustained injuries such as broken

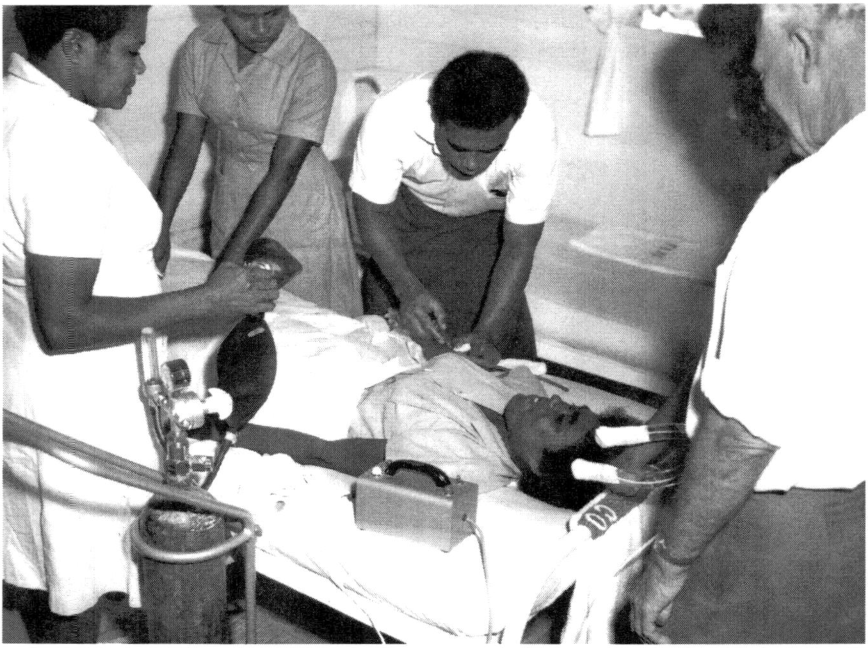

Figure 6.5. Mock ECT, St Giles Hospital, 1965 with Dr. M. Vuki, deputy head orderly, Asena Ranadi, and head orderly, Charlie Sachs. Source: Neg. no. G7245, NAF.

teeth and bones. Memory loss and trauma were possible; in 1968, a patient remained unconscious for three hours following convulsions from ECT.[123] The rationale for such intervention was treatment, but oral and written evidence indicates that the new technologies were also methods of control and punishment.[124] The medical superintendent's handwritten reports during the early 1950s show that ECT was "given to rowdy patients" to pacify them.[125] For example, "J. violent but had a good reaction to shock."[126] Shock therapy appears to have been widely administered to patients with a wide range of conditions: mania, postpuerperal psychosis, depression, anxiety, and epilepsy. Records indicate that patients were separated according to their suitability for ECT, as was a very confused female patient in 1949: "Case appears a good subject for shock therapy." She was still bewildered after treatment.[127] Mrs. D. V. underwent several ECT sessions during the 1960s, which led her general physician to wonder whether her headaches and earaches were caused by the shocks. Despite this and extensive drug therapy during more than forty admissions from 1947, Mrs. D. V. was mostly treated as an outpatient and was able to travel overseas.

Insulin

At least seven patients were administered modified insulin coma therapy when it was introduced into St Giles in 1955.[128] Elsewhere, ICT involved lower doses of insulin (usually 30 to 50 units) than those used to induce comas (around 100 to 150 daily units) and was recommended for the treatment of neurotic disorders and anorexia nervosa.[129] At St Giles, much higher doses were given to treat schizophrenia and, in at least one case, epilepsy. The latter case was a Fijian teacher who finished a course of seventeen treatments at 180 daily units, after which he was considered improved although he did not teach again.[130] Partly because of the potentially life-threatening risks, ICT required close medical attention. It is unclear whether trained nurses and a doctor were always present during treatments, although, by the mid-1950s, the medical superintendent, Dr. H. W. Conran, did have a diploma in psychiatric medicine, and his wife, who was a nursing sister, also worked at St Giles. ICT was offered to only a few, selected patients in Fiji, probably because of the higher costs and labor demands.[131]

On August 4, 1955, Mrs. S. B. began her first course of seventeen insulin treatments, administered intramuscularly over nineteen days. She had been diagnosed as a schizophrenic paranoid and asserted that she worked for the government, "straightening out the world, stopping floods, earthquakes and so on by cutting wires with a diamond ring," claiming that her hair was affected by atomic radiation. Mrs. S. B. came from a more affluent background than most patients and submitted orders for tinned food, biscuits, lipsticks, nail polish, perfume, writing materials, cigarettes, and clothes.[132] For nineteen days, at 7 a.m. after a night's fast, she would be administered insulin, starting at 10 units and rising to 70. The insulin lowered her blood sugar to induce sweating, while she was sleeping or drowsing, for two to four hours. When woken, she was usually offered a syrup drink, then breakfast, after which she might fall asleep again. That was on a "good" day, because her nursing notes reveal that she did not always sleep but instead became disorientated, was uncoordinated, sweated profusely, and shivered:

> 16 Aug 1955: 7am 70 units . . . 9.15 excitement, talk, nonsense and noisy, retching & ataxia [lack of coordination]. Interrupted with sweet drink . . . had meal in bed. At 12 midday doubling up in bed shivering with cold. Warmth & hot bottle applied.
> 22 Aug 1955: Insulin 70 units 8am. Slept. 9.30 Noisy & disorientated. Pulse 80. Gradual loss of responses to speech 8 or 9.45. Absence of responses to stimulus (visual, tactile, & auditory). COMA for 15 minutes. 10am. Interrupted with 60cc. 33% Dextrose intravenously. Immediately roused & awake after. Glucose by mouth was also given.

She fell dangerously into a coma—not intended with modified ICT because it could lead to brain damage or death. During the next day's treatment, she was somnolent and stuporous while sweating profusely before falling into another coma. The treatment was stopped, also because the nasal tube had been introduced through her trachea. No mental changes were observed at the end of this course of insulin treatments but Mrs. S. B. had gained weight, and her blood pressure was elevated. Between September 9 and 30, she was placed on a course of Raudixin (reserpine) two to three times a day. Raudixin was more commonly prescribed as an antihypertensive medication, but it was trialed in Fiji, as elsewhere, as a treatment for chronically mentally disturbed patients.[133] Mrs. S. B. underwent a second round of twenty-eight insulin shock treatments from October 11 to November 12, 1955. On November 1, she experienced a seizure and the following day was administered combined ICT and ECT. Another seizure followed the next day, but combined treatments resumed two days after that. She was discharged the day after and then readmitted, staying in the asylum from November 1956 to October 1961. It would seem that the shock therapies she received made little difference to her mental condition, nursing notes suggesting that she had not "altered much over the years—has to be constantly watched with personal hygiene; very non-cooperative and demanding at times—constant stream of fantastic delusions—paraphrenia fantastica—paranoid delusions."[134]

Deep Sleep and Acid

"Deep sleep" or Pentothal (thiopentone) narcosis was briefly trialed at St Giles. Sleep therapy, where patients were put into continuous sleep for several days, was a practice in many psychiatric hospitals during the first half of the twentieth century.[135] Pentothal narcosis was administered to a severely depressed patient diagnosed with schizophrenia in 1947 during her sixth hospital admission. Records do not indicate how long she was under, but nine days later she was still depressed and anxious. After a few weeks, she was discharged but the following year was readmitted.[136] Pentothal was used on a few other patients at the hospital and as a course of treatment, probably as a powerful sedative.

A small number of patients at St Giles were selected for succinic acid treatments in 1954.[137] In Australia, experimental trials of this "revolutionary drug," used to treat schizophrenia and manic depression, were reported prominently in newspapers, and the news quickly spread to Fiji.[138] Dr. Conran cited the *Australian Post* when he sought permission from Mani's father to treat his son with succinic acid.[139] When Conran asked Esau's father for consent, he pointed out that Esau had undergone several courses of ECT "without effect."[140] It is unclear whether acid treatment provided any relief because both of these patients, diagnosed as schizophrenic, were readmitted several times in the decades that followed. This points to the controversy surrounding "acid treatment." According to Dr. Peter Whyte, its success, if any, correlated with patterns of remission common in mental illness. He attributed the value of the treatment to the extra attention and specialized nursing patients received—a similar pattern could be observed in those selected for insulin therapy.[141]

By the 1940s, some patients received a different type of "acid treatment." Nicotinic acid (niacin or Vitamin B3), glutamic acid, and other vitamins were given to treat confusion, delirium, pellagra, and alcoholism.[142]

Escaping Madness

The ultimate form of resistance to the asylum was escape, which ranged from simply walking through an open gate to suicide. Mills suggested that "perhaps the most dramatic evidence of resistance strategies involving the body of the individual resisting is in patient suicides."[143] Although very few patients committed suicide or are recorded as attempting it in St Giles, several were suicidal before admission or had to be closely watched because of their "suicidal tendencies."[144]

When Robert Gaius Anderson, the chief warder, locked Hector in his room on the evening of December 22, 1913, he did not regard him as suicidal, although Hector said he would not be there in the morning. Hector was a former patient at Goodna Asylum in Queensland, employed by a trading company in Fiji. One day, Hector caught a launch from Rewa to Suva, stripped his clothes off, attempted to jump overboard, struck an Indo-Fijian, was arrested, appeared before the court, and was sent to Suva Gaol. His manic behavior there resulted in his being transferred to the asylum. The night of December 22, Hector smuggled something into his room and asked Anderson to close the shutters. He died from asphyxia in a fire that was presumably deliberately lit.[145] The coroner ruled that Hector's death was accidental, although Anderson was found guilty of failing to fulfill his duties and patient neglect.[146]

The meaning of suicide and whether it is a form of resistance remain highly contentious.[147] Moreover, it is impossible to know whether this final act was primarily a response to being incarcerated. Two Fijian men who committed suicide by hanging in 1887 and 1934 had been sentenced to life imprisonment for murder.[148] Both men were in their early twenties when they were committed to the asylum. They hanged themselves soon after. Other tragedies before 1964 were two older Indo-Fijian men who hanged themselves in their rooms with their *dhoti*.[149] One was diagnosed in 1953 as a mental deficient, and the other in 1948, when he was about seventy years old, with senile dementia. The latter was a Muslim who had been a beggar and had attacked a Muslim religious leader with a stone. According to a police sergeant, he had refused food for up to a week. In the three years he lived in hospital before his death, he "was quiet and always appeared depressed—did no gardening or other work nor spoke to anyone." His two sons attended his funeral.

Molly, already mentioned, threatened to commit suicide immediately on admission to the hospital in 1948. Eight days later, she wrote an insightful letter to Dr. K. R. Steenson detailing her personal despair and reasons for her depression. Her father had died suddenly a few years earlier, and his sudden death seemed to have precipitated her depression. She complained about overwork and her difficult marriage to an alcoholic husband. Molly clearly was distraught at being separated from her infant daughter and begged Steenson to allow her to leave the same day that she penned her letter. She wrote that she became "tongue-tied" when meeting the doctor on his ward visit and apologized for her rowdy behavior, saying, "I am sorry for the trouble I have caused these willing workers here and apologize deeply for the noise I have caused the neighbours." Molly begged to be discharged, stating, "I am not insane." She was not released that day, and a few weeks later she tried to escape from the hospital.[150]

Institutional controls did not prevent determined patients like Molly from escaping. Michael announced his intentions to escape to the medical superintendent on November 12, 1910. He made several attempts by "rushing" the guards, but an opportunity finally came when an attendant fell asleep and Michael was able to climb over a gate.[151] Pita's escape, during the night of June 6, 1913, would have particularly concerned, not only asylum staff, but also colonial authorities because of his recent seditious activities at Daku, where he had threatened Europeans. He stole a small boat from the nearby prison, but the following day the master of the cutter *Amy* rescued him from the ocean between the mainland and Beqa. Pita was returned to the asylum.[152] A few other patients physically confined in a "cell" or a "strong room" managed to bend wires or remove iron bars. Raghu did this and released another patient when he escaped in December 1946 by scaling the concrete walls, erected in 1926, that surrounded much of the asylum. Warders caught Raghu later that day in the town of Navua, around thirty-six kilometers (twenty-two miles) from the hospital.[153]

Most opportunities were seized when warders were distracted or asleep and escapes were generally short lived. In 1914, when two warders fell asleep at 10 a.m. in the male yard, "a lunatic took the key from above their heads & walked out."[154] Orderlies were playing cards with patients in 1966 when one was able to walk past unnoticed and escape, much to the patients' amusement.[155] Such staff negligence might invert the institutional hierarchy of control, whereby patients disciplined staff by occasionally reporting staff breaches of security and care. During the 1960s, a patient, Temesi, wrote a letter to Head Attendant Charlie Sachs, dated 3:30 a.m., reporting Josua, a warder, who "paid no attention to his duty" and "sleeps when he should be on guard." This breach enabled Temesi and another patient to escape. Temesi was found by Sachs in town enjoying a cigarette with a watchman; police located the other patient in nearby Tamavua-i-wai village and returned him to the hospital. In his letter, Temesi wrote, "Dr—you shouldn't employ this hopeless man" and threatened to contact Ratu Kamisese Mara if his complaints were not considered. An Indo-Fijian patient also reported that Josua was asleep while on night duty. Josua was dismissed. Although Temesi had written a rational complaint, another letter on the reverse revealed his inner world. This letter contained details of war maneuvers and was written to Lieutenant Colonel Prendergast from the Eighth Army headquarters on behalf of Field Marshal Bernard Montgomery on April 2, 1944.[156]

Private Struggles, the Asylum, and the Community

This chapter opened with a rare glimpse into a patient's perspective on life in the asylum. Syljeseth's letters are among the few documents concerning the treatment of psychiatric patients in colonial Fiji. Although officials were dismissive of most patients' letters, they recognized that writing could be therapeutic, which returns to the question raised in chapter 5. How seriously did medical personnel take the concerns patients voiced, especially in a cross-cultural clinical setting?[157] We return to patients' letters—in two very different forms—one written by Grace during the early 1960s and the other by Hanif in 1970.[158] These examples show that it was not only Europeans who wrote complaints or communicated about the mental and social trauma that brought them to St Giles. Grace was Kailoma, about twenty-two years old; Hanif an Indo-Fijian and about forty-one. Their audience was different, and the content of their letters is difficult to interpret. Their letters and the context in which they were written bring together the private struggles with madness in the asylum and the community. The lines could be porous between patients and the outside world. Individual struggles within the institution could reflect troubled lives before admission and sometimes patients' fears about returning to these lives.

When I read Grace's admission papers, they had not been opened since they were filed away in the 1960s.[159] As I unfolded them, I was surprised to find sheets of delicate, clean toilet tissue on which Grace had penciled semi-legible remarks. These comments were addressed to Mr. Fenn, the assistant head attendant, and to the police. She wrote these remarks before she underwent various therapies, including twenty electroshocks combined with 900 millograms of Largactil per day. Grace was then allowed to return home following a positive assessment: "alert & questions are answered *humbly & relevantly*. No worsen of delusions now. She is a good worker" (emphasis in the original). She was readmitted and in

1964 wrote a detailed eight-page letter to Sachs and the police. She made serious allegations about prominent Europeans in Fiji, claiming that they had photographed her when she was younger. She also suggested that, when she was a patient, she was sexually abused by a doctor for whom she did housework:

> one day he wanted me to open up. I had nothing to hide from him. Then it went on that way. Sometimes he does it to me sometimes he only wants to have a look, then one day I told him I don't want to work anymore. The next day he went to the hospital and he came back within an hour . . . He told me to take my pantie off and lie on the bed.

It is impossible to assess the truth of these claims, given that other delusions, notably being married to a local European, were incorrect. Doctors termed Grace's claims delusional and said that her inability to distinguish truth from reality showed a lack of insight. Her testimony shows that she interacted with different ethnic groups and understood the nuances of local idioms. Within her delusions and fantasies are detailed accounts of everyday life as well as references to events that would have made an impression on many Fijians at the time, such as Queen Elizabeth's visit in 1963. Grace also consulted her "book of omens" and mentions an Ouija board. It is not my role to assess retroactively the truth of testimony left by a patient diagnosed with schizophrenia, and her disjointed phrases make the content difficult to follow. Grace's letters may have been a form of accommodation to the limited means of expression within the hospital. Did she write on toilet paper because it was the only material available, or was it because she was inscribing her thoughts on an intimate material? The letters she later wrote were probably therapeutic and a plea for someone to understand her private world both in the asylum and the community. She challenged this world through her words and her madness, but the record of this challenge remained confined to her case notes.

In contrast, Hanif publicly drew attention to the plight of patients at St Giles, which was "run like a 12th century Roman slavery camp" and "virtually run like a prison." Under the pseudonym "A Sick Patient," Hanif wrote a letter to the editor of the *Pacific Review,* who published it on August 29, 1970, with an article headlined, "Are Mental Patients At Suva Subjected To Cruelty? A CORRESPONDENT SAYS 'YES' "[160] Hanif spoke out against those sites of resistance at St Giles covered in this chapter. He presents the hospital as a place of violence—"cruelty and savagery is rampant everywhere"—attributing the worst patient abuse to the orderlies. This abuse could be direct or through punishment, such as withholding food or spatial (often solitary) confinement in Bua Ward. Hanif's observation that confinement in this ward (for the most acutely disturbed and sometimes violent patients) would drive a sick patient insane reiterates the long-standing problem at St Giles of patients with widely differing mental conditions sharing the same ward as well as the use of space as an institutional form of control. He mentions work as a contested struggle between patients and staff where patients who refused or were unable to work would be punished. Like Syljeseth, Hanif takes on the role of patient advocate:

> A common source of fun for SOME ORDERLIES is "Charlie" and "Safique". These two unfortunate patients have been inmates of this institution for some time. These poor unfortunate beings are treated like punching bags. One orderly takes pleasure in punching Charlie everytime he passes him.
>
> Poor Charlie simply steps aside trembling. If someone else speaks for Charlie, the orderly tells him to "shut up" and mind his own business. It is no use complaining to the visiting doctor or anyone else. They simply ignore us and accept the words of the Orderly. . . . Some orderlies excite other patients to violence and when the patients start fighting among themselves, the orderlies appear to derive sadistic pleasure out of it and simply stand and watch and actually kick some of the patients and provoke them to fight. This, of course, does not happen every day.

Hanif's own story runs through the letter. He refers to "some of us who through unfortunate circumstances, nervous tension frustration, had become mentally ill and found ourselves confined" yet had been "useful citizens," which reflects his former successful career in the civil service and mental deterioration following a cerebral hemorrhage in 1959. Hanif was first admitted to St Giles for two months in 1962 and 1963 then readmitted in January 1970. This readmission occurred after he had made suicide threats in a letter to a magistrate; in this letter, Hanif detailed the various employment and domestic crises he had faced during the 1960s that he said precipitated him to steal from his employer. He expressed shame at being sent to prison and remorse for his behavior:

> Do you think I have been given a fair break in life? Do you think I love doing this thing? Do you think I like to bring disgrace upon my family for the love of it? Can you give me one reason I should not commit suicide?[161]

The bigger picture and the timing of the letter's publication are significant—less than six weeks before Fiji's independence from Britain on October 10, 1970. It was given prominence in the *Pacific Review,* the main rival newspaper to the *Fiji*

Times that supported the pro-establishment Alliance political party.[162] By 1970, the *Pacific Review* was aligned with the National Federation Party and, under the editorship of Ratu Mosese Varesekele, critically monitored the governance and functioning of the civil service. Ratu Varesekele was circumspect in his commentary, writing, "It is well known that the St Giles Mental Hospital in Suva is a humane institution with warm and understanding staff." He reiterated that, although considerable care was taken before a person was certified for mental treatment, the discharge process was more complicated and thus sometimes patients remained in mental hospitals. He posed this question about his correspondent,

> Is he one of the SANE ones who is caught in the unwitting arms of the law? If his coherent letter is the product of an unsound mind the content of the letter does not betray this. But let readers judge his letter and we hope those in authority view it with sympathy and understanding keeping in mind that there is nothing in the world easier than to condemn a SANE plea from a "certified person."[163]

We do not know how readers judged the letter, but medical authorities reacted swiftly. Remarks in Hanif's file show that he was identified as the culprit, "a delusional" patient who had made allegations that were "quite untrue." Hanif was assessed as a

> Psychopathic Character—feel the world is against him and that he will improve the lot of the patients—St Giles (See article written by him—Pacific Review) all absurd allegations are lies & fabrications.

Dr. Ram Narayan, the medical superintendent, wrote in large letters, "Do Not Admit this Pt as Voluntary in Future." This was the reaction behind the scenes. D. W. Beckett, the acting director of medical services, publicly gave a more muted response in *Pacific Review,* denying the "cruel charge," defending St Giles and its staff, and suggesting that the allegations could deter some mentally ill people from seeking treatment. But his final sentence summed up the unsympathetic stance toward patient complaints:

> It should be understood that a common symptom of mental disease is the desire to make complaints and cause trouble out of sheer maliciousness and this must always be considered when reading letters written by patients in a mental hospital.

Among his parting comments on completing his term as medical superintendent at St Giles, Macgregor expressed disgust at the way some staff abused patients there and how government handled this abuse. He stated, "things go on every day in this hospital which would blow the whole edifice sky-high if it were not for the incessant vigilance and disciplinary pressure of the Head Attendant." Macgregor referred to the 1961 Royal Commission of Inquiry into the cruelty and neglect of patients at Callan Park Hospital in New South Wales and said that Fiji was not immune from a similar scandal.[164] He warned that brutality to patients had to be seen as dealt with by instantaneous dismissal. Otherwise, he continued, there would be no defense when the warder

> or others like him get up to their old tricks again? One enterprising reporter, one indiscrete medical officer, one knowledgeable member of the Board of Visitors even one patient with an elementary knowledge of his legal rights would be enough to bring about a scandal that would set back progress in psychiatry for many years.[165]

Hanif's letter would not cause such ripples. It certainly could have, especially because it was published in a newspaper opposed to the government. But the letter was published during a period of excitement at certain nationhood when the country faced a multitude of wider political, economic, and social issues. Fiji was on the brink of a decolonized future. What would this mean for psychiatry and people with mental disorders in the new Fiji?

CHAPTER 7

Conclusion

Recolonizing Mental Health in Postcolonial Fiji?

In the 1880s, newspapers in Fiji shocked readers with reports of two instances of madness in the island colony. For different reasons, Qaqa and Sukudaia became objects of fascination and would be among the first patients admitted to Fiji's newly established lunatic asylum. Qaqa was a homicidal maniac who had savagely attacked a white woman and a fellow prisoner. Sukudaia was regarded as a public nuisance, a vagrant who behaved indecently and possibly manically, which marked her as insane. The new colonial order faced the problem of how to remove dangerous and difficult subjects from the community while treating them with a modicum of humanity, the latter being a mark of civilization, even if it was colonization that determined the new parameters and management of madness.

During the mid- to late nineteenth century, asylum building was in its heyday, not only in Europe and North America, but also in the imperial outreaches of Australia, New Zealand, and Fiji. The decision to establish a lunatic asylum in Fiji and to introduce legislation to control and treat the insane was unique within the Pacific Islands during the 1880s. Few colonial institutions globally would have the longevity of Fiji's small asylum.

That asylum became St Giles and still functions as a key psychiatric institution in the postcolonial Pacific. Most of its patients have not attracted the public attention of Qaqa, Sukudaia, or—in the new millennium—Apete Kaisau. Neither were St Giles's patients subjected to the intense examination that Kaisau was by the medical superintendent of St Giles, Dr. Shishram Narayan, and by renowned Melbourne forensic psychiatrist Professor Paul Mullen. In 2001, the "crime that shocked the country"—a double murder, at the heart of which was madness in Fiji—brought unprecedented local and international scrutiny.[1] Global media coverage included a book, written by the brother of one of the victims—*Deep beyond the Reef: A True Story of Madness and Murder in the South Pacific*—and a documentary—*An Island Calling*, released in 2008.[2]

Since the Kaisau tragedy, two other alarming cases concerning people with mental disabilities in postcolonial Fiji sparked media interest. Unlike Kaisau,

Sujit Kumar and Nur Nisha were not dangers to the community, but the community failed them nonetheless. Both were confined for years for reasons that remain unclear. Sujit was never diagnosed with a mental illness, but had epilepsy, which may have been induced through the abuse inflicted on him; abuse had probably caused him to exhibit bizarre behavior and to never learn to speak. Nur, diagnosed with schizophrenia in 1987, was confined in a shed by her family in a rural settlement for around forty years.

Sujit, known as the Chicken Boy, had been confined by his parents in a chicken coop, probably since he was a baby. After his mother committed suicide in 1977 and his father was murdered in 1979, his elderly grandfather was responsible for him.[3] At about age eight, he was found in the middle of the road at night. Social welfare staff placed him in the Samabula Old People's Home—his home for the following twenty-two years. Staff frequently tethered him to a bed or to the wall with cotton sheeting, where he was left in filthy conditions. Elizabeth Clayton, who "rescued" Sujit, observed that he pecked at his food and crouched, "as if roosting. His fingers turn inward from scratching around in the dirt, he communicates by making a rapid clicking noise with his tongue and he seems detached from much that goes on around him."[4] Clayton met Sujit in 2002 when she was president of the Rotary Club of Suva; she became his guardian and tried to rehabilitate and "humanize" him. According to tests run by international experts, Sujit had normal brain function; later tests confirmed that he had epilepsy.[5]

Sujit's story created sensational headlines in the international media and was followed through television broadcasts and a documentary. It also drew attention to the neglect of unwanted and abused children, some of whom were intellectually impaired.[6] Sujit's plight highlighted the dearth of information about the trauma many of these children had endured, and, as lawyer John Rabuku declared, Sujit's life was virtually untraceable, and "He was a non-person."[7]

Chapter 2 of this book referred to "lost souls," many labeled as destitute, whose lives remained a mystery. Although Sujit was not declared mentally ill or committed to a psychiatric institution, Narayan spoke to the media about a similar patient at St Giles "whose behaviour was also imprinted with traits common to fowl." She had spent ten years around chickens: "All her hands and legs were contracted, she could hardly stand and walk. It was like she was crawling . . . She could not eat with her hands, she would spread food around and pick from there." Narayan said the patient had made some progress, but "there is no one to take her back."[8]

As elaborated in this chapter, community and family neglect of people with mental disorders remain a problem in postcolonial Fiji. In 2013, a newspaper report about Nur Nisha in the *Fiji Times* quickly drew a television crew from New Zealand to film her crouching under a blanket in a filthy shed, where she slept on the concrete floor, ate, and went to the toilet. Nur received medication and her family was allocated ninety dollars per month for her care, but they told the media that they did not know how to restrain her from wandering naked around the settlement. Her sister said that Nur became violent and uncontrollable around the age of eight and her condition worsened over the years. Families during the colonial era made similar observations when some women and children were committed to the asylum. Nur's situation reveals that, although biomedical treatment was ostensibly available to mentally disordered people living in the community in postcolonial Fiji, the quality of care and understanding of mental illness was sometimes deplorable.[9] The institutional solution to managing madness—the asylum—was slowly dismantled but not inevitably augmented with effective forms of care.

These three media cases emerged decades after colonial rule ended in Fiji, yet they highlight key issues in the colonization of madness. These issues include the meaning and construction of madness, the management of mental disorder, and the rights of mentally ill individuals and those of the community. Judge Justice Salesi Temo raised some of these dilemmas in 2014 and 2015 when Kaisau sought to be discharged from St Giles.[10] Although the use of medication in the management of mental illness was far more entrenched than when the hospital had been founded, Temo was still concerned about the protection of society as well as patients' rights and welfare. Further, Kaisau's possible discharge depended on the efficacy of psychiatric care in the community. In the decades after colonial rule ended in 1970, decentralized mental health services had developed slowly and intermittently. This chapter traces some of the problems mental health services face in contemporary Fiji, not least of which are economic development and political turmoil, especially since the first coup d'état in 1987.

This book has explored how the colonization of madness was distinctive in Fiji and accordingly has traced the patterns and practices of how mental disorder was constructed and treated in the cultural and historical context of the colony. It has shown how the institutionalization of colonial madness was entangled not only with specifics of race and gender in the Pacific colony, but also with universal psychiatric discourses and practices. This global legacy did not disappear when Fiji was declared an independent nation on October 10, 1970. Indeed, in the lead-up to independence, development and political discourse in Fiji promoted modernity. Health was a key indicator, as proclaimed by C. H. Gurd, the secretary of health in 1970: "medicine in Fiji is on the march."[11] Mental health, however, was pushed down the list of priorities, just as it had been in colonial Fiji. In postcolonial Fiji, the ideals of development and modernity soon encountered economic and political tensions, and other needs were prioritized.

Although mental health provision continued the colonial model of biomedicine that was highly centralized, custodial, and framed within "a master narrative called 'the development of modern medicine,'" attempts were made, beginning in the 1960s, to break down the image of the isolated asylum.[12] This final chapter outlines these attempts. It examines how, with the use of new psychotropic medications, greater emphasis was placed on the outpatient management of mental illness. It shows how the resources for this approach were far from adequate and how the application of biomedical concepts of mental disorder still met with indigenous, religious, and cultural understandings of madness. It discusses how communities might offer alternative explanations and treatments, yet can also reinforce stigma and neglect those with mental disorders. To an extent, madness had been colonized in Fiji, and the asylum was central to that process. Although health experts called for and sometimes instigated shifts in the care and treatment of patients in St Giles and in the outside community, the process of change was uneven and painfully slow during the first three decades after independence.

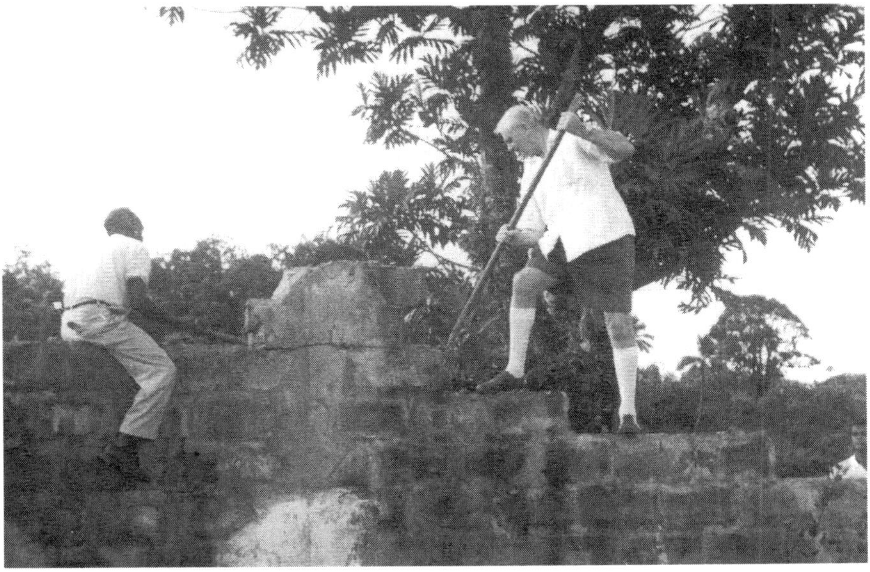

Figure 7.1. Dr. Duncan Macgregor leading demolition of St Giles's walls. Source: Robert Macgregor.

Breaking Down the Walls

In 1966, it gave Dr. Duncan Macgregor great satisfaction to lead a party of patients and orderlies in demolishing most of the concrete wall that encircled St Giles.[13] This act symbolized some of the changes, in line with modern psychiatric practices in the United Kingdom, that Macgregor sought to bring to Fiji. During the ten years prior to his appointment at St Giles in 1964, he had been medical superintendent at Carlton Hayes Hospital in Leicester, where community care and an open door policy were in place. Macgregor came to St Giles in an era when a new drug regime enabled patients to be treated and discharged more rapidly than before. He believed that breaking down the walls gave patients a sense of freedom, in keeping with the emphasis he placed on patient dignity and respect from the staff caregivers. Actually, some of the stone walls at St Giles remained, and wire fences replaced those that had been destroyed—albeit out of sight—below the hospital. Almost thirty years later, Alison Cupit, chair of St Giles' Board of Visitors, deplored the arrangement, saying that the buildings "may be best described as prison camps without the elaborate fencing."[14] Institutional confinement in these old buildings would continue, but during the late 1960s initiatives were launched for patients to become part of the outside community. Macgregor hoped that greater visibility might reduce the stigma associated with the place and the patients. His successor, Dr. David Sell, confirmed this, saying, "The mental hospital has stood for too long in isolation with its inhabitants out of sight, out of mind and socially stigmatized."[15]

Staff training and professionalism were further outcomes of Macgregor's commitment to modern psychiatric practice. They were a necessary corollary of the localization of medical staff and essential to the decolonization of the civil service in Fiji.[16] Two full-time Indo-Fijian doctors, Issac Karim and Ram Narayan, were hired in 1962 and 1967, and an indigenous Fijian doctor, M. Vuki was appointed in 1962.

It was during the early 1960s, that Narayan, the newly appointed deputy superintendent of Labasa Hospital, received a telephone call from Dr. David Bookless, Fiji's deputy director of medical services, encouraging him to pursue postgraduate studies in psychiatry because of the probable withdrawal of expatriate staff with decolonization. Narayan was among the early Fijian citizens to train in medicine overseas, completing a medical degree at the University of Otago in 1955 and an internship in New Zealand. Narayan followed Bookless's advice and studied psychiatry in Sydney. In 1970, he became the first local superintendent and acting consultant psychiatrist at St Giles. Overseas study called him again, and after gaining a diploma of psychological medicine from Otago in 1972, he returned to Fiji as medical superintendent of St Giles in 1973.[17]

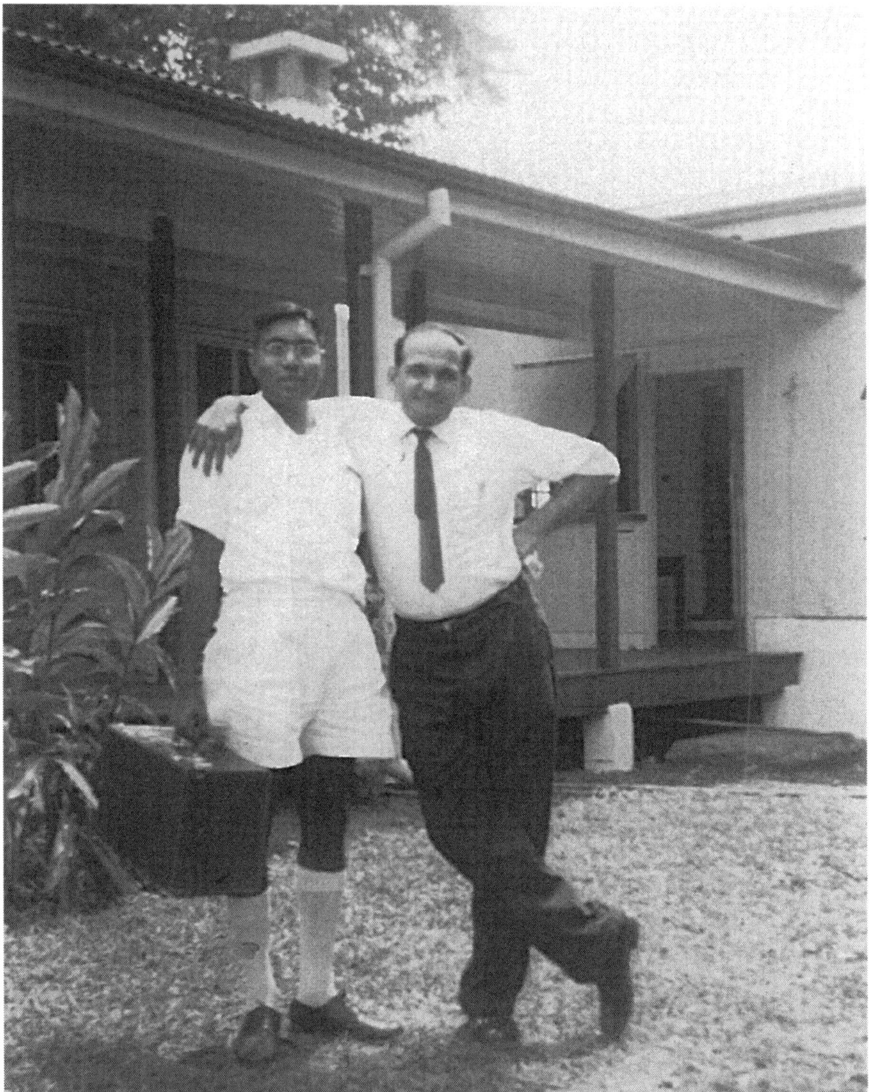

Figure 7.2. Dr. Ram Narayan and Dr. Shiu Chand Ramrakha, Labasa Hospital, 1963. In 1970 Narayan was the first Fiji-born medical superintendent (acting) and consultant psychiatrist at St Giles. Source: Ranjana Narayan.

Macgregor's aims had been supported by Charles Cochrane Sachs, known to staff as Charlie or Chas and to the patients as Daddy.[18] As head attendant, Sachs was appointed to a role that became the precursor of that of hospital matron, vested with the responsibility to implement hospital management and oversee patient care. One of his first tasks was to ensure that more Fijians and Indians were employed as orderlies, a need earlier pointed out to government by Fiji's Great Council of Chiefs in 1940.[19] Until then, most orderlies were Samoans, but by the 1960s, very few Samoans were employed at St Giles. Despite the high proportion of Indo-Fijian patients, an Indo-Fijian attendant, Ashok Kumar, was not appointed until 1966.

From Warders to Nurses

Sachs's dedication to improving nursing and physical conditions in the hospital may have contributed to the radical decline in St Giles's death rates. According to Macgregor, prior to 1951, 10 to 30 percent of patients died within two years of their admission, but by 1961, after Sachs's arrival, this rate fell to 1 percent.[20] Patients' physical condition was also increasingly screened, and new biomedical knowledge and medications (including penicillin) contributed to falling death rates. Sachs energetically worked with the new psychiatric drugs and technologies, which enabled patients to be discharged much earlier than before. Before 1961, only 35 to 65 percent of patients were discharged within two years, but after the new drug regime was implemented in 1961, 97 percent left.

The introduction of psychotropic drugs and shock therapy necessitated a shift in expertise among orderlies. They trained on the job and had a primary role as nurses in shock and drug therapy, witnessing both immediate and long-term side effects. In 1965, Macgregor advocated renaming and upgrading the post of head attendant to chief nursing officer to reflect that the head attendant's role had shifted from being primarily an administrative officer to being a nursing officer with responsibility for general management.[21] Although Sachs had created this role, it was not until after he retired in 1969 that the position of senior supervisor was approved. A qualification in psychiatric nursing was deemed essential. Nursing sister Qamrul Nisha Mohammed was appointed to that position in 1972.

Macgregor's attention to localization and professionalization focused on the orderlies, who provided the bulk of primary mental health care; however, unprofessional behavior persisted. As discussed in chapter 5, by the end of his contract, Macgregor was disillusioned with the unprofessional attitudes and violent behavior of some staff toward patients despite his efforts to train staff in less coercive methods.[22] Incidents of violence and unnecessary force by orderlies persisted in the decades that followed. As we have seen, Hanif's allegations of staff brutality made newspaper headlines in 1970. In 1977, a patient complained that an orderly had rudely shouted, provoked, and punched a very ill patient several times in the stomach; the witness begged, "Don't punch him. Don't punch him."[23] The medical superintendent reported this incident to the permanent secretary of health, who laid charges against the orderly under the 1974 Public Service Commission (Constitution) Act. Complaints about orderlies' behavior, poor nursing standards, and patient neglect continued into the 1980s and drew severe reprimands from Karim and Matron Mohammed.[24]

Continuing the efforts Macgregor had started in the 1960s, senior nurses during the 1980s advocated training in modern methods and basic nursing for orderlies to improve patient care.[25] On February 1, 1988, at her first meeting with the orderlies, Acting Matron Jane Erasito stressed the need to work in cooperation with patients and to not leave them alone. Erasito was a psychiatric nurse who was eager to apply the knowledge she had gained while attached to Nelson Polytechnic in New Zealand in 1980. She discussed modern psychiatric practices around confinement and listening to what patients say about how their medication is affecting them.[26] Some orderlies later explained that they learned from and appreciated Erasito's psychiatric nursing expertise and firm but gentle ways of relating to patients.

In that 1988 meeting, Erasito stressed that the registered nurses were there to supervise the orderlies; however, as the number of nurses employed at St Giles rose, tensions between nurses and orderlies increased as well. In 1982, the ratio was twelve nurses to sixty-four orderlies; by 1991, the number of nurses had increased to around twenty, and these were assisted by as many as thirty student nurses.[27] On the one hand, professional qualifications and general nursing experience did not always equate with the hands-on knowledge that many orderlies had acquired through years of nursing the mentally ill. On the other hand, stubborn insistence on keeping to entrenched and sometimes harsh methods was not in the patients' interests and ran counter to modern psychiatric nursing. By the 1990s, many orderlies had embraced new methods, such as one-on-one interaction with patients so that patients could "learn the inside" and have more self-awareness of their disorder.[28] Not all orderlies wanted to change, and for many years tensions between staff factions, including divisions between and within groups of nurses and orderlies, were a problem at St Giles, sometimes threatening to spill into industrial action during the 1970s and 1980s.[29]

The Dark Clouds on the Horizon

The secretary of health presented an optimistic report in 1970 on the future of medical services in postcolonial Fiji, but the prognosis for mental health was far gloomier. St Giles's medical superintendent warned that although Fiji had not yet reached the dimensions of psychiatric diseases experienced in developed countries, "the dark clouds are gathering on the horizon and there is no room for complacency in the matter."[30] This warning could have referred to the immediate issues that independence posed to Fiji's psychiatric services. Admissions of indigenous Fijians to St Giles were increasing relative to those of other ethnicities, and existing psychiatric services did not have the capacity to cope with the rising numbers of inpatients and outpatients.[31] The dark clouds could also have referred to the negative social and psychological effects of urbanization and modernization that would come with postcolonial development. Leading Pacific psychiatrists—Macgregor from Fiji, Burton G. Burton-Bradley from the Territory of Papua and New Guinea, and Georges Zeldine, a psychiatrist with the French military in New Caledonia—had identified links between pathological mental states, urbanization, and modernity and the rise in mental disorders in the 1960s in their areas.[32] They identified such contributing factors as

> over-urbanization, interterritorial migrant rootlessness (anomie), discriminations, educational and accultural disparities of spouses, problems of retirement, intergenerational conflicts, faulty race relations, and certain deleterious consequences, on the psychiatric level, of tourism.[33]

Delinquency, alcoholism, and prostitution were also correlated with mental illness; later, Henry Murphy added the burdens of decolonization on the elite to the list of psychological stress factors.[34] Experts did not, however, foresee how extensively poverty would hit Fiji and many other Pacific countries during the late twentieth century. Economic deprivation and unemployment could accentuate or be conducive to mental disorders, and poor communities might struggle to provide material support for those with mental illness.[35] As chapter 2 emphasizes, many patients in St Giles in the early years were considered vagrants, and by the end of the twentieth century, homelessness was a problem for many mentally ill people. In 2008, the St Vincent de Paul Society received a grant from the state to assist its night shelter for the homeless, who were mostly former patients from St Giles.[36] The society's night shelter was in Toorak, near the place where Sukudaia and her child were given temporary shelter by the state during the early

1880s. The night shelter was established in 1989 in the aftermath of two military coups in 1987 that had precipitated immense economic and social dislocation in Fiji. At the time of Fiji's decolonization, psychiatrists and social scientists could not anticipate the trauma and insecurity that later political upheaval would bring, including the impact on those who were psychologically vulnerable and "left behind" by sustained emigration after 1987.

Patient Turnover

Macgregor had been enthusiastic about the potential for improved care and conditions for psychiatric patients in St Giles, but his successor, Sell, was more negative about the hospital's capacity to cope with increased admission numbers. Although patient death rates fell during the 1960s and many patients spent shorter periods in hospital than before, Sell conservatively estimated in 1969 that admissions would rise from 208 at the end of 1970 to 315 by the end of 1975. He advocated for a new psychiatric hospital on another site to accommodate around five to six hundred patients. His vision for a hospital included a maximum-security wing for the "criminally insane and violent" but also expansive grounds for outdoor recreation and villa-type accommodation to house quieter patients.[37] Sell's prediction was never realized. The bed capacity in 1979 was 170.

During the 1970s, Murphy and Narayan painted a more positive picture of St Giles. They found that "mental hospitalisation rates in Fiji were exceptionally low, and the mean duration of stay in hospital lower than in many other countries, without the hospital being overcrowded and without discharged patients rapidly needing readmission."[38] They cautiously attributed the lower rates to the care provided for mentally disturbed people in the community. Murphy and Narayan also warned that more psychiatric services were likely to be required because tolerance of the chronically mentally ill was probably waning.

Although mental hospitalization rates in Fiji were relatively low relative to elsewhere, mental health services continued to be plagued by problems. Some of these problems were common in the general health sector: difficulties identified by the 1979 Select Committee of Inquiry into Fiji's Health Services included inadequate resources, drug and staffing shortages, inadequate training, administrative mismanagement, and political interference.[39] Unreliable supplies of psychiatric drugs were especially critical in outlying areas and could be the reason patients "defaulted" on their medication. St Giles lacked specialists: in 1979 one consultant psychiatrist and two doctors were responsible for all psychiatric care, which included 3,713 outpatient consultations. Locally based training in psychiatric medicine and nursing was piecemeal: postgraduate nurses and doctors

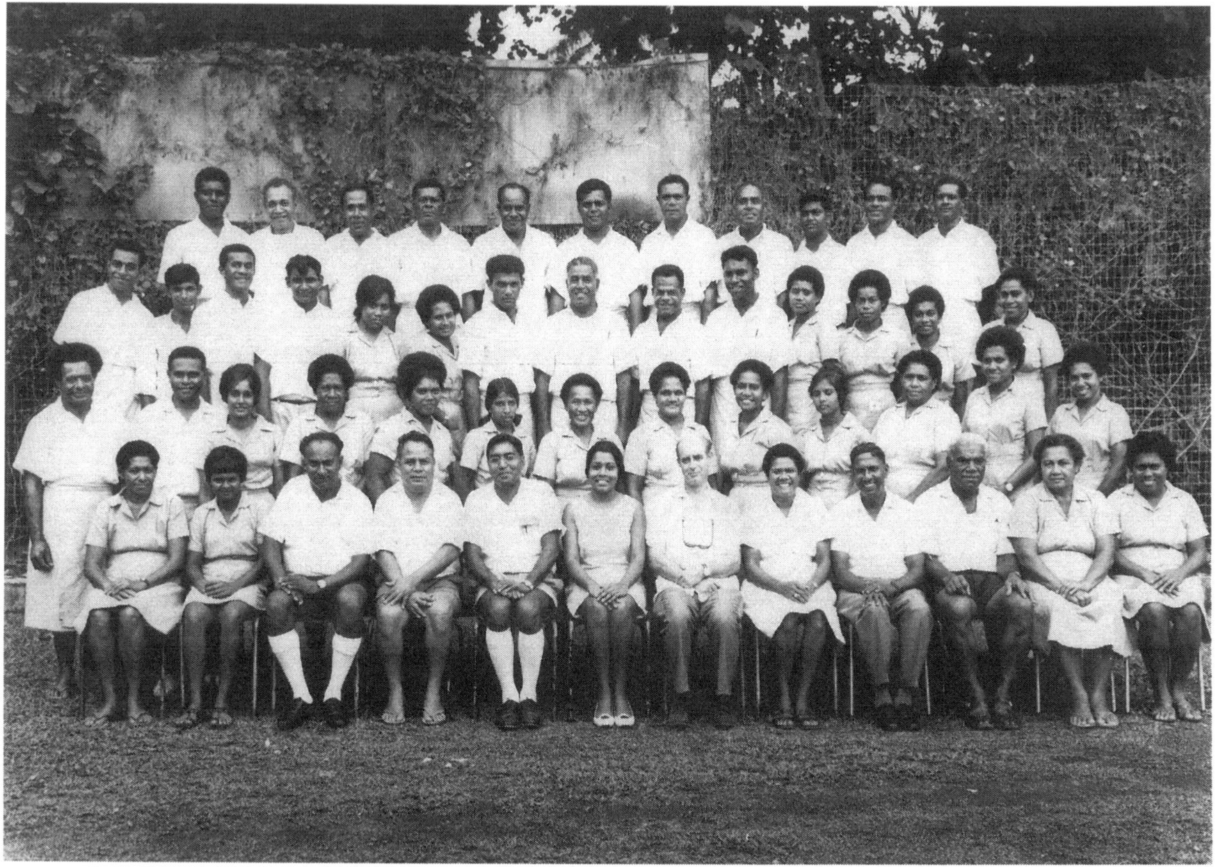

Figure 7.3. Staff, St Giles Hospital, 1970. Bottom row, fourth from left to right: K. Taratai, Dr. Ram Narayan, unknown, Dr. David Sell, Asena Ranadi, Dr. Issac Karim, V. Suliano. Source: Ranjana Narayan.

began to train in mental illness from 1966, and by independence a new syllabus in nurse training included mental illness.[40] In the 1980s, some medical students in Fiji were taught modules in psychiatry through externally based degrees.[41] It was not until 2006 that public health nurses were trained in mental health and James Cook University in Australia offered nurses in Fiji a post-basic nursing certificate in mental health. Postgraduate qualifications for mental health professionals in the Pacific commenced at the Fiji National University in 2012.[42]

Murphy and Narayan highlighted how the care that families and communities in Fiji provided was a key factor in keeping admission rates down, but that hospital policies were responsible for rapid patient turnover. As discussed in chapter 6, psychotropic drugs offered the potential for severely disturbed patients to live in the community, even if they were not "cured." In 1965, about 70 percent of patients admitted to St Giles were discharged within the following three months. Nearly two-thirds of admissions were patients readmitted for the second or subsequent time.[43] Narayan admitted to the permanent secretary of health in 1975 that he had been able to keep a lid on patient numbers only by admitting patients when necessary and discharging patients prematurely, adding, "this is an unsatisfactory state of affairs from relatives [*sic*] point of view and I must admit that I feel very guilty about this."[44] He estimated that approximately half of patients suffered a deterioration in their mental health due to the lack of outpatient aftercare and should have been under continual outpatient supervision, just as Macgregor had pointed out a decade earlier.[45]

After independence, fewer new patients than before spent long continuous periods of their life in the institution. One female, for example, lived as a patient for forty-five years between 1949 and 1996. In contrast, Vilisi was first admitted to St Giles in 1971, and over the following decades was readmitted almost annually and sometimes several times a year. Between admissions, she lived with kin in her village, cared for her children and those of her siblings, and did domestic and farm work. Her mother checked that Vilisi took her medication, but when Vilisi stopped taking it her disordered behavior invariably led to a readmission. Like Shankar, discussed shortly, this behavior included wandering and sometimes living on the streets.

In the hospital's eagerness to discharge patients—patients who ostensibly could function as long as they took their pills—little consideration was given to providing outpatient care in the community. As Nur's story reveals, a biomedical solution did not necessarily extend to community care. Patient follow-up, let alone support, was nonexistent for many years, and only some former patients were able to attend clinics at St Giles; those who could usually depended on family or friends to take them there. Other patients were expected to visit their local health center for check-ups and to be issued with medication. Medical officers and district nurses outside Suva had no formal psychiatric training but were at the front line of biomedical care in the community. Patients were expected to take their drugs, but clearly many did not; families might assume responsibility to oversee drug "compliance," but in practice this could be difficult to enforce. Not all families were supportive either.

Vijay's predicament is reminiscent of the breaking point families could reach in rural Fiji (as with Biman in chapter 2), but it also indicates neglect and cruelty. Vijay had been discharged to the care of his father and extended family in 1975 and prescribed medication to control his "fits." He worked unpaid on the family's small cane farm, although Ram Narayan was informed that the family could not clothe or feed him. If excessive demands were made of him, Vijay would become irritable, which provoked family members to assault him and tie him up. His drug supplies had to be obtained from the district hospital, but in 1978 his brothers refused to fetch new supplies. When Vijay was prevented from leaving the farm to obtain his drugs, he reacted by assaulting his father with an ax handle. Narayan believed that Vijay was not suffering from mental illness, even though his family called him mad; a district nurse was therefore asked to visit Vijay regularly and deliver his drugs.[46]

The initiative to seek medical intervention was placed on patients and their families. They were issued with instructions to follow doctors' orders, to take medication, and to turn up for medical checks. Families did not or could not always fulfill this responsibility and had little control over a family member who "wandered." Shankar was nineteen when he was first admitted to St Giles in 1955 after assaulting people and wandering about "raving." He was diagnosed with schizophrenia and by 1991 had been admitted eleven times. During those years, he worked intermittently as a cane laborer and lived with his father and kin. He continued to be violent and would not remain at home. As an elderly man, Shankar ambled around an urban area, where he begged and annoyed people. His appearance was very dirty, his feet became septic, and he urinated and defecated in public places. A medical officer despaired that he did not know what to do with Shankar, who needed someone to care for him.[47]

Shankar's family had taken responsibility for him but could not control his mobility; in other instances, families, who regarded having a member committed to St Giles as irrevocable, did not readily accept discharged patients. As noted, in earlier times communal support was also not always forthcoming when patients were discharged from the hospital. The stigma associated with having been committed to St Giles could persist. In other cases, contrary to the families' expectations, individuals were not fully cured, or the side effects of their medication could be as alarming as the original disorder; rather than returning a person to "normality," the side effects often accentuated difference and inhibited acceptance into the community. Patients might forget or refuse to take medication because of its side effects, or dislike the overall effect of the medication on their mental state (for example, feel constantly "flat"). If patients suddenly ceased taking high levels of psychotropic drugs, they could experience a relapse, possibly enhancing the primary mental condition. Failure to take drugs could also be because supplies were irregular, especially in outlying districts.

Education about medication effects was usually absent. Families did not always understand that, even if a former patient appeared normal, medication should be continued. Although the family might have welcomed the docility some drugs induced, this particular effect could limit the patient's active contribution to family and community life and work.

The Social Climate

Doctors at St Giles had long regarded lay views as a hindrance to the acceptance of biomedical management of mental illness. In 1963, when doctors were optimistic that the new drug therapy would lead to shorter hospital stays, the medical superintendent observed, "it is becoming apparent that in the less sophisticated social climate of Fiji, a more conservative attitude is required."[48] He was referring to attitudes toward mental illness in Fiji's cultures, along with public ignorance about psychiatry, patient treatment, and rehabilitation. His statement also suggests stigmatization toward St Giles and those with mental illness, which inhibited patient treatment and rehabilitation. Derogatory names for St Giles were common. Macgregor would have been disappointed that the tin fencing he erected to open up St Giles would lend itself to the slang for the hospital: *bakava,* which also became an adjective meaning crazy, silly person.[49] Stigma stopped some patients and families from seeking biomedical treatment, as social worker Janice Smith pointed out in 1986: "An institution for 'mad' people, and westernized medical care can be frightening to some people and will prevent their coming."[50] Ohaeri also emphasized that the public did not understand the biomedical approach to mental illness and the use of medication.[51]

The stigma attached to mental illness and being a patient at St Giles is a key reason families abandoned some patients there. Sometimes kin would refuse to accept discharged patients back into the family because of economic hardship and the extra labor entailed in caring for a recovering patient or because of the perception that mentally ill people were unproductive. Ohaeri suggested that abandonment was a recent trend in Fiji's post-coup economic climate.[52] Neglect by some families was similar during colonial times, however, though probably to a lesser extent. Sodhi, introduced in chapter 5, who first came to St Giles at age twelve, had twenty-two admissions by 1997 but had always been discharged to her mother's care. When Sodhi's mother died, however, her brother refused to accept her back into the family.

In the twenty-first century, some staff and former patients spoke out publicly about the effects of stigma. They described how stigma prevented former patients from securing a livelihood, forming social relationships, and being accepted outside St Giles. The removal of stigma was a major goal of psychiatric support groups, and this advocacy has been essential to recent mental health reforms in Fiji.[53] A survey in 2004 in Suva indicated that community attitudes toward people with mental disorders were changing for the better.[54] Yet community attitudes in Fiji have been and remain contradictory and complex.[55]

Traditional understandings and responses to mental disorder are still quite strong in Fiji's communities. Cultures and religions, which may offer compassion and caring for mental illness, can give space to beliefs that madness is a punishment for past or present wrongdoing. The families of Nur and Sujit may have regarded them as being possessed by an evil spirit.[56] One of Nur's nephews told reporter Barbara Dreaver that "It's probably a demon that is in her, that has ruined her and is ruling and commanding her."[57] Many patients believed that their illness or strange behavior was caused by witchcraft (*draunikau*) or a malevolent force. In 1975 Ram Narayan described Mr. A., of Indo-Fijian and Solomon Islands parentage, diagnosed with paranoid schizophrenia.[58] Mr. A. believed that, after a trip to the Solomon Islands, he had been possessed by three spirits that had given him special powers for healing up to three hundred people in Fiji. He became certain that an evil force was penetrating him with electric shocks in order to dispossess him of his healing powers. When Mr. A. was admitted to St Giles, he was considered a danger to the community because, it was feared, he might commit homicide. Once he was under medication, he was discharged to the care of his wife, but his healing powers had gone.

Chapter 3 traced how Christian beliefs could become entwined with mental disorder. A diagnosis of religious insanity is no longer used, but religion remains part of many patients' worlds and is fundamental to community responses. In postcolonial Fiji, as before, religious delusions are entwined with the broader social context. An alternative interpretation of the Bible in one community might be the norm in another, and religious extremism intensified with the assertion of religious ethnic nationalism in post-coup Fiji.[59] The night before he killed John

Scott and Gregory Scrivener, Kaisau had discussed the Bible with his cousin and referred to the killing of beasts as sacrifices. A note written by Kaisau and found in a Bible suggests that he had been taken over by a spirit and guided toward the murders:

> Calm as the sea on a sprinkling rainy day was my heart when dawn came. It cruised on, drifting slowly deep into my own galaxy of freedom and rights when suddenly it was moved. Deeply, moved that a SPIRIT took over me
>
> I was fearless of anyone under earth at point moment
> So bold was I like a lion going for a prey
> Anger of the highest level
> Anger to destroy
> Anger to kill
> Anger for my freedom I can say.
> Anger for the "path of the truth" to make access and entry.[60]

Kaisau told Mullen that "he was not mad, but anointed and doing God's will."[61] Kaisau had earlier reputedly said, "I don't like gays. They should be dissolved on Earth. They should not be alive."[62]

Religion remains a powerful way of treating mental disorders in Fiji. Families often seek help from mainstream religious counselors or other faith-based healers before turning to biomedical intervention. Prayer meetings are held at St Giles, and, for many discharged patients and their families, spiritual participation is an important part of healing, although health workers have raised concerns over this practice:

> Some religious groups that advocated prayer as the elixir to cure all ailments and actively discourage the use of medication. The power of these organisations are such that many of our patients succumb to their influences repeatedly. . . . Our message should be "Pray and take your medicines."[63]

Traditional healing also plays a significant role and is legal in postcolonial Fiji. Although indigenous and Indo-Fijian remedies using plants, diet, or massage might be classified today under complementary medicine, these remedies can be dismissed in popular discourse as witchcraft or black magic. Local doctors have recognized the dual use of traditional and biomedical healing but have been skeptical about the efficacy of traditional healing for mental illness. Ram Narayan observed, "The element of suggestion plays a large part as it is done in western medicine; and an intelligent doctor recognises this and uses it to make his treatment more effective."[64] Karim told me that witchcraft made the "treatment of patients much more difficult. When patients become sick the first thing is they think it is from witchcraft. Then go around consulting witch doctors, faith healers and so forth." He suggested that this belief shifted the blame and the potential for cure for the illness away from the individual and onto other people: "I think it's much easier to say oh this is from witchcraft, rather than say oh this is mental illness."[65] Narayan observed that families consulted native healers before and after treatment in St Giles; after such consultations, families might delay seeking biomedical help, and, once discharged, patients might be advised to stop taking medication.[66] A 1996 workshop was concerned that some relatives lacked understanding about patients' delusions and hallucinations, leading to relatives taking patients to traditional healers, who reinforced beliefs about possession and sorcery.[67] Attitudes toward traditional healing and the primacy of supernatural causes in mental illness are diverse and evolving in Fiji's communities.[68]

Community Care

When Erasito encouraged staff to take patients on excursions outside St Giles during the late 1980s, she said, "we have to introduce them back to society." Erasito regarded patient reintegration into the community as an important therapy, otherwise, patients would struggle when they returned to their communities. As she explained, "they will find everything strange because they never went out. So we have to introduce them back to society, so they see normal things, normal people, so they enjoy the things they used to enjoy."[69] Twenty years earlier, when Macgregor drew attention to the high rates of readmissions to St Giles, he identified wider causes outside the asylum: inadequate medical follow-up and a lack of social services and community support for the rehabilitation of those with mental illness, "inseparable from the organisation of a developing country."[70]

Services were inadequate in two associated areas: the care of people, especially children, with intellectual disabilities and the care of older people suffering from dementia. Chapter 5 indicates how, in the past, intellectual impairment and dementia were commonly confused with other mental disorders. Some patients with intellectual disabilities were admitted to the asylum because suitable institutions were absent or families could not cope. As Sell advised the director of medical services in 1969, families were unwilling and unable to care for old people or young mentally defective children.[71] During the 1970s, several families asked Narayan whether the hospital could take in very young mentally ill children who were unmanageable at home.[72] Some "difficult patients" were accommodated at the Samabula Old People's Home, St Giles staff providing some oversight.[73] In 1979, Ayesha's parents requested that their daughter, in her mid-thirties, be sent to the Old People's Home after her discharge from St Giles.[74] After the former leprosy hospital, St Elizabeth's Home, became part of St Giles in 1977, patients with severe intellectual disabilities began to be accommodated there.

Independence did not improve state and community support for former patients and those living with mental illness in the community. In 1999, at the National Health Conference, Jude Ohaeri emphasized that "the challenge for mental health care delivery in the new millennium, is how to link up effectively treated severely ill patients with community resources for rehabilitation, so as to curtail the chronic psychosocial disabilities consequent to these illnesses."[75] He also identified the need to assist families supporting former patients, to assure the public that treated patients are safe, to convince employers to hire former patients, and to find shelter for homeless patients whose family may have abandoned them or emigrated.

Macgregor may have been in favor of "breaking down the walls," but this step did not extend to the deinstitutionalization of psychiatric care. Although by the 1970s large mental hospitals were on the way out in the United Kingdom, New Zealand, Australia, and many other countries, hospitalization remained the primary focus for mental health care in Fiji.[76]

Community care and services developed slowly, unevenly, and inadequately in Fiji through outpatient services in Suva and district home care. After the introduction of widespread drug therapy and a policy of more rapid discharges from St Giles from the early 1960s, outpatient services became essential if patients were to have their prescriptions renewed. Outpatient provision gave medical care to more people who had mental disorders without certifying and hospitalizing them. Outpatient resources were also being used more because of stress disorders, an increase by 1968 linked to development.[77] Relative to other ethnic groups, Indo-Fijians had a proportionately high usage of outpatient services, which is perhaps unsurprising given that they have long been more accustomed to accessing health services than indigenous Fijians.[78] Outpatient figures were first published in 1963, when total consultations numbered 1,265.[79] By 1970, that figure had risen to 1,859.[80] The dramatic increase indicates the extension and incorporation of biomedicine in Fiji, a further colonization of madness.

Although St Giles provided highly centralized psychiatric services that continued to be inadequately resourced and staffed, greater integration with general health services was required.[81] Outside Suva, district nurses and assistant medical officers (AMOs) remained responsible for acute psychiatric intervention and supporting chronically ill patients. In 1968, a domiciliary care program for mental illness was introduced, though it is not clear how effectively this operated in practice. Through this program, drugs for mental and neurological disorders were dispensed by the medical superintendent and sent to regional health centers for registered patients. Health officials communicated by radio-telephone, but letters were still important. In 1961, Dr. Helen Rushton issued radio broadcasts to AMOs on schizophrenia and manic depression. An AMO in Lakeba might have listened to Rushton read out the lengthy article "Sedatives and Tranquillizers" by William Sargant of the Department of Psychological Medicine at St Thomas's Hospital in London. She said that the broadcast would offer AMOs "insight . . . because even in places where life is as comparatively easy as it is in the Pacific Islands the use of sedatives has increased."[82]

Community psychiatric nursing (CPN) did not get under way until 1993, and even then it was directed from St Giles and covered only the Suva area. Although CPN had impressive goals—to provide community psychiatric care, support affected families, decrease hospital admission and readmission rates, prevent new admissions, educate the public and health professionals, raise the profile of mental health, and promote community mental health within the hospital and wider community—it was hampered by limited resources and a vast array of social and economic problems.[83]

In 1997, the St Giles Day Care Centre for therapy and rehabilitation was established.[84] In previous years, similar efforts had come under programs of occupational therapy or work therapy, offering activities that included sewing and craft work, such as making doormats, quilts, and weaving mats, fans, and baskets. Items were sold to the public when "open days" were held at the hospital. Proceeds went into a Patients' Comfort Fund, initiated by Charlie Sachs, which along with donations collected by the Board of Visitors paid for necessities that families might not provide (for example, soap), recreation equipment, excursions, visits to the cinema, social evenings, dances, celebrations, and special feasts. Other therapy schemes operated from the 1960s to early 1990s. *Diwali* is a major festival in Fiji, and in 1980 patients celebrated by lighting candles in colorfully decorated wards, eating sweets, and enjoying a feast before being taken on a bus ride to view the festive lights in Suva. For varying periods, schemes included a craft center, women's workshop, book-bindery, social therapy center, art therapy, and a canteen.[85] The Day Care Centre, which opened in 1997, differed from these former occupational therapy schemes, focusing on discharged patients and encouraging their integration into and employment in the community.

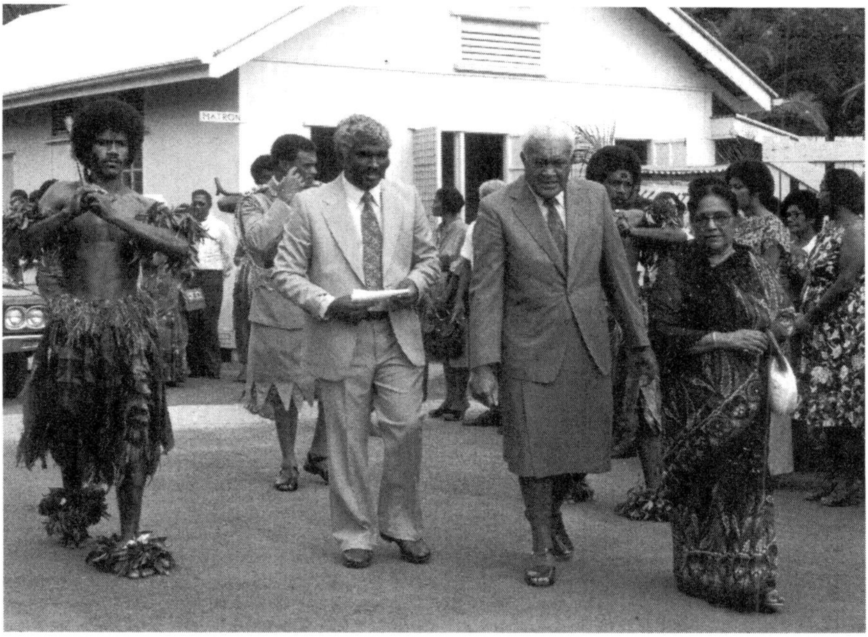

Figure 7.4. Medical Superintendent Dr. Balram Iyer shows Governor General Ratu Sir George Cakobau and Mrs. Grace Deoki, chair, Board of Visitors, around St Giles at the Open Day, 1981. Source: Neg. no. MB5655, NAF.

Change in the New Millennium: Local, Regional, and Global Networks

Local, regional, and global networks helped shape mental health reform and the management of mental illness. As Fiji overhauled its mental health legislation and services in the early twenty-first century; it had to deal with the tensions that arise when managing mental illness, tensions between offering secure confinement, especially for those deemed by society as dangerous and homicidal, humanely treating people with severe mental distress and illness, and protecting patients' rights. In the nineteenth century, colonial "webs" had forged the style of medical management that would take root in Fiji. In the new millennium, global and regional networks shaped the reform of mental health legislation and policies. During both eras, local contingencies were important in determining the management of mental illness—a reiteration of the interface between asylum and community,

It is beyond the scope of this book to provide many details of recent mental health reforms in Fiji.[86] The four key areas tackled were legislation, prevention and treatment of mental disorders, integration of mental health into general health services, and decentralization of mental health care. Although the 1884 Public Lunatic Asylum Ordinance had long been superseded by the Mental Health Act of 1940 and the Mental Treatment Act of 1978, legislation still centered on certification, custody, and treatment in a psychiatric facility.[87] This legislation did not include preventative measures, mental health promotion, rehabilitation, or explicit references to human rights. Nor did it establish any framework for dealing with increasing social and psychological issues in the new millennium, such as "the welfare of vulnerable groups (women, children, elderly, and people with disabilities); natural disaster responses; the mental health consequences of HIV infection and AIDS; and the effects of the use of the newly emerging psychoactive 'recreational' drugs."[88] In 1997, a Technical Working Party on Mental Health was established; it was followed by the National Advisory Council for Mental Health in 1999.[89]

Ohaeri played a leading role in these bodies and the improvement of mental health services, including drafting the St Giles Mental Health Plan for 1998 to 2002. He highlighted mental health issues in academic publications and the media and engaged in proactive public outreach, to improve community relations and tackle the stigma of mental illness.[90] Ohaeri energetically lobbied government and donors for resources, such as new medications, and improved patient and community facilities for the mentally ill. Ohaeri, a Nigerian psychiatrist, advocated a globally informed biomedical approach to psychiatry, but he also sought local solutions and called for further research as a basis for mental health reform.

The presence of the World Health Organization (WHO) in Fiji and in other Pacific nations became more visible in the twenty-first century. In 2003, WHO sponsored a mission to Fiji to discuss a review of mental health legislation with the Fiji Reform Commission. Another review in 2004 examined the Ministry of Health's role in the care, treatment, and rehabilitation of the mentally ill in Fiji.[91] Local initiatives, such as those of psychiatrist Dr. Odille Chang, furthered the development of new mental health legislation, the expansion and decentralization of community care, advanced training for mental health professionals, and awareness campaigns about mental health. Equally important in the groundswell of change were new patient advocacy groups, such as the Psychiatric Survivors' Association, established in 2004, and the Youth Champs for Mental Health, set up in 2007.[92] Suicide prevention was a crucial part of grassroots initiatives, and the National Committee for the Prevention of Suicide was formed in 2003. In 2010, the Fiji Alliance for Mental Health was set up to coordinate research and public awareness concerning mental health.

Despite delays in the implementation of mental health reforms, partly because of another coup in Fiji in 2006, the Fiji Mental Health Decree was implemented in 2010.[93] This measure was far more extensive than previous legislation. For example, it defined behavior that did not constitute a mental disorder, outlined principles for patient treatment and review, and identified objectives, which included the prevention of mental disorders, mental health awareness, and the development of rehabilitative and community psychiatric services. This legislation facilitated the establishment of general hospital psychiatry through the creation of Stress Management Wards in Fiji's main divisional hospitals in Suva, Labasa, and Lautoka. The new discourse of stress aimed to destigmatize any association with madness and was inclusive of mental disorders such as depression, anxiety, and substance abuse, although Stress Management Wards have dealt with severe emergency situations. Nur, who had schizophrenia, was admitted to the Lautoka Stress Management Ward after her neglect in the community was highlighted in the media. Community rehabilitation centers and stress management clinics were also established. The new legislation enabled the creation of a Mental Health Review Board to review inpatient and community treatment orders and appeals against involuntary treatment orders.

Given the recent reforms in Fiji, it is tempting to conclude this study of the colonial extension of the medicalization of madness and mental disabilities on a high note, and to suggest that the barriers between asylum and community have been removed. The reforms are a cumulative result of decades of small incremental changes since independence as part of the progression from earlier "breaking down the walls" of the asylum. By the end of the twentieth century, Fiji was taking a leading role in the Pacific region when WHO invited Fiji to initiate a regional action plan for mental health.[94] In 2009, Fiji was recognized internationally by the Asian Federation of Psychiatric Associations of the World Psychiatric Association with an award of excellence for improving mental health services through training.[95] In 2013, Dr. Neil Sharma, Fiji's minister for health, announced plans, endorsed by other Pacific ministers of health, to open the region's first mental health facility in Suva.[96] The choice of Fiji to lead this regional center is not surprising given Fiji's established role as one of the few Pacific island nations to offer psychiatric care, and Suva is the headquarters of WHO's Western Pacific Regional Office.

This book has discussed the colonization of madness in the context of the entanglement of local cultures with colonial and medical hegemony, so it is appropriate to refer briefly to new global initiatives in mental health that are shaping developments in Fiji today. Mental health reforms in Fiji have taken root during the era of the Global Mental Health (GMH) movement, which aims "to make

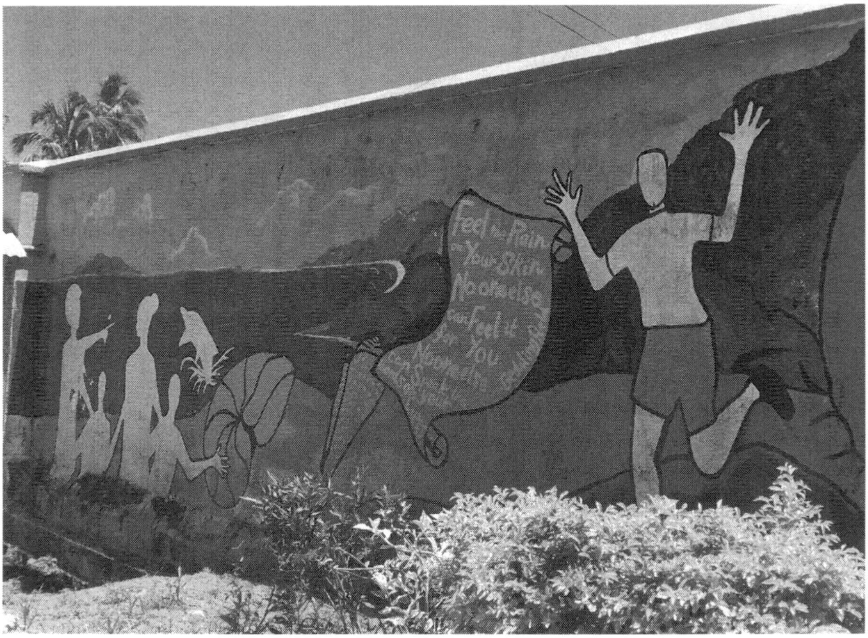

Figure 7.5. New life to St Giles's walls in 2010. Mural (detail) by artist John Mausio, staff, patients and members of Youth Champs for Mental Health. Source: Author.

mental health for all a reality."[97] GMH invokes a moral argument to act and is based on universals—those of human rights but also people's shared biology and common suffering from mental disorders.[98] Professor Vikram Patel emphasizes that GMH is based in global health, not psychiatry.[99] GMH nonetheless aims to "scale up" mental health care through pharmacological and psychosocial interventions using cost-effective evidence-based health practices to reduce the psychiatric "treatment gap" within developing countries and between developed and developing countries.[100]

GMH discourse quickly became engrained in mental health circles in Fiji. In 2009, a press release from the Ministry of Health identified a treatment gap of approximately 90 percent for mental disorders, given that only about 10 percent of adults with a mental illness received treatment.[101] These estimates embrace a much broader definition of mental illness than that discussed in this book or for which the asylum was established. Fiji has also been part of regional (albeit globally driven) initiatives, such as the Pacific Islands Mental Health Network (PIMHnet), which comprises eighteen countries. PIMHnet was established in 2007, the same year the GMH movement took off.

GMH has attracted considerable criticism, and especially pertinent here are assertions that GMH is a form of recolonization, whereby a global model and power structures are said to be imposed on local and indigenous communities. Derek Summerfield equates GMH with medical imperialism, presenting a universalism in which the "colonised were typically spoken for and unable to control the way they were represented."[102] This criticism also places GMH within the expansion of the biomedical model of psychiatry.[103] Summerfield argues that GMH is set against a "Western cultural backdrop" with "a relentless rise in the medicalisation and professionalisation of everyday life," which echoes LiPuma's description of the colonial encompassment of Pacific societies.[104] Beginning in the late nineteenth century, a Western framework of medical services became embedded in Fiji, but this framework met with resistance and had to be adapted locally. Suman Fernando's criticism of GMH referred to the colonial suppression of indigenous understandings of mental health and practices of healing.[105] This colonial pattern applied to Fiji, but, as several examples in this book show, indigenous beliefs about madness and healing persisted.

Fernando also argues that GMH is a neo-imperial form of oppression because it is dominated by powerful agencies, such as WHO, and pharmaceutical corporations promoting Western psychiatric knowledge.[106] As chapter 6 outlines, psychotropic drugs and foreign pharmaceutical interest were already features of psychiatry in Fiji during the later colonial era. Indeed, although policies around deinstitutionalization and discharging patients changed in Fiji, reliance on medication in the management of mental disorders never abated. For several decades in Fiji, Largactil was the mainstay in the treatment of psychiatric conditions. In the 1970s, lithium carbonate was introduced into Fiji for the treatment of bipolar disorder.[107] During the late twentieth century, developments in global pharmacology produced new antipsychotic (such as Olanzapine and Risperidone), antidepressant, and anti-anxiety drugs that did not have the same adverse side effects of earlier medications. So the use of Western medicine by Fijians is hardly new. But, as discussed, although psychotropic drugs enabled shorter periods of hospitalization and allowed people with mental illness to function in the community, patient resistance to medication was considerable, families were not always supportive, and drug supplies were often inconsistent. Some of these problems may be overcome with the recent decentralization of psychiatric services in Fiji, but issues of inadequate funding and resources for mental health services remain. Patients and communities will undoubtedly continue to access a range of healing strategies.

The attack on GMH, on the grounds of its being a form of global hegemony, can sideline local and regional initiatives in the Pacific, even if driven by WHO.

Such initiatives include PIMHnet, set up to advance mental health legislation, policy, and delivery but which has to tackle environmental and economic constraints unique to the environments and cultures of the Pacific Islands. Pacific governments endorsed PIMHnet as a new mental health network, and a regional donor, the New Zealand Aid Programme, provided the first three years of funding.[108] Mental health workers are few on the ground in the Pacific, but some work with both biomedical and Pacific cultural frameworks. For example, Tongan psychiatrist Dr. Mapa Puloka sought to indigenize Western psychiatry and translate it into Tongan concepts, but he did not reject biomedical intervention.[109] GMH may be an expansion of what China Mills calls a psychiatric "creep" across geographical borders, but biomedicine and psychiatry had been transferred to Fiji well before GMH; as chapter 5 outlines, changing psychiatric classifications and diagnoses were played out in the colony. It remains to be seen whether this latest effort to decolonize and decentralize mental illness services in Fiji will enable a more participatory engagement that embraces Fiji's diverse cultures or become another recolonization of mental illness.

Perennial Issues, Care, Control, and Community

The colonization of madness in Fiji centered on sequestering people who were legally certified as insane, diagnosed with a mental illness, and treated as patients until they were discharged or died in the hospital. These cases were real people, people who had lived in communities and were variously loved, accepted, cared for, rejected, teased, or feared. They had sometimes been treated by indigenous healers for varying degrees of mental distress that might be called madness, whether expressed in English or in other languages. From a contemporary vantage point, it is tempting to see St Giles as representing the extension of biomedicine to the colonization of "mad" bodies and minds and as colonial hegemony over difficult or incomprehensible colonial subjects. Yet only a tiny proportion of those who were mentally ill were confined in the asylum, and, until the 1960s, biomedical intervention and psychiatry were applied only to some patients. Warders provided most patient care, and treatment centered on instilling in patients the regular daily regimes described in chapter 6. Embodied practices were as much at the core of restoring normalcy as drugs and coercive or invasive treatments were.

We conclude by returning to Kaisau, because the outcome of his high profile trial raised unresolved questions and dilemmas over mental illness, shown in other examples in this book. One concern has been the state's responsibility for dangerous mentally ill prisoners, which was one of the reasons an asylum was established in Fiji. In both the nineteenth and the early twenty-first centuries, prison officers did not want to take responsibility for mentally ill prisoners, their care and confinement remaining a dilemma in the twenty-first century as it was in the nineteenth. In 2005, Deputy Commissioner of Prisons Opeti Laladidi asserted that "prisoners are not our responsibility when they are being referred to St Giles." Conversely, Medical Superintendent Chang warned, "There is a risk of the prisoners escaping because Saint Giles is a hospital not a prison."[110] Earlier medical superintendents had raised the need for a separate secure facility for patients confined on the governor's orders.

When Kaisau was sent to St Giles, questions concerning its role as a place of incarceration or as a hospital resurfaced. Even before Kaisau became a patient, Shishram Narayan revealed to the court that he had been threatened by Kaisau, that he feared for his safety, and that St Giles was not a unit for the forensically insane.[111] Kaisau briefly escaped from the hospital in November 2001.[112] According to the New Zealand media, he was released two years later, raising alarm over the secure confinement of a mentally ill patient who had admitted to committing two murders.[113] Did the judge's ruling of not guilty by reason of insanity mean that effective treatment could allow Kaisau's readmission into the community? His rehabilitation and therapy included weekend leave to visit his parents, which was queried by Mick Beddoes, leader of the opposition.[114]

In 2015, Kaisau returned to court to challenge the validity of his original sentence under the 1978 Mental Health Act.[115] The 2010 Mental Health Decree was now in place, and the director of the Legal Aid Commission, Sunil Sharma, argued that the presidential committal custody order on the grounds of insanity against Kaisau no longer existed. Judge Temo was concerned about Kaisau's recovery and the safety of his living in the community.[116] Dr. Peni Biukoto pointed out that Kaisau already had access to potentially dangerous implements, such as cane knives and forks, while doing farm work at St Giles, and if he continued to take his medicine, he could be productive in the community.[117] The assistant director of public prosecutions asked Biukoto whether Kaisau had expressed any remorse about his actions; according to Biukoto, Kaisau had not. This response poses the dilemma that though insanity may be diagnosed and treated as a medical illness or disease, society may still expect the recovered individual to take moral responsibility for their actions. These issues are much the same as when Qaqa was sent to the asylum in 1884, though today medication allows mental illness to be managed. Kaisau's lawyer maintained that Kaisau was "cured," and that he would be under family care.[118]

Kaisau's support networks contrast with those of Sujit and Nur and many of the patients discussed in this book, for whom the community had been remiss in the care of those with mental or neurological disorders. As we saw in Sukudaia's narrative, social and broader pressures, such as the dislocation of migration, may have engendered what experts diagnosed as a mental disease or what society called madness. In colonial Fiji, distinctive patterns and practices of framing and treating madness were entangled with universal and colonial psychiatric and lay discourses and practices. In postcolonial Fiji, this legacy was challenged over time. Although recent reforms in mental health legislation, services, and patient rights appear to be breaking with the past, it remains to be seen how these changes will fit with global agendas in mental health, local political and economic pressures, and local conceptions of illness, well being, and healing.

Glossary

bakava	slang term for St Giles; also crazy, silly person
Bose Levu Vakaturaga	Great Council of Chiefs
Brahmin; Brahman	highest Hindu caste; specialist priests or teachers
buli	head of the Fijian administration at the district level
bure	Fijian indigenous house
Dakuwaqa	Fijian snake god
Degei	Fijian ancestral snake god
dharma	duty (Hindi)
dhoti	garment worn by male Hindus, tied around waist and covering the legs
draunikau	spell, curse, witchcraft (Fijian)
filo' raksa'a	"bad head" (Rotuman)
girmit	indenture contract; also Indian indenture experience
girmitiya	Indian indentured laborer
hawa	illness caused by malevolent spirits
i-Taukei	indigenous Fijian(s); "owners of the land"
jahaji bhai, jahaji bhen	Indian men and women who were shipmates
jaurara	half witted, silly, stupid, delirious (Rotuman)
kaci yalo	mental illness (Fijian)
Kailoma	peoples in Fiji of mixed ethnic ancestry
koko	foolish, silly, mad, naughty (Rotuman)
koro	village (Fijian)
Largactil	sedative and antipsychotic medication
lialia	mad, silly, childish, crazy; can be used in jest (Fijian)
luveniwai, kalourere	spirit possession to gain invulnerability in war (Fijian)
manumanuisoni	epilepsy; also *laquiqui* (Fijian)
mangiti	presentation of food (Fijian)
mate ni vakasama	thought illness (Fijian)
mataqali	Fijian landholding and patrilineneal descent group
matiruku	someone periodically insane, usually at low tide (Fijian)
maulvi	Islamic scholar
meke	Fijian dance
narak	hell, referring to the oppressive nature of *girmit*
orjah, ojha	Indian healer
pagaali	mad, crazy woman (Fiji Hindi)

pagalaa	mad, crazy man (Fiji Hindi)
pagla, paagal	crazy, mad (Fiji Hindi)
pandit	Brahmin scholar
puja	prayer (Hindu)
pujari	Hindu temple priest
purdah	seclusion and modesty
ratu	Fijian male chief
roko	provincial head of the Fijian administration
sese	wandering in a physical and mental sense; also term for madness (Fijian)
setan (shaitan)	evil spirit
sirdar (sardar)	plantation overseer; also *sahib*
sulu	cloth worn by Fijians as a skirt
Taukei	indigenous Fijian
tevoro	devil
turaga ni koro	Fijian village headman
vaidya	ayurvedic physician
vakamatei koya vakai koya	suicide; also *rika i savu* (Fijian)
vakarokoroko	deference (Fijian)
vakaturaga	respect within the presence of a person of high status (Fijian)
veidokai	respect for others (Fijian)
veiwasei kei na veikauwaitaki	sharing and caring (Fijian)
vu (kalou)	ancestral spirits or gods (Fijian)
yagona	drink from root of *Piper methysticum*; known as grog, kava
yalo	spirit or soul (Fijian)
vuniwai vakaviti	Fijian healers
yalololoku, yalolailai	depression (Fijian)
yavusa	larger tribal Fijian descent group

Notes

Chapter 1: Introducing the Colonization of Madness into Fiji

1. From Auckland, Murray was serving twelve years in jail for attempting to murder his estranged wife and attempting suicide. *Marlborough Express,* 1883; *Grey River Argus,* 1883. Unless stated, personal information is from admission papers, usually cited as a patient's first admission number (PN), and, if data is available, the hospital register and case notes, all at St Giles Hospital (SG). Some personal information is from CSO files (Fiji National Archives) and the *Blue Book of Fiji* (BB), 1884–1940. Colonies were required to submit annual blue books of statistical and other information to the Colonial Office. The books included a section on lunatic asylums, but also had sections on the colony's finances, population, education, imports and exports, agriculture, land, prisons, hospitals, charitable institutions, banks, transportation, and government employees.

2. Outwards Correspondence of Colonial Secretary (CS), CSO 84/1178.

3. CS to Superintendent of Prisons, CSO 84/888.

4. He was certified insane on August 4, 1884 (PN 6).

5. Scott 2004. Kaisau's case resumes in chapter 7.

6. Judgment, Judge Nazhat Shameem, High Court of Fiji, Criminal case no. HAC0018 of 2002, *State v. Apete Bauleka Vakananumi Kaisau,* August 6, 2003, http://www.paclii.org/cgi-bin/sinodisp/fj/cases/FJHC/2003/197.html.

7. Kate 2015.

8. For histories of Fiji, see Lal 1992; Scarr 1984.

9. People sometimes use the words "mad" and "madness" in derogatory and offensive ways. The application of such discourse is discussed throughout this book. I have retained terms such as "mad," "lunatic," or "imbecile" as used in the original texts. I use the terms "mad" and "madness" not in a negative or offensive way, nor to pass judgment on people or their behavior. The words have sometimes been adopted by people with a psychiatric illness.

10. LiPuma 2000, 24.

11. Kailomas are the descendants of unions between indigenous Fijians, Europeans, Indo-Fijians, and other Pacific peoples. Terminologies included part-Fijian, part-European, half-caste, Euronesian, and mixed race. See de Bruce 2007.

12. PN 1.

13. PN 3.

14. PN 2. Sukudaia is the name on her admission certificate. She is recorded as Sudaia on CSO minute paper (MP) 82/2287 and as Sookdaie on CSO 84/241. Her emigration pass is no. 79 (Department of Immigration 1879–1916).

15. PN 5.

16. Sadowsky 2003.
17. Ibid. 1999, 8; also Scull 2015, 10.
18. Copy of medical journal entry, September 24, 1883, CSO 83/2549.
19. *Fiji Times,* November 29, 1883.
20. Scott 2003.
21. As depicted in TV One's "Saints or Sinners" (2001b) and "Double Lives" (2001a).
22. Mills 2000, 146; Sadowsky 1999, 50.
23. Vaughan 1983, 219; see also Comaroff and Comaroff 1992, 155–178.
24. See, for example, Anderson 2008; Bennett 2006; Buckingham 2011; Buckingham and Luker 2017; Cavert 2016; Denoon 1989; Douglas 1998; Guthrie 1979; Fowler 2000; Hattori 2004; Inglis 2013, 2014; Jolly 1998; Lewis and MacPherson 2008; Lukere 2002; Lukere and Jolly 2002; McLane 2012; Rubinstein 1999; Stuart 2006a, 2006b; Sykes 2016; Widmer 2010.
25. Goddard 1988, 1992, 2011; Leckie 2004a, 2004b, 2005a, 2005b, 2007, 2010, 2012; Leckie and Hughes 2017; Mouchenik 2001–2002; Roberts 2017; Robillard 1987; Rubinstein and White 1983.
26. On colonial asylums and colonial psychiatry, see Bhugra and Littlewood 2001; Ernst and Mueller 2010; Mahone and Vaughan 2007; Minas and Lewis 2017; Porter and Wright 2003. For a comparative essay of British and French colonies, although the Pacific is not discussed, see Keller 2001. On colonial Africa, see Bell 1991; Beuschel 2001; Deacon 1996, 1999; Jackson 1999, 2005; Jackson 2013; Keller 2007; Marks 1999, McCulloch 1995; Parle 2007; Sadowsky 1999; Swartz 1995a, 1995b, 1995c, 2015; Vaughan 1983, 1991, 100–128; on Malta, see Cassar 1995; on India, see Ernst 1991a, 1991b, 1997, 1998, 1999b, 2013; Mills 2000, 2001. Minas and Lewis provide histories of mental health in several countries in Asia. On the Caribbean, see Jones 2008; Smith 2014.
27. See Brookes and Thomson 2001; Coleborne and MacKinnon 2003; for an excellent summary of the literature on colonial psychiatry in Australasia, see Coleborne 2010, 15–42.
28. Brookes 1992, 1994; Coleborne 1997; Garton 1988; Labrum 1992, 1994.
29. Barry and Coleborne 2011; Coleborne 2010, 38.
30. Coleborne 2015; McCarthy 2015; see also Dawson 2013; Labrum 1992, 2005.
31. Tucker 1887, 1492. He was superintendent of Bayview Asylum in New South Wales and surveyed more than four hundred asylums worldwide. See also Cody 1974, 208; Kimmich 1956.
32. Leckie 2010; Mouchenik 2001–2002.
33. For an outline of the development of psychiatric facilities in the Pacific Islands, see Leckie and Hughes 2017.
34. Smith 2014, 49–74.
35. Jones 2008, 71–72; Swartz 2010.
36. Vaughan 1983, 220. Oahu Insane Asylum's first six patients came from the Honolulu jail (Cody 1974, 208).
37. Board of Visitors Annual Report (AR) 1881, CO 83/29.
38. Dispatch 185 to CO, December 30, 1881, CO 83/29.
39. Secretary of State for the Colonies (SS), outward letters, May 11, 1882, CSO 82/849.
40. CSO 84/1178.
41. September 21, 1883, CSO 83/2549. The writer's name is indecipherable.
42. *Feilding Star* 1884.
43. On moral management and moral therapy, see Shorter 1997, 18–22.

44. Superintendent of Prisons, memo, July 17, 1884, CSO 84/1574.

45. Address to the LC, December 28, 1881, CO 83/27.

46. Submitted by MacGregor, December 6, 1883.

47. Lal 2000.

48. Dispatch 122 to CO, October 20, 1883, CO 83/34.

49. *Suva Times* 1881, 1882; see Mishra 2012.

50. To CS, February 20, 1882, CSO MP 82/568.

51. Acting Agent General Immigration to CS, April 4, 1882, CSO MP 82/568.

52. Extract, prison medical journal, July 4, 1884, CSO 84/1340.

53. April 9, 1883, CSO 83/968. Allen returned to New Zealand as an elderly destitute "in his second childhood," "not fit to take charge of himself" (*North Otago Times* 1883).

54. Joyce 1971, 39–65.

55. CSO MP 82/568; dispatch 122 to CO, October 20, 1883, CO 83/34.

56. Corney, Acting CMO, to Administrator, "Prisoner Labour," February 28, 1885, CSO 85/598; Corney to CS, "Move to New Asylum Site: Additional Pay Requested for Staff," April 15, 1885, CSO 85/1047.

57. Joyce 1971, 25. On NMPs, see Guthrie 1979; Hoodless 1947; Montague 1930. In 1928, the school became the Central Medical School. The term NMP was replaced by AMP (assistant medical practitioner) in 1951, AMO (assistant medical officer) in 1956, and MO (medical officer) in 1964.

58. On early Scottish psychiatry, see Davis 2008, 43–82; Halliday 2003; Walmsley 1991.

59. Ballantyne 2012, 24–47.

60. *Fiji Royal Gazette*, "An Ordinance to Provide for the Care and Maintenance of Lunatics and Idiots," March 1884. A lunacy ordinance based on 1838 French colonial law was introduced in Tahiti on December 28, 1885 (Berne 1960).

61. PN 100. Michael is a pseudonym. Because of Fiji's small population, pseudonyms are used unless referring to individuals in the public domain. Throughout the colonial period, Indians and other indentured laborers, and to a lesser extent Fijians, often had only one name recorded on admission certificates, in contrast to Europeans and Kailomas, who usually had a full name recorded. Complete names for Fijians were usually recorded after World War II. Indo-Fijians who were not *girmitiyas* usually had full names recorded.

62. Sue Heydon, personal communication.

63. Brunton 2001; Lewis 1988, 1–31; Melling 1999; McCarthy 2015, 21–34.

64. Scull 2006, 115; on British colonial asylums in the Caribbean, see Smith 2014, 173–174.

65. Vaughan 1991, 8; Swartz 2010, 161.

66. Cohn 1987, 136–71.

67. Suzuki 1999, 116–117.

68. Coleborne 2015, 2, 84–113, 139–163; 1997, 48, 57–80.

69. On the few records found for pauper lunatics in nineteenth-century Britain and Ireland, see Bartlett 1999.

70. "An Ordinance to Provide for the Care and Maintenance of Lunatics and Idiots," CP (Council Paper) 28/36; "Public Lunatic Asylum (Management) Regulations 1928," MP 28/2614.

71. I refer to these as Case Books (CB) but they are not detailed individual cases. Those I located at St Giles, dated intermittently from December 2, 1903, to 1953.

72. Lipphardt and Widmer 2016, 3.

73. Smith 2014, 127 referring to Mills 2000, 67–68.

74. See Ballantyne 2012; on transcolonial history, see Ghosh and Kennedy 2006.

75. *Fiji Royal Gazette*, "To Amend Ordinance No. III of 1884 Instituted an Ordinance to Provide for the Care and Maintenance of Lunatics and Idiots," January 1885.

76. Ernst 1999a, 82–87. The Natal Government Asylum, which opened in 1880, accommodated Africans, Indians, and Europeans (see Parle 2007, 4–5).

77. Angela McCarthy argues that Catharine Coleborne and I each elided over the ethnicity of European patients (2015, 171). Birthplace was occasionally noted but the ethnic categories of Europeans were not usually evident in the records I consulted. It would be more relevant to analyse the tribal affiliation of i-Taukei and the regional background of Indian migrants, but such details were rarely recorded in the asylum papers.

78. Foucault 1965; see also Porter 2003, 1–5; Scull 1989, 2006.

79. Fanon 1952.

80. Coleborne 2001, 106; see also Mahone and Vaughan 2007; for a critical review of this debate, see Ernst 2007.

81. Porter 1987, 235

82. Vaughan 1991, 8.

83. Jackson 2005, 188.

84. Goddard 1992, 55; 2011,15–40.

85. Mills 2000, 147.

86. Keller 2007, 89; Smith 2014, 152.

87. Sadowsky 1999, viii.

88. Finnane 2003, 24; see also Finnane 1985, Suzuki 2006.

89. Wright 1997, 139.

90. See Coleborne 2010; McCarthy 2015. On other colonies that stress the community, see Edington 2013; Parle 2014; Swartz 2015.

91. Ernst 1999a, 95; 2007, 509.

92. Ibid. 1991a, 159.

93. Harper to CS, August 19, 1927, CSO 27/3359.

94. Marks 1999, 270; Vaughan 1991, 120.

95. See Mahone and Vaughan 2007, 14; Sadowsky 1999, 115.

96. "Messy entanglements" is from Quanchi and Talu 1995; see also Crick 1997.

97. Jolly 1998; Thomas 1990.

98. See, for example, Jackson 2005,188; Smith 2014; McCulloch 1995, 44; Parle 2007, 17; Sadowsky 1999; Vaughan 1991,101.

99. Melling and Forsythe 2006, 2.

100. LiPuma 2000, 6. Warwick Anderson discusses how colonial medicine was entangled, appropriated, or ignored in the local context (2004, 294–295).

101. *Fiji Royal Gazette*, "Report of BOV for Year 1896," 1897.

102. In 1891, Europeans made up 1.7 percent of the total population (Fiji Bureau of Statistics 2012).

103. Ibid.

104. Fiji Government 1916, 12; 1961, 23.

105. Karim 1996.

106. On Samoans in Fiji, see Tuimaleali'ifano 1990.

107. Fiji Government 1884–1940, 7.

108. "Head Attendant (Anderson) Public Lunatic Asylum to Medical Superintendent: Sanitary Arrangements at the Asylum," CSO 27/2216.

109. August 19, 1927, CSO 27/3359.

110. Data on the certificates was in notes. I usually retain the original shorthand and grammar in quotations.

111. For example, in 1902 there was confusion over the name of PN 185: her name appeared differently on her indentured emigration pass, police records, and admission papers. The MS wrote that "inaccuracies of name frequently occur." The patient was also recorded as having a single marital status, but in 1903 the CMO ordered her to be discharged to her husband.

112. Today the terms "Indo-Fijians," "Fiji Indians," or "Fijian Indians" are used by people of Indian descent in Fiji. "Indians" is still widely used and was common in the colonial period, but in this book I mostly use "Indo-Fijian."

113. Rotumans are Polynesian but are indigenous to Fiji because Rotuma was incorporated into the state in 1881. Usually, when indigenous Fijians are referred to in this book, the reference includes Rotumans (especially in statistics), whereas i-Taukei are ethnic Fijians who are predominantly Melanesian.

114. Between 1865 and 1911, contracts for Pacific Islanders totaled 27,027. This figure includes workers who reengaged (see Munro 1990, xlviii). Between 1884 and 1916, approximately twenty-nine patients in the asylum were Pacific laborers from outside Fiji.

115. Guthrie 1979, 34. Margaret Guthrie was the daughter of the medical superintendent David Hoodless. See also "Mental Hospital—Reports and Recommendations by the Board of Visitors," F48/10/pt 1; MS to Deputy MS, December 16, 1935, F82/1/8.

116. See, for example, Lewa 2002. I use the names asylum, mental hospital, the hospital, and St Giles throughout this book. These terms are usually aligned with the historical context in which they were used, but St Giles can refer to the hospital before the name was officially adopted.

117. See LiPuma 2000.

Chapter 2: Displaced Minds

1. April 21, 1886, CSO MP 86/84.

2. Parts of this chapter were originally published in *Migration, Ethnicity and Mental Health: International Perspectives, 1840–2010,* edited by Anglea McCarthy and Catharine Coleborne (see Leckie 2012; McCarthy and Coleborne 2012b).

3. Cited in Lal 2000, 162; for a revision of MacGregor's role in the *Syria* rescue, see Chand 2017.

4. From PN 1270.

5. Lal 2000, 143–151.

6. CSO 84/241.

7. Emigration pass no. 87. Where possible, emigration passes of insane *girmitiyas* were checked, but numbers are not cited unless publicly known.

8. Department of Immigration 1879–1916.

9. CSO 84/241.

10. *Suva Times,* October 29, 1881, 2.

11. Ibid., November 5, 1881, 2.

12. CSO MP 82/568.
13. Gillion 1962, 190–197. Families were supposed to accompany rejected *girmitiyas* to India.
14. PN 580.
15. Angela McCarthy and Catharine Coleborne consider whether the ease with which migrants adjusted overseas was the result of prior experiences or the new environment (2012a; see also Coleborne 2015; McCarthy 2015).
16. Gillion 1962, 82–90; Naidu 1980; for a *girmitiya*'s account, see Sanadhya 1992.
17. Gillion 1962, 29–36; Lal 1983, 28–33.
18. See Lal 1998, 49–94. The surgeon superintendent was responsible for the welfare of *girmitiyas* on the ship (see Gillion 1962, 60–63).
19. PN 70.
20. PN 38.
21. Laing 1889, cited in Lal 1998, 39.
22. PN 152.
23. PN 72.
24. PN 286.
25. PN 71.
26. PN 161.
27. PN 391.
28. During the first fifteen years of the twentieth century, Indo-Fijian suicide rates were the highest among all Indian labor-importing colonies in Africa and the West Indies and much higher than in India: 0.780 per thousand in 1900 and 0.831 per thousand in 1910 (Lal 2000, 216).
29. PN 429; PN 720.
30. Andrews and Pearson 1916; Garnham 1918.
31. Lal 1985, 136.
32. CP 28/1910.
33. Lal 1985, 137. In 1912, for every forty-three Indian females were one hundred males.
34. CP 21/1908.
35. Parle 2009, 156–177.
36. Lal 1985, 138.
37. Lal 1985, 154–155.
38. Lal 1985, 148.
39. May 23, 1905, CSO MP 05/2281.
40. Lal 1985, 150–151.
41. Magisterial enquiry into cause of death of Manesa no. 6750, CSO MP 90/1346.
42. Lal 1985, 146.
43. A. R. Coates, Agent-General of Immigration, CP 21/1905; CP 21/1908.
44. SM, Lautoka, CSO 10/8542.
45. Coates, CP 48/1912.
46. Lal 1985, 152–153.
47. Coates, CP 21/1905.
48. See, for example, Wells and Joseph 1993, 273–275, 293. Kay Saunders qualifies suicide as the "effects of defeat" rather than of agency (1979, 181).
49. Lal 1985, 155.

50. SM Rewa to CS, May 12, 1889, CSO MP 90/1346.
51. CP 39/1916; MP 4098/1916. Reg. no. 58557.
52. CP 39/1916; MP 4098/1916. Reg. no. 43264.
53. Coates, CP 48/12.
54. PN 444.
55. PN 316.
56. PN 104.
57. PN 513.
58. PN 332, accused of malingering, spent twenty-six years in the asylum.
59. CSO 85/2886.
60. PN 27.
61. CSO 89/940.
62. PN 51.
63. CSO MP 16/1045.
64. CSO MP 09/8312.
65. PN 570.
66. PN 37.
67. Noted by Coleborne 2010, 47–51.
68. PN 680.
69. PN 249.
70. PN 113.
71. These figures include repeat admissions.
72. *Auckland Star* 1915.
73. Gillion 1962, 106.
74. See Lal 1992.
75. Gillion 1962, 142.
76. PN 553.
77. PN 555.
78. PN 585. In Fiji, bush could mean a heavily forested tropical rainforest.
79. Lynette Jackson uses the term "surfacing up" for when African pre-patients came to the attention of the state in colonial Southern Rhodesia (2005).
80. Fiji Indian Indenture Ordinance no 1. of 1891 (reproduced in Lal 1998, 49–94; for tickets of leave, see 72–74).
81. PN 246.
82. PN 248.
83. PN 186.
84. PN 151; CSO MP 99/5057.
85. MP 3409/1901, cited in PN 817.
86. Gillion 1962, 190–197.
87. CSO 97/5066. Reg. no. 6295. Musai arrived in 1886 on the *Bruce*.
88. PN 1041; BB 1934.
89. PN 1387.
90. See Jinna and Mangubhai 2008.
91. PN 1312.
92. PN 1530.
93. PN 1520.

94. PN 503. His father was Daleepa, PN 316.

95. PN 589; PN 671. Although called orphans, some children at Dilkusha had parents who were still alive. Dilkusha was established in 1906 by Reverend John Burton of the Indian (Methodist) Mission in Fiji (Newman 2018).

96. PN 1318.

97. MS, Mental Hospital to DMS, AR 1938, January 14, 1939, F48/4/5.

98. See Hare 1998, 131–132. This disease was once associated with psychiatric institutions when patients refused to eat.

99. Verified by Pearce in 1935, cited in Ross 1950, 921; PN 445; PN 493; PN 533; PN 671.

100. PN 1361.

101. Susan Heydon, personal communication.

102. Analysis of BB, 1884–1940 and patient admission papers.

103. BB, 1884–1940; Duncan 2000, 292. Fijians also died from phthisis (for example, PN 295, PN 324, PN 460).

104. PN 889.

105. Fowler 2000.

106. *Girmitiya* patients included two who died from hookworm infection, PN 363 and PN 388.

107. Buchanan et al. 1979, 369–376.

108. Sethi, Robilotti, and Sadan 2004.

109. Gillion 1962, 107.

110. F. E. Montague, MS, PLA to DMS, AR 1932, F48/4/5; see Lambert 1946.

111. Wilson 1921, 10.

112. PN 683.

113. PN 496.

114. Gillion 1962 130–135; Jinna and Mangubhai 2008.

115. PN 394; CSO MP 15/759; CSO MP 15/6370.

116. For Indo-Fijians after indenture, see Gillion 1977; Ali 1980; Kelly 1991; Jayawardena 1975a, 1975b; Mayer 1973.

117. As asylums became established, the number of chronic long-stay patients rose (Busfield 1986, 263–265).

118. No. 18600.

119. PN 244.

120. PN 513; death inquiry, F48/28/16.

121. But see Gill 2010; Singh 1986, 57–88.

122. Gill 2010, 136, 395.

123. Thanks to Jan Tent for providing these Fiji Hindi terms. *Paagalkhaanaa* refers to an insane asylum.

124. See also Mayer 1973, 84–86. His original fieldwork was in 1951.

125. Gill 2010, 136.

126. See, for example, Fabrega 2009; Kakar 1982.

127. PN 509; PN 536.

128. PN 409.

129. PN 1636. *Shaitan* is usually associated with Muslim beliefs. The word may have been a misinterpretation of *setan*, which means “evil wind.”

130. See chapter 3.

131. PN 1195. The original note-taker could have mistakenly written "devils" as *devis* (goddesses).

132. On the diversity of ritual healing in contemporary India, see Sax 2014, 829–849.

133. Sanadhya 1998, 106.

134. Gill 2010, 75–78, 100–106.

135. Narayan 1974.

136. Gill 2010, 77, 111–112, 112, 115–117; see also Price and Karim 1975; Haynes 1987.

137. Narayan 1974; see also Singh 1986. A short sacred text was washed in water to dissolve the ink into the water, to convey the text's power. This water was drunk as part of a healing ritual. William Sweetman, personal communication.

138. Gill 2010, 77–78.

139. Narayan 1975, 275–276.

140. Quotations on Qawa from Randall 1969, 4–5; other details from Sell to DMS, November 25, 1968, St Giles Hospital file (STG) 1/5; Leckie 2004b; Parke 1995.

141. Largactil was a powerful sedative and antipsychotic medication (see chapter 6).

142. This test was used to identify suggestibility and the so-called female hysteric personality (see Moss and McEvedy 1966). In its November 1996 issue on epidemic hysteria, the *British Medical Journal* had a remarkably similar discourse to Sell and Randall's accounts, suggesting that the Fiji doctors probably read this issue.

143. PN 1651.

144. PN 1260; PN 1291.

145. PN 1542.

146. PN 2687.

147. PN 1767.

148. PN 1926.

149. The same was true of indentured workers in Natal and Zululand (Parle 2009, 159).

150. Macgregor 1967, 4–5.

151. Haynes 1984, 1987; Morris and Maniam 2000; Karim and Price 1973; Price and Karim 1976; Ree 1971.

Chapter 3: Lialia? Indigenous Fijians, Community, and "Madness"

1. Brewster 1922, 126–129. Joske later changed his name and published his memoirs as Brewster.

2. See Nicole 2011, 45–69; Kaplan 1995.

3. PN 13; CSO 85/988.

4. Brewster 1922, 127, 128–129, 128.

5. CSO 85/988.

6. CSO 90/530.

7. PN 47.

8. Thomas 1997, 58–60.

9. See, for example, Coleborne 2010, 65–87; Parle 2007, 165–202; Smith 2014, 126–152; Swartz 2015, 89–115; Wright 1998.

10. Hazlewood 1872, 67; Capell 1941, 120. Hazlewood's 1855 Fijian-English dictionary was based on missionary accounts and later edited by James Calvert. It was revised by Capell, who gave prominence to the Bauan dialect and excluded many words from Fijian dialects.

11. Gatty 2010, 138, 42.

12. Citing Jean-Marie Neyret's 1935 Fijian-English and English-Fijian dictionary (typescript in NAF), Price and Karim 1978, 228; Capell 1941, 143.

13. Gatty 2010, 319.

14. Capell 1941, 143.

15. Hazlewood 1872, 199.

16. PN 119.

17. Hazlewood 1872, 80.

18. Churchward 1940, cited in Rensel and Howard 1997, 23.

19. Capell 1941, 173.

20. Gatty 2010, 165.

21. Resolution no. 13, Council of Chiefs, Lomaloma, May 19, 1892, CSO 93/2659. Penalties proposed were up to six months' imprisonment plus being whipped; see also J. K. M. Ross, Acting Resident Commissioner, "Evidence in a Death Enquiry," CSO 82/2925; SM Savusavu to Assistant CS, September 5, 1892, CSO 92/3080; minute paper [writer's name indecipherable], "Inquiry into the Death of Mere," August 24, 1894, CSO 94/3128.

22. Hazlewood 1872, 59.

23. See Weaver 2009.

24. See, for example, Brewster 1922; Thomson 1908; Williams 1982. Ronald Derrick stated that sickness and insanity were the work of malignant spirits (1950, 15).

25. Native Regulation no. 5 of 1887 in regard to Luveniwai, Kalourere and Other Similar Practices. See Brewster 1922, 236–248; Kaplan 1989, 349–371; Kasuga 1994, 43–44; Marzan 1987, 37–47. *Luveniwai* and *kalourere* were originally forms of spirit possession and rituals to gain invulnerability in war, and after being banned they became forms of resistance (see Nicole 2011, 134–140).

26. Kasuga provides extensive historical and ethnographical references to *draunikau* (1994; see also Roth 1935, 1953, 39–40; Spencer 1941, 34–45; Thompson 1940, 130; Vakatawa 1940).

27. PN 2690.

28. Gluckman 1969. He wrote a thesis on *makutu* or witchcraft among Māori.

29. Thompson 1940, 125.

30. Spencer 1941, 68; see also Vakatawa 1940, 522.

31. Becker 1995, 104; see also Harthorn 2005; Katz 1999.

32. Narayan 1974.

33. PN 659; PN 663.

34. PN 1558.

35. See Lukere 1997.

36. *Cyclopaedia of Fiji* 1984, 47.

37. Attempts to ban native healing were common in many colonies. On the suppression of Māori healing, see Dow 2001.

38. Lukere 2002, 11; Narayan 1974.

39. Quain 1948, 69–70; Spencer 1941.

40. Ravuvu 1988, 34.

41. PN 1550.

42. See Katz 1999; Sahlins 1962, 358–359; Spiegel 1983; Thompson 1940, 124–131; for Rotuma, see Howard 1979.

43. Kasuga 1994, 42, referring to Toren 1990, 104–107.

44. Thompson 1940, 126–127.

45. An exception to the lack of research on the relationship between mental disorders and women's role in traditional medicine is Barbara Herr Harthorn's in Lau on anxiety and depression (2005).
46. On women's traditional roles in Fijian medicine, see Lukere 1997, 159–164.
47. Thompson 1940, 126.
48. PN 135.
49. PN 1136.
50. PN 1138.
51. PN 1511.
52. PN 1138.
53. Harper 1916, 678–679; see also chapter 5.
54. Lukere 1997, 158; see also Inglis 2014.
55. See, for example, Vakaruru 1937.
56. Berne 1959b, 312; see also 1959a.
57. Ravuvu 1987, 18. Anne Becker refers to *vikawaitaki, viqwaravi,* and *vilomani* and the enactment of care as a core Fijian value (1995, 75–78).
58. See, for example, Belshaw 1964, 123–125; Quain 1948; Sahlins 1962, 266; Spate 1959; Toren 1990.
59. Bayliss-Smith et al. 1988, 63–65.
60. CS to DMS, July 26, 1939, CSO F48/175.
61. PN 42; CSO MP 89/982.
62. PN 908.
63. PN 61.
64. Fiji Government 1912, 13.
65. PN 413; PN 427; PN 428.
66. PN 879.
67. For example, PN 1542; PN 1767.
68. PN 67; SM Lau to CS, September 29, 1891, CSO 91/3044.
69. PN 233.
70. H. C. Monckton, September 17, 1939, CSO F50/6, cited in Macnaught 1982, 70.
71. PN 142.
72. PN 80.
73. PN 682.
74. PN 529.
75. Brewster 1922, 129. Joske was referring to Nacoulauli.
76. Under native regulations, Fijians required their chiefs' permission to be absent from their village for longer than sixty days, but after 1912 absenteeism was no longer an offence for men (Macnaught 1982, 101–102).
77. Nayacakalou, 1963; see also Griffin and Monsell-Davis 1986.
78. CSO 96/317 on PN 112. *Na Mata* was a Fijian language newspaper.
79. Peck 1963. Fiji's first telephone line was laid in 1904 between Suva and Levuka. Lines in Fiji were quite difficult to maintain. Radio-telephone became available in many parts of Fiji after World War II, which made medical communications easier.
80. Reference to man named Taniela who committed assault on a Polynesian and Sergeant of Police, April 8, 1895, CSO 95/1448; assault committed by Taniela mad Tongan on 7th inst., April 9, 1895, CSO 95/1465.

81. Epileptiform resembles epilepsy. PN 103.

82. PN 741.

83. Quain 1948, 69–70.

84. Lukere 2002, 112–113. See *The Native Medical Practitioner*, published 1930–1940 by the Central Medical School.

85. Roth 1935.

86. Vakatawa 1940, 524.

87. Scull 1993, 13.

88. Roth 1953, 145–149.

89. Ravuvu 1987, 18.

90. Ravuvu 1983, 104–105, 109–110.

91. Michael Goddard found that the Kaugel people accepted crazy behavior but not when it was violent or when social obligations were ignored (1998, 63; see also Rensel and Howard 1997, 28).

92. PN 212.

93. PN 1928; PN 3027.

94. PN 64.

95. PN 520.

96. PN 282.

97. PN 1326.

98. For example, on nudity, Ravuvu 1983, 111; see also Toren 1999, 132–139.

99. PN 230.

100. PN 1122; PN 1198.

101. PN 454.

102. PN 324.

103. In some colonial documents, the term "town" was used for village.

104. PN 44.

105. Spiegel 1983, 29.

106. Hazlewood 1872, 220.

107. PN 146.

108. PN 1682.

109. PN 1218.

110. On the maintenance of spatial (and social) order under the colonial administration, see Macnaught 1982, 104–105.

111. Kaplan 1990, 12.

112. Sahlins 1962, 440–441, 127. It is not clear whether this man had a mental disability or the term *lialia* was conflated with laziness.

113. See Rensel and Howard 1997, 31, 26–27; see also Noricks 1981.

114. PN 710.

115. Bartlett and Wright 1999, 9–10.

116. PN 386; PN 387.

117. PN 824.

118. This is a reference to Sailosi Ratu (Brewster 1922, 253).

119. CSO 83/43.

120. Nayacakalou 1975, 92, referring to the 1950s.

121. PN 148; CSO 18/63; Brewster 1922, 253–254; Thomas 1997, 52–56.

122. Brewster 1922, 253. Queen Victoria died in 1901.

123. Joske, SM Colo North and East to CMO, February 20, 1899, CSO 99/919.

124. June 6, 1899, CSO 99/919.

125. Adolf Brewster states that Sailosi was in the asylum for twelve years, but the asylum records show no evidence of this (1922, 253–254).

126. Nicole 2011, 79–97.

127. "Sailosi Confined to Lunatic Asylum," April 15, 1918, CSO 18/63.

128. CSO 18/63. A note on the document said that Tola men take in the produce for Suva.

129. Brown to CS, "Comments on Movement Organised by Sailosi," April 12, 1918, CSO 18/44.

130. April 12, 1918, CSO 18/44.

131. March 30, 1918, CSO 18/33.

132. Martha Kaplan and John Kelly discuss disaffection law (1994, 124–125).

133. Barwick to CS, April 20, 1918, CSO 18/63.

134. PN 530.

135. April 15, 1918, CSO 18/44.

136. Brewster 1922, 254.

137. Filariasis is an infection caused by roundworms and transmitted by infected mosquitos. It can lead to elephantiasis, lymphoedema, and hydrocele.

138. Acting Provincial Commissioner, Colo East to Secretary for Native Affairs, "Seventh-day Adventist Religion—Villages of Naraiyawa and Wainimakutu in Namosi Province Adopting," September 2, 1919, C39/1919.

139. PN 997; PN 1092; CSO F48/61/7. On the conflict associated with Ravoka and Verata, see Macnaught 1982, 71–74.

140. Cited in Macnaught 1982, 72.

141. To DMS, May 18, 1936, CSO F48/61/7.

142. Memo in CB, December 16, 1935.

143. May 28, 1936, CSO F48/61/7.

144. CSO F48/61/7. Robert Nicole sees Ratu Peni's arrangement as exile (2006, 249n113).

145. Native Commissioner (NC) and Inspector General of Police to CS, "Conduct of One Pita and his Followers at Nadroga," August 21, 1913, CSO MP 13/6052.

146. CSO MP 13/3317.

147. Maurice Brown cited seventy to eighty Fijians, but newspaper reports suggested twenty-six (*Brisbane Courier* 1913).

148. *Cumberland Argus and Fruitgrowers Advocate,* 1913. This report in a Parramatta newspaper exaggerated Maurice's account and named Oscar as Colin.

149. To CS, July 10, 1913, CSO MP 13/6052.

150. NC and IGP to CS, August 21, 1913, CSO MP 13/6052.

151. September 3, 1913, CSO MD 13/2735.

152. NC and IGP to CS, August 21, 1913, CSO MP 13/6052.

153. Garrett 1973, 58; 1997, 240.

154. Ibid. 1973, 59.

155. PN 1506.

156. Snow 1997, 247–248.

157. DMS to CS, September 14, 1951, on PN 1506.

158. Memo to MS, February 18, 1947.

159. Chairman BOV to CS, March 6, 1947, F48/10, part 1. The chairman was also the AG.

160. Snow 1997, 248.

161. See Garrett 1973, 59.

162. Snow 1997, 248.

163. Nayacakalou 1975, 88.

164. Alan Tippett, "Report on the Activities of Ratu Emosi of Daku, at the Church Gathering Held at Nasautoka, Wainibuka, during the Week of July 1955," cited in Garrett 1997, 241.

165. PN 1984.

166. See Mills 2000, 146; Porter 1987, 231; Sadowsky 1999, 50.

167. PN 112.

168. PN 223; PN 275.

169. Murphy and Narayan 1979, 4–11.

170. Macgregor 1967, 4.

171. On changes for Fijians during the war and afterward, see Belshaw 1964, 270–280; Macnaught 1982, 148–164; Spate 1959.

172. Bayliss-Smith et al. 1988, 79; Griffin and Monsell-Davis 1986; Nayacakalou, 1963.

173. For the impact of changes on the periphery during the late colonial years, see Bayliss-Smith et al. 1988, 76–80.

174. Fiji Government 1969, 9.

Chapter 4: Mad Woman

1. See Lal 2000, 143–151.

2. CSO 84/241; quotes for Sukudaia are from PN 2. Ozeeari's emigration pass is no. 406. Department of Immigration 1879–1916.

3. There was confusion over Janki's gender. CSO MP 82/2287 states that Janki was a woman. Janki is usually a woman's name. PN 3, also called Janki, was recorded as a male in the asylum.

4. *Suva Times,* November 5, 1881, 2.

5. PN 2158.

6. Sections of this chapter were previously published based on conference papers (Leckie 2000, 2002a, 2003, 2005b, 2007). I am grateful to feedback from Michèle Dominy, Jean Mitchell, and Jeanette Mageo, who initially urged me to consider how madness was embodied through gender. This analysis was also informed by Catharine Coleborne (1997, 53–57).

7. See, for example, Laing 1960; Szasz 1961.

8. Tomes 1994, 354; see also Chesler 1972.

9. Showalter 1985.

10. Busfield 1988, 536; Russell 1995.

11. On revisions, see Busfield 1996; Marland 2004; Tomes 1990, 1994; Wright 2004; see also Coleborne 2007, 2010, 2014; Coleborne and MacKinnon 2003; Ernst 1996; Jackson 2005; Labrum 1992, 2005; Leckie 2005, 2007; Parle 2007; Swartz 1999.

12. Coleborne 2014, 470.

13. CB, December 23, 1904. The month is unclear.

14. To DMS, September 1, 1936, CF 48/5.

15. Compare Coleborne 2007, Gittins 1998.

16. Meeting, BOV, September 27, 1892, CSO 92/2961.

17. CMO to CS, September 6, 1892, CSO 92/2961.
18. CSO 14/8621.
19. CSO 15/3916.
20. PN 1050.
21. *Fiji Royal Gazette* 1907.
22. CSO MP 09/9771.
23. BOV Report, 1914, CSO MP 14/8621.
24. CSO 14/6232.
25. BOV Report, 1914, CSO MP 14/8621.
26. Acting MS to CMO, October 27, 1914, CSO MP 14/8621.
27. BB, 1885.
28. Fiji Government 1884–1940. Daily rates for first-class patients were ten shillings for the first three months then six shillings eightpence, and for second-class patients two shillings for the first three months then one shilling sixpence. The 1913 *Blue Book* allocated rations under the categories of Europeans and natives.
29. CSO MP 14/8621.
30. MS to DMS, January 14, AR 1939, F48/4/5.
31. Coleborne 1997, 57; 2007, 112–113.
32. CW to CMO, reports, August 1896.
33. CB, March 1, 1952; Public Lunatic Asylum, April 3, 1914, CP 15/1914.
34. Brookes 1998; Coleborne 2014; Ernst 1996; Labrum 1992, 127–128; Swartz 1999. Wright 2004 found that women were not confined disproportionately to men during the Victorian era in Buckinghamshire.
35. These patterns were from my database, compiled from admission papers, BB, and the Mental Hospital Register, where patient outcomes are known within a five-year band of admission dates.
36. PN 174. The pills were hyped as "a remedy for many female ailments" (*Kansapedia*, "Pink Pills for Pale People," Kansas Historical Society, July 2002, accessed July 26, 2014, https://www.kshs.org/kansapedia/pink-pills-for-pale-people/10240).
37. PN 891.
38. On hysteria among young Indo-Fijian women, see Leckie 2004b.
39. PN 1809.
40. PN 2333.
41. Tomes 1990, 145.
42. See also Coleborne 2010; Wright 2004.
43. Garton 1988, 140.
44. PN 102.
45. PN 785; PN 894.
46. See Hare 1998.
47. PN 18.
48. PN 1113.
49. See chapter 5.
50. Compare Coleborne 2015, 153–154; Ernst 1996, 362.
51. PN 875.
52. PN 900.
53. PN 75.

54. PN 177. Between 1876 and 1911, only 3.2 percent of Solomon Island recruits to Fiji were women (Siegel 1985, 54).
55. See, for example, Coleborne 1997, 47–68.
56. PN 74. On the history of gender, class, and psychiatry, see Andrews and Digby 2004.
57. PN 1383.
58. PN 1546.
59. PN 811, testimony from DC Taveuni and patient's employer.
60. PN 613.
61. Nabobo-Baba 2006, 27.
62. PN 436.
63. PN 522.
64. PN 217.
65. PN 166. The sisters' brother was also an asylum patient (PN 219). Their mother became a resident of Cottage House in Suva, as Anne later did when Emily was in the asylum. Cottage House was a private institution for elderly Europeans.
66. PN 1392.
67. PN 3110.
68. PN 86.
69. PN 1633.
70. PN 119. A *meke* is a Fijian song and dance.
71. PN 891.
72. McClintock 1995; Stoler 1991, 1995, 1997.
73. PN 217.
74. PN 242.
75. PN 256.
76. Levine 2003, 183–184, 188–191.
77. "Volubility" can refer to being highly articulate, but in medical discourse it was considered a sign of mania. A similar term in St Giles records is "loquacious."
78. PN 185.
79. PN 52.
80. PN 145.
81. Lal 1992, 66, referring to CP 52/1923 and CP 50/1926.
82. PN 128.
83. Leckie 2002b.
84. Aucoin 1990, 23–42.
85. Lukere 2005, 369.
86. See Lateef 1990, 44–48; Kelly 1991, 236–237.
87. Sue Carswell, personal communication, August 1997.
88. PN 1265; PN 1373.
89. PN 566.
90. PN 1804.
91. PN 30. Thanks to Catharine Coleborne for copies of Eliza's records in New Zealand.
92. Jackson 2005, 92–128.
93. PN 241.
94. PN 367.
95. Sanadhya 1992, 44–45.

96. PN 636.
97. PN 1286.
98. Garton 1988,145.
99. Confidential file, SG.
100. "Evidence in a Death Enquiry," CSO 82/2925.
101. SM, Savusavu, to Assistant CS, September 5, 1892, CSO 92/3080.
102. "Inquiry into the Death of Mere," August 24, 1894, CSO MP 94/3128.
103. Tomes 1990, 152–153, referring to madness.
104. Jaworski 2014, 102.
105. "Inquiry into death of Fijian female prisoner," CSO 90/1275.
106. See Aghanwa 2004b, 63–69; Hawton 2000, 484–485; Jaworski 2014.
107. PN 55.
108. Insufficient data makes it difficult to plot earlier suicide trends in Fiji (see Booth 1999; Haynes 1984; Morris and Maniam 2000, 46–48).
109. Haynes 1987, 25.
110. Karim and Price 1973; Price and Karim 1975.
111. Ree 1971.
112. Regional Inspector of Immigrants Lautoka to Agent-General of Immigration, February 1, 1909, CSO 09/1571.
113. Busfield 1996, 143–165; Showalter 1985, 55–59.
114. Cited in Busfield 1996, 143.
115. Busfield 1996, 165.
116. Wright 2004.
117. CB, 1914.
118. Sell to DMS, November 25, 1968, STG 1/5.
119. Yee-Chief 2000. However, this study was of well-educated, employed women in 1998.
120. PN 1072.
121. PN 667.
122. PN 1657.
123. PN 1536.
124. Becker 1995, 184n10; 1998, 431.
125. Marland 1999, 144; see also Marland 2004, 35.
126. PN 1411.
127. Marland 1999, 144.
128. Acting Agent General Immigration to CS, April 4, 1882, CSO MP 82/568.
129. Compare Marland 1999, 143.
130. PN 10; Marland 1999, 139.
131. From the title of Marland 1999.
132. PN 138.
133. CMO, reports, 1896.
134. St Giles correspondence, 1967. This example raises issues of consent for mentally disordered women who have suffered physical and mental trauma connected to childbirth. Thanks to Ruth Fitzgerald for alerting me to this.
135. PN 2855.
136. PN 406.
137. PN 607.

138. PN 1379.
139. PN 1290.

Chapter 5: Diagnoses and Discourse of Mental Disorders

1. Suzuki 1999, 125.
2. Sadowsky 1999, 50.
3. Douglas 1966, 97.
4. David Wright emphasizes the community's role in certification (1998).
5. Schedule F, Asylum Register, "An Ordinance to Provide for the Care and Maintenance of Lunatics and Idiots," *Fiji Royal Gazette,* 3/1884.
6. On stereotypes of race and madness, and how the Other is perceived as mad, see Gilman 1985, 129–130.
7. PN 792; PN 1532.
8. PN 153; PN 968.
9. PN 150; PN 857.
10. PN 124.
11. PN 1966.
12. PN 728.
13. Sander Gilman refers to the correct and meaningful use of language as a marker of normality (1985, 129).
14. PN 304.
15. PN 659.
16. See chapter 3; PN 103.
17. See MacKinnon 2003, 73–82.
18. On the limitations of the psychiatric interview in a colonial and cross-cultural context, see Sadowsky 1999, 167.
19. PN 115; see Tent 2001, 209–245.
20. PN 397.
21. PN 2172.
22. PN 230.
23. PN 927.
24. PN 821. On the history of leprosy in Fiji, see Buckingham 2011.
25. PN 1395.
26. PN 386.
27. PN 308; PN 449.
28. PN 64.
29. PN 1142.
30. PN 1542.
31. PN 1395.
32. PN 508; PN 1493.
33. PN 29.
34. PN 1383.
35. PN 414; PN 700.
36. PN 533.
37. The cleanliness issue is not just about dirt and hygiene (see Douglas 1966).

38. Thomas 1990, 149–170.
39. PN 97.
40. PN 195.
41. PN 57.
42. PN 543.
43. PN 12; PN 29; PN 41; PN 74; PN 84.
44. PN 937; PN 314.
45. PN 438.
46. PN 175.
47. PN 902.
48. PN 1437.
49. PN 876.
50. PN 1248. On the modern psychiatric discourse of "insight" at Ingutsheni Asylum in colonial Zimbabwe, see Jackson 1997, 266–267.
51. PN 1204.
52. For the history of European psychiatric understanding of delusions from the second half of the nineteenth century, see Berrios 1996, 104–139.
53. PN 1194.
54. PN 550.
55. PN 240.
56. PN 516.
57. PN 895.
58. PN 2206.
59. PN 1668.
60. PN 940; PN 1359.
61. PN 786.
62. PN 501. DMO's testimony.
63. PN 662.
64. PN 748.
65. See Dawson 2012.
66. PN 1195; PN 1231.
67. Berrios 1996, 428–429; Dowbiggin 1991.
68. Schedule F, Asylum Register, "An Ordinance to Provide for the Care and Maintenance of Lunatics and Idiots."
69. PN 398; PN 790.
70. Clark 1981, 273.
71. See Busfield 1986, 47–48.
72. Knapman 1986, 63, 69; PN 124; PN 162; PN 169; PN 180; PN 239.
73. See Knapman 1985, 68.
74. PN 329.
75. See Hare 1998, 146–173.
76. On the use and effects of *yagona* in Fiji, including intoxication ("grog doped") and kava hangovers (*lomoloma ca*), see Aporosa 2012, 177–184.
77. PN 45.
78. PN 1248.
79. PN 1787; PN 2136.

80. PN 109.
81. PN 202.
82. PN 557.
83. Eves 2005, 1999. Will Jackson discusses loneliness among insane Europeans in colonial Kenya (2003).
84. PN 524.
85. PN 1090.
86. Coleborne 2015, 118.
87. PN 1223; PN 1225.
88. PN 979; PN 1249; Yeo and Blong 2010, 657–683.
89. PN 28.
90. For example, PN 148; PN 224; PN 789; PN 1500.
91. PN 148.
92. McLane 2012, 77–182.
93. In the asylum, fifteen of seventy people contracted influenza; seven died, three of whom were warders (Fiji Government 1919).
94. See Ayers and Yellowlees 2008.
95. PN 556.
96. PN 134.
97. PN 566.
98. PN 909.
99. Mercier 1902, 111, cited in Clark 1981, 286.
100. For a contemporary summary of the many forms of dementia, see Edwards et al. 2014, 184–187.
101. PN 472.
102. PN 743.
103. Löckenhoff et al. 2009, 941–954.
104. PN 969.
105. PN 2122.
106. PN 1260. Discussed in chapter 2.
107. PN 132.
108. PN 1255.
109. See Leckie and Durutalo 2015, 283–310.
110. MS to DMS, AR 1944, F48/4/5.
111. PN 1247.
112. PN 1301.
113. PN 1322.
114. PN 1448.
115. Leese 2001, 411–415.
116. PN 803; PN 1036.
117. PN 1391; CB, December 6–8, 1943.
118. PN 1277; PN 1332; PN 1340.
119. Most American troops with war trauma in Fiji were treated by Dr. Theodore Litz at the Army Hospital (Lidz 1946, 193–213).
120. PN 1833. The Emergency (1948–1960) was imposed when the Malayan Communist Party attempted to overthrow the British colonial administration.

121. Swartz 1995a, 401.
122. See Berrios and Porter 1995.
123. Busfield 1986, 42.
124. BB, 1922–1923.
125. Presumably based on Royal College of Physicians of London, *The Nomenclature of Diseases*, 3rd ed., 1896 (https://archive.org/details/nomenclatureofdi00roya).
126. Puerperal insanity is discussed in chapter 4.
127. See, for example, Healy 2008, 83. German Berrios traces the transformation of notions of melancholia and mania during the second half of the nineteenth century into today's classifications of depression and mania (1996, 298–300).
128. PN 429; PN 720; PN 927.
129. PN 734; PN 1446.
130. PN 772; PN 837; PN 834.
131. See Berrios 1995; Porter 1995.
132. Kleinman and Good 1985.
133. Swartz 1995b; Sadowsky 1999, 108.
134. MS, Mental Hospital, to DMS, January 14, 1939, AR 1938, F48/4/5.
135. Guthrie 1979, 33–34.
136. See Berrios 1996, 188–190; Berrios, Luque, and Villagrán 2003.
137. PN 684.
138. PN 751.
139. For example, PN 75.
140. PN 2; BB, 1886.
141. PN 79.
142. See Berrios 1996, 172–207.
143. Ohaeri 1997a, 263.
144. PN 2354.
145. PN 2583; PN 2720.
146. PN 366.
147. PN 1548.
148. Estimates varied greatly from 45 percent in parts of Europe, to 20 percent in New York during the early twentieth century to 5 percent at Denbigh Mental Hospital in Wales (Braslow 1997, 74; Ernst 2013, 107).
149. Fiji Government 1911a, 3.
150. BB, 1890; PN 541.
151. PN 2721.
152. Davis 2012, 267; Clouston 1911, 243–245.
153. PN 450; Harper 1916; Clouston 1911.
154. PN 253.
155. On theories about GPI in the nineteenth and early twentieth centuries, see Davis 2008; Hare 1959; O'Connor 2015; Thompson 1988.
156. Buck 1900, 87.
157. See O'Connor 2015; Dawson 2013.
158. PN 357. One of the doctors in this case was Lynch.
159. Harper 1916, 679.
160. Campbell 1928.

161. Lambert 1929, 433.

162. See American Public Health Association 1917, 1587.

163. William MacGregor described the postmortem of a patient with GPI in 1871 when he was a medical assistant at the Royal Lunatic Asylum of Aberdeen (1872).

164. Lambert 1929, 433. Rheumatic fever was common in Fiji and could lead to degenerative heart disease.

165. Harper 1916, 678; Lambert 1929; Lynch 1917; Manson-Bahr 1954; Miles 1997, 56–58. Endemic treponematoses are difficult to distinguish from each other.

166. Manson-Bahr 1954, 244. But Dr. Arnold, the district medical officer for Labasa, reported a Fijian, previously with yaws, contracting syphilis in 1910 (Fiji Government 1911a, 12).

167. See, for example, Chapple 1921; Harper 1917; Lynch 1917.

168. Montague 1914, 12; Harper 1917. On salvarsan as a therapy for GPI, see Davis 2008, 168–173. Arsenical treatments were replaced by penicillin, which destroyed treponemal spirochaete, during the 1940s.

169. Chapple 1921, 30–31.

170. Harper 1916, 678; also 1917.

171. Harper 1916.

172. Lynch to Special Committee to Report on Syphilis to the Congress, November 11, 1913, reproduced in Australasian Medical Congress 1916, 112.

173. PN 710.

174. PN 1020; PN 374. Gayle Davis notes that "final diagnosis" near to death was important in GPI because this was often the only time when characteristic mental and physical symptoms were exhibited (2012, 270).

175. Philip Manson-Bahr, for example, states that with yaws the nervous system was never seriously affected (1928, 53).

176. Roman and Roman 1986, 767.

177. Manson-Bahr 1954.

178. MS to DMS, January 14, 1939, AR 1938, F48/4/5.

179. See, for example, Coleborne 2015, 120; Holloway 2001, 163–164.

180. See Scarr 1980, 188–189.

181. PN 344.

182. See Steele 2011, 84–88.

183. PN 769.

184. PN 192.

185. PN 1062; PN 1065; PN 1883; PN 1943; PN 2159; PN 2650.

186. PN 329.

187. Stuart 2006a, 139.

188. According to Deryck Scarr, Governor Thurston informed Walter Carew that Ratu Alifereti Ravulo was sent to the Lunatic Asylum following alcohol abuse during the "X'mas orgies" of 1888 (1950, 203). There is no record of an admission.

189. PN 1478.

190. Quoted in Stuart 2006a, 139.

191. Anne Digby discusses differing terminology and shifting legal definitions of mental disability in English history, including the separation of mental disability from lunacy during the twentieth century (1996, 2; see also McDonagh 2008).

192. The observation of manic depression refers to PN 1514.

193. Berne 1959a, 105. Only the 1911 census separated lunatics from imbeciles and feeble minded.

194. Gatty 2010, 89.

195. For example, in 1911 only one European was reported as an imbecile (Fiji Government 1911b, 29).

196. Price 1979, 49. For a review of attitudes and services for people with disabilities in Fiji since the 1960s, see Denholm, McGowan and Tatham 1996.

197. MS to DMS, January 14, 1939, AR 1938, F48/4/5.

198. PN 1032.

199. PN 1557.

200. "St. Giles Hospital Annual Report 1967," unpublished typescript, SG.

201. See Kale 1997; Temkin 1971.

202. PN 1346.

203. PN 375.

204. PN 863.

205. Kendler 1995, 368; Lewis 1970.

206. See Shorter 1997, 296–297.

207. PN 774.

208. PN 1141.

209. PN 977. The hospital register recorded the disorder as manic depressive.

210. PN 973; PN 1477. Cathy had several admissions, including a period at Avondale Hospital in Auckland, New Zealand.

211. Fiji Government 1957.

212. Price and Karim 1976, 155–157; Murphy and Narayan 1979.

213. Jackson 2005, 171–172.

214. Price and Karim 1976.

215. Fiji Government 1966.

216. MS to DMS, "Psychiatric Services, Annual Report for 1968," February 20, 1969, typescript, SG.

217. Micale 1995, 109.

218. *New Zealand Herald* 1907.

219. PN 706.

220. Busfield 1986, 48–49.

221. PN 2108.

222. See Micale 1995.

223. PN 1570.

224. PN 323. Her brother-in-law said that she had been a patient in a mental asylum in Wellington twenty years earlier.

225. PN 1113. See also chapter 4.

226. MS to DMS, "Psychiatric Services," AR 1968.

227. Wilson, 1965, 364.

228. Kleinman and Good 1985; Littlewood and Dein 2000a; Yap 1974.

229. See Goddard 1998, 61; Kleinman 1988.

230. Berne 1960.

231. Berne 1959a.

232. Fiji Government 1966, 78.

233. Ibid., 10.
234. On culture-bound syndromes, see Littlewood and Dein 2000b, 14–17.
235. Price and Karim 1978, 228.
236. Dr. Isaac Karim, interview, June 23, 1999.
237. Price and Karim 1976.
238. Murphy and Narayan 1979, 4.
239. Karim, interview.
240. Duncan Macgregor, letter to doctor at CWM Hospital, December 15, 1967, SG.

Chapter 6: Struggling with Madness

1. CSO MP 23/1111.
2. Syljeseth to Neill, March 23, 1923, CSO MP 23/1111.
3. Harper to CS, October 7, 1927.
4. PN 2134.
5. Syljeseth, age about thirty, left London for Wellington on the *Gothic* on January 20, 1897 (*UK, Outward Passenger Lists, 1890–1960,* BT27, Records of the Commercial, Companies, Labour, Railways and Statistics Departments, Board of Trade and successor and related bodies, The National Archives, United Kingdom). An advertisement on the first page of the *Auckland Star* dated July 2, 1941, inquired after the whereabouts of Syljeseth, formerly of Green Lane, Auckland.
6. PN 525.
7. PN 722.
8. Syljeseth to Neill, March 23, 1923, CSO MP 23/1111.
9. Ibid., March 10, 1923.
10. September 17, 1922, CSO MP 23/1111. Syljeseth backdated the letters that were included in his letter to Neill on March 23, 1923, so that he provides letters from himself as Dr. Jenner and "Castor God." Unless stated, all the following quotations by Syljeseth/Jenner are from this letter.
11. September 17, 1923, CSO MP 23/1111.
12. Prisoner no. 82/22; PN 705.
13. CS to CMO, March 27, 1923.
14. PN 1227.
15. Sadowsky 1999, 154.
16. Coleborne 2007, 105–119.
17. Historiography has critiqued the binary of resistance/no-resistance, to stress accommodation and coping (see Munro 1993).
18. See, for example, Hereniko 1995; Mageo 1998. On humor in psychiatry in Tonga, see Poltorak 2007, 2013.
19. PN 25.
20. Porter 1987, 231.
21. On women, madness, and resistance, see Ussher 2011, 185–220.
22. Biopolitics and biopower is used in this book to denote state and institutional control over bodies, the internalization of this regulation by the normal (and recovered) individual, and the construction of "mad" bodies through statistical and expert information (Foucault 1978, 140–144; see also Fanon 1952).

23. Keller 2007, 111.
24. Mills 2000, 2.
25. PN 329; CB, September 7, 1910.
26. Patients' Property Book, St Giles Hospital, June 1926–December 1968.
27. CB, November 5, 1905.
28. CB, March 31, 1948.
29. PN 117; CB and Reports on Mrs. J. at SG. The reports were mostly by Smith, CW to the CMO.
30. CW to CMO, July 28, 1896.
31. PN 232; CB, July 9, 1905.
32. Ralph de Boissiere, Acting MS to CMO, August 11, 1914, CSO MP 14/7315.
33. In practice these hours may have been much longer. CP no. 15 Public Lunatic Asylum April 3, 1914; CSO MP 14/7315. Tell-tale clocks were used in institutions like prisons and asylums to ensure that warders checked on prisoners or patients.
34. CB, April 6, 1951; PN 1673.
35. Steenson, MS to the Public Trustee, September 17, 1948, on PN 1506.
36. CB, May 19, 1948; PN 1537.
37. Unpublished AR on Mental Hospital 1954, SG.
38. DMS to CS, complaints re treatment of patients, October 4, 1955, F48/524.
39. Board of Visitors (BOV) Reports, March 6, 1951, F48/10, part 2.
40. Unpublished AR on Mental Hospital, 1954.
41. Karim interview; DMS to Consultant Psychiatrist, SG, February 9, 1971, CMD, 4/3/3-III, SG.
42. Harper to CS, "Issues Raised Following Report of Chief Police Magistrate into Death of Sarjudei, 10 August 1927," August 19, 1927, CSO MP 27/3359; see PN 848. A sanitary gang from the jail removed buckets daily from the asylum's closets and from the Korovou Indian Immigration Depot. Buckets were often mixed up, which increased the transference of diseases transmitted through feces. A septic tank was installed in 1928 (Fiji Government 1928, 23–24).
43. Montague to CS, January 3, 1928, CSO MP 27/3359. Montague had been medical superintendent since 1912.
44. CB, August 15, 1905.
45. CB, CW to CMO, July 30, 1896.
46. CB, September 21, 1914.
47. Mills 2000, 115.
48. For example, PN 1362.
49. CB, December 17, 1906.
50. BB 1894, 83.
51. PN 1402.
52. During the early twentieth century, nasal feeding was typically one pint milk, one ounce whisky, and one egg dissolved, through a tube, three times daily.
53. PN 1494.
54. PN 1447; prisoner 393/44; CSO F109/127.
55. PN 817; prisoner 378/16.
56. CSO MP 27/4290 on PN 817.
57. PN 1285.

58. Daniel Bower, interview, January 2002.
59. *Pacific Review*, 1970.
60. MS to DMS, January 14, 1939, AR 1938, F48/4/5.
61. See Ernst 2016.
62. AR 1887, December 16, 1887, CSO 87/3847.
63. Corney, Acting MS to CW, January 14, 1888, SG.
64. March 22, 1916, CSO 16/2206.
65. For example, Montague, MS to DMS, AR 1932, F48/4/5.
66. Commented on in several annual reports, for example, AR 1897, CSO 98/96; AR 1938, F48/4/5.
67. AR 1938, F48/4/5.
68. Bower, interview.
69. As Grace, discussed later in this chapter, was selected. Dorothy Sachs recalled patients working in staff houses in the 1960s (interview, January 17, 2002).
70. PN 117; CW to Dr. Finucane, August 19, 1896.
71. Public Lunatic Asylum, Regulations for Management and Direction of the Public Lunatic Asylum, April 3, 1914, CP 15/14.
72. CSO MP 27/4290 in PN 817.
73. CSO 29/5191. Question asked in Legislative Council, October 30, 1929.
74. DMS to CS, June 2, 1941, F48/10 part 1.
75. Macgregor to DMS, November 27, 1966, MS 19.
76. PN 693; PN 737; CSO 24/1059.
77. PN 220.
78. Shula Marks discusses the frustrations and violence in the asylum among nursing staff in colonial South Africa (2007).
79. PN 596.
80. CB, August 24, 1906; PN 233. Ananaiasa was diagnosed with GPI.
81. 1887 Lunatic Asylum Regulations, CP 4/87.
82. AR 1887, December 16, 1887, CSO 87/3847.
83. CP 15/14.
84. PN 117, CW to CMO, July 26, 1896.
85. AR 1887, December 16, 1887, CSO 87/3847.
86. Ibid.
87. Alena, interview, June 18, 1999; Bower, interview.
88. PN 1635.
89. PN 327. The postmortem gave the cause of death as exhaustion and tuberculosis peritonitis.
90. PN 688.
91. The *Blue Book* of 1938 has a discrepancy, with all patients under seclusion apparently male, but showing twenty-seven instances of females being restrained.
92. AR 1946, January 24, 1947, F48/10, part 1.
93. Visitor to CS, February 15, 1944, DMS F48/353.
94. MS to CS, February 23, 1944, DMS F48/353.
95. November 4, 1967, STG 4–5, SG.
96. Macgregor, MS to Chairman, Public Service Commission, "The Machinery of Discipline," October 16, 1967, STG 4–5, SG.
97. "Machinery of Discipline," November 4, 1967, STG 4–5, SG.

98. *Pacific Review* 1970.

99. Leckie 2005a.

100. Although most of the cases of shock therapy in this chapter are women, it was not possible to accurately breakdown gender. Others have emphasized that women were more likely than men to receive shock therapy (see, for example, Showalter 1985, 205–207; Ussher 2011, 74).

101. See Shorter 1997, 196–203.

102. See López-Muñoz, Ucha-Udabe, and Alamo 2005.

103. Shorter 1997, 198.

104. PN 1386.

105. CB, March 14, 1955; see also Healy 2002, 77–101; Shorter 1997, 248–255.

106. Fiji Government 1962, 10.

107. See, for example, Gittins 1998, 210–211. A former SG staff confirmed that drugs were used to restrain patients.

108. PN 2456.

109. PN 117, Memo to CMO.

110. PN 817; PN 1285.

111. PN 1929. So, too, did Grace refuse. For the disturbing effects reserpine could have, especially when used primarily to treat hypertension, see Healy 2002, 113.

112. Healy 2002, 117; 117–124. With the exception of one female, who had been ill for two months before admission and who was diagnosed with catatonic schizophrenia ("Report of a Small Trial of Serance," December 6, 1963; AMO Vuki, "Clinical Trial on Serance," SG).

113. Rowe to Macgregor, November 8, 1965, MTU/902, SG.

114. PN 1515.

115. See Shorter 1997, 207–224. Edward Shorter and David Healy locate shock therapy within a positivist framework: "one can actually do something for people with schizophrenia, melancholia, and manic-depressive illness—that turns a page in the history of psychiatry" (2007, 14). Psychiatric survivor and activist Leonard Frank offers a radically critical perspective (1978).

116. On the history of Metrazol therapy, see Shorter and Healy 2007, 21–30.

117. Kalinowsky 1959, 1500.

118. PN 1522.

119. Letter in nursing notes, circa 1973. I found no evidence of any patient deaths from Cardiozol therapy or injections.

120. AR 1949, F48/10, part 2.

121. Fiji Government 1950; unpublished AR 1951, SG.

122. Bender 2013.

123. MS to Magistrate, Sigatoka, memo, April 2, 1975, RN/mb, File no. C107.

124. Compare Braslow 1997, 104–111.

125. CB, December 30, 1950.

126. CB, February 26, 1953.

127. PN 1595.

128. For a history of ICT, see Shorter and Healy 2007, 11–21.

129. Ackner 1964, 302–303.

130. PN 1887.

131. Akihito Suzuki discusses the economics of ICT in Japan (2010, 128–132).

132. British psychiatrist Harold Bourne, argued that if ICT worked at all, it was because ICT patients were an elite group, chosen for their good prognosis, and given special treatment (1953).

133. Holt et al. 1955. Elsewhere, Raudixin was implicated in causing hypertensive patients to become mentally ill and severely depressed (see Mukherjee 2012).

134. PN 1929. Paraphrenia was considered slightly different to schizophrenia as patients maintained "a well-preserved personality and affective response" (Roth 1955, 283).

135. Healy 2002, 44–45; López-Muñoz, Ucha-Udabe, and Alamo 2005.

136. PN 1477.

137. CB, 1954.

138. Westmore 2003, 214–215.

139. PN 1778; Hellier 1954.

140. PN 1761.

141. Whyte 1954.

142. Ferraro 1959, 1041. Healy discusses experiments to treat schizophrenia with nicotinic acid. PN 2099 was treated for alcoholism with nicotinic acid (2002, 184–186, 190–192).

143. Mills 2000, 171.

144. PN 713.

145. PN 392.

146. CSO MO 1288/14. Anderson was charged with "failing to properly search a patient, inadequate observation of a patient, improperly causing shutters of room to remain closed." Hector is a pseudonym.

147. See Weaver 2009.

148. PN 34; PN 1016.

149. PN 1530; PN 1826.

150. PN 1537.

151. CB, December 26, 1910.

152. "Reward for the Capture of Pita," June 20, 1913, CSO MP 13/5279.

153. CB, December 2, 1946; BOV report, January 24, 1946.

154. CSO MP 14/7315.

155. MS to DMS, November 30, 1966, "MS. 56.2 Incidents" file, SG.

156. Confidential files, MS; PN 2471; PN 2783. Josua is a pseudonym.

157. Jackson 2005, 154.

158. Both pseudonyms.

159. Her first admission was in 1958. PN 2134.

160. *Pacific Review* 1970; PN 2633.

161. Hanif to Senior Magistrate, Suva, December 26, 1969, in PN 2633.

162. See Lal 1997, 121–124.

163. *Pacific Review* 1970.

164. See Cummins 1979.

165. "Machinery of Discipline," November 4, 1967, STG 4–5, SG.

Chapter 7: Conclusion

1. Scully 2002.
2. Scott 2003; Goldson 2008.

3. The Sujit Kumar Happy Home Trust, http://www.thehappyhometrust.com/sujit-kumar.

4. Forsyth 2004.

5. See Vallis and Stinson 2004; Masters 2008.

6. TV One 2005. Other attention-grabbing media headlines included "Civilising the Chicken Coop Wild Boy" (*Dominion Post* 2005), "'Chicken Boy' Test Case for Humanity" (Fynes-Clinton 2007), and "Flying above a Life with the Chickens" (*New Zealand Herald* 2008).

7. Fynes-Clinton 2011.

8. Vallis and Stinson 2004.

9. OneNews 2013. Fiji media reported similar cases, such as a mother chaining her son and two daughters at their home (Vakarewakobau 2004). Two "mentally retarded brothers" near Labasa, were tied to posts beneath their house (*Fiji Times* 2007).

10. Judgment, Judge Salesi Temo, High Court of Fiji, Criminal Miscellaneous Case no. HAM 071 of 2014S and Miscellaneous Case no. HAM 101 of 2015S, *Apete Vakananumi Kaisau v. State and Attorney General of Fiji,* October 2, 2015, http://www.paclii.org/cgibin/sinodisp/fj/cases/FJHC/2015/712.html; Chand 2014.

11. Fiji Government 1972, 14.

12. Anderson 2004, 299.

13. Fiji Government 1968, 9; *British Medical Journal* 1984.

14. Newsletter, "Friends of St Giles," 1992, STG 1/3–I.

15. Fiji Government 1969, 10.

16. On localization in Fiji's public service, see Leckie 1997, 41–42, 67–70.

17. Ranjana Narayan's photo collection, Fiji Museum. Ranjana Narayan is Ram Narayan's daughter.

18. Information from his daughter-in-law, Dorothy Sachs, January 17, 2002.

19. Extract, Proceedings Council of Chiefs 1940, resolution 4, F29/159.

20. Macgregor 1967, 2.

21. MS to DMS, "Duties of Head Attendant St Giles. Draft Estimates 1966," April 15, 1965, MS 564, SG.

22. MS to DMS, "The Machinery of Discipline," November 14, 1967, STG 4–5. SG.

23. STG (confidential). The orderly's employment was terminated in January 1988.

24. "Orderlies Meeting," October 3, 1984 through January 16, 1989. Foolscap book at SG.

25. As recommended in a meeting of the Nursing Staff Board; PS, Health and Social Welfare, to Matron, memorandum, September 15, 1985, STG 1/19.

26. "Orderlies Meeting," February 1, 1988; "Orderlies Meeting," March 14, 1988; Jane Erasito, interview, December 11, 1996.

27. Notes on STG 1/19; STG 1/3–I (BOV), staff profiles, 1991.

28. Bower, interview.

29. See, for example, "Organisational Review Report, St Giles Hospital," prepared by Sarita Mani, senior assistant secretary, Management Services, Public Service Commission, n.d., probably early 1980s.

30. Fiji Government 1972, 11.

31. Fiji Government 1969, 9.

32. Burton-Bradley 1973, 1975.

33. Burton-Bradley, Macgregor, and Zeldine 1967, vii; also Sell to DMS, March 7, 1969, STG 2/7.

34. Murphy 1978, 39–40.

35. See Patel et al. 2010, 115–134.

36. Narayan 2008.

37. MS to DMS, "Projected Numbers of Inpatients at Mental Hospital 1971–75," March 7, 1969, STG 2/7.

38. Murphy and Narayan 1979, 10.

39. See Leckie 1997, 101–103; "Report of the Select Committee of Inquiry into Fiji Health Services," Parliamentary Paper no/ 28/79.

40. Fiji Government 1972, 11.

41. See curriculum by Dr. Kippax in 1987, FSM.

42. Foster et al. 2009, 179–186; Chang, Allen, and Pandit 2015.

43. Fiji Government 1966, 73–74.

44. November 19, 1975, STG 1/3.

45. Fiji Government 1966.

46. MS to Magistrate, November 9, 1978, SG.

47. PN 1913.

48. AR 1963, SG.

49. Gatty 2010, 11; Alison Cupit, Chair of BOV, Newsletter, "Friends of St Giles," 1992, STG 1/3–I.

50. Smith, "Social Work Report," AR 1986, SG, appendix 2, 5.

51. Ohaeri 1999a.

52. Ibid.

53. Nabukavou and Teaiwa 2008; Nabukavou et al. 2013.

54. Aghanwa 2004a.

55. Pointed out by Murphy and Narayan 1979, 10.

56. Lewis 2011.

57. TVNZ 2013.

58. Narayan 1975.

59. For example, Tomlinson 2013.

60. Cited in Scott 2004, 378.

61. Scott 2004, 381.

62. Kaisau apparently said this to his host on a trip to New Zealand while watching the coup on television and seeing Scott praised as a "white angel." Goldson's documentary, discussed in Chisholm 2008.

63. Smith 1996, 4.

64. Narayan, "Native Healing," March 7, 1974, typescript, STG 2/3.

65. Karim, interview.

66. Dr. Ram Narayan, "Domiciliary Service to the Mentally Ill," c. 1973, STG 1/3—I/54; Narayan, "Native Healing"; also Chang 2011, 75; Narayan 2012 [2003].

67. Smith 1996, 6.

68. See Aghanwa 2004.

69. Erasito, interview.

70. Fiji Government 1965.

71. Sell to DMS, March 7, 1969, STG 2/7.

72. Narayan, MS, to PS, Health, September 19, 1977, STG 2/7. Disability services were established by nongovernment organizations in Fiji during the late 1960s and 1970s but were

uncoordinated. The government has since provided some services (see Price 1996, 85–87; Denholm, McGowan, and Tatham 1996, 100–125).

73. MS to DMS, November 2, 1967, STG 2/7. In 1999, the Father Law Home had nine St Giles' patients, including a thirty-four-year-old (MS to Chairman, BOV, Father Law Home, December 24, 1999).

74. PN 2687. See also chapter 2.

75. Ohaeri 1999a, 529.

76. See Kritsotaki, Long, and Smith 2016.

77. Fiji Government 1969, 10.

78. Noted by Murphy and Narayan 1979, 4.

79. Fiji Government 1965, 11.

80. Fiji Government 1972.

81. See also Pridmore 1993, 9–12.

82. Transcripts of broadcasts at FSM, nos. 3/61/128, 3/61/129.

83. Smith 1996.

84. Gounder and Brugnoli 1998; AR 1997, STG 1/9; Alena, interview.

85. For example, notes on STG 1/3-I; STG 1/15; OT department, STG 2/3/7; memories of former staff, for example, Vasiti, who started at SG in 1966, interview, January 11, 2002; also Sachs, interview.

86. See Roberts, Leckie, and Chang 2017.

87. Mental Treatment Act, Chapter 113 (February 28, 1940, rev. 1978).

88. See Roberts, Cruz, and Puamau 2007, 108.

89. National Health Promotion Council 1998.

90. See Ohaeri 1997a, 1997b, 1998, 1999a, 1999b, 1999d, 1999e.

91. Cruz 2004; Roberts, Cruz, and Puamau 2007.

92. Nabukavou and Teaiwa 2008; Nabukavou et al. 2013; Clery 2012.

93. Mental Health Decree 2010 (Decree no. 54 of 2010), *Republic of Fiji Islands Government Gazette* 11, no. 119 (2010).

94. See Ohaeri 1999c.

95. See Singh et al. 2013, 7.

96. ABC 2013.

97. Patel et al. 2011, 90.

98. See Bemme and D'Souza 2014, 859–860.

99. Patel 2014.

100. For details and debates about GMH, see Bemme and D'Souza 2014; Mills 2014; Whitley 2015.

101. *Fiji Times* 2009; Singh et al. 2013, 23.

102. Summerfield 2013, 3509.

103. Campbell and Burgess 2012; Fernando 2011; Summerfield 2012.

104. Summerfield 2012, 520.

105. Fernando 2014.

106. Ibid., 89–91, 121–129.

107. This medication required regular monitoring of lithium serum levels; only possible for outpatients who could regularly visit St Giles.

108. See Leckie and Hughes 2017; Allen and Laycock 1997.

109. Poltorak 2013.

110. Biumaiono 2005. Laladidi's comments followed the death by hanging of a prisoner, Private Iliesa Liganivai, in Korovou Prison. Liganivai was serving a sentence for mutiny; his parents allege that his mental health was affected by beatings from the military.

111. Scott 2004, 378.

112. Scully 2002.

113. Chisholm 2005.

114. *Fiji Times* 2005.

115. Kate 2015a.

116. Kate 2015b.

117. Deo 2015.

118. Chand 2014.

References

ABC. 2013. "Fiji to Open Region's First Mental Health Facility." http://www.abc.net.au/news/2013-07-17/fiji-to-open-the-regions-first-mental-health-facility/4825588.

Ackner, Brian, ed. 1964. *Handbook of Psychiatric Nurses*. London: Ballière, Tindall & Cox, Royal Medico-Psychological Association.

Aghanwa, Henry Stephens. 2004a. "Attitude toward and Knowledge about Mental Illness in Fiji Islands." *International Journal of Social Psychiatry* 50, no. 4: 361–375.

———. 2004b. "The Determinants of Attempted Suicide in a General Hospital Setting in Fiji Islands: A Gender-Specific Study." *General Hospital Psychiatry* 26, no. 1: 63–69.

Ali, Ahmed. 1980. *Plantation to Politics: Studies on Fiji Indians*. Suva: University of the South Pacific and *Fiji Times and Herald*.

Allen, John S., and Jennifer L. Laycock. 1997. "Major Mental Illness in the Pacific: A Review." *Pacific Health Dialog* 4, no. 2: 105–118.

American Public Health Association. 1917. "Accuracy of Certified Causes of Death: Its Relation to Mortality Statistics and the International List." *Public Health Reports* 32, no. 39: 1557–1632.

Anderson, Warwick. 2004. "Postcolonial Histories of Medicine." In *Locating Medical History: The Stories and Their Meanings*, edited by Frank Huisman and John Harley Warner, 285–306. Baltimore, MD: Johns Hopkins University Press.

———. 2008. *The Collectors of Lost Souls: Turning Kuru Scientists into Whitemen*. Baltimore, MD: Johns Hopkins University Press.

Andrews, Charles Freer, and W. W. Pearson. 1916. *Indian Indentured Labour in Fiji: An Independent Inquiry*. Calcutta: Star Printing Works.

Andrews, Jonathan, and Anne Digby, eds. 2004. *Sex and Seclusion, Class and Custody: Perspectives on Gender and Class in the History of British and Irish Psychiatry*. Amsterdam: Editions Rodopi.

Aporosa, S. 2012. "Yaqona (Kava) and Education in Fiji: Investigating 'Cultural Complexities' from a Post-Development Perspective." PhD thesis, Massey University.

Auckland Star. 1915. "Island News." September 7.

Aucoin, Pauline McKenzie. 1990. "Domestic Violence and Social Relations of Conflict in Fiji." *Pacific Studies* 13, no. 3: 23–42.

Australasian Medical Congress. 1916. *Transactions, Tenth Session, Auckland, February 1914*. Wellington: John Mackay, Government Printer.

Ayers, Kathleen, and Peter Yellowlees. 2008. "Mental Health Considerations during a Pandemic Influenza Outbreak." *Internet Journal of Rescue and Disaster Medicine* 9, no. 1, https://ispub.com/IJRDM/9/1/8275.

Ballantyne, Tony. 2012. *Webs of Empire: Locating New Zealand's Colonial Past.* Wellington: Bridget Williams Books.

Barry, Lorelle, and Catharine Coleborne. 2011. "Insanity and Ethnicity in New Zealand: Māori Encounters with the Auckland Mental Hospital, 1860–1900." *History of Psychiatry* 22, no. 3: 285–301.

Bartlett, Peter. 1999. *The Poor Law of Lunacy: The Administration of Pauper Lunatics in Mid-Nineteenth Century England.* London: Leicester University Press.

Bartlett, Peter, and David Wright. 1999. "Community Care and Its Antecedents." In *Outside the Walls of the Asylum: On Care in the Community in Modern Britain and Ireland,* edited by Peter Bartlett and David Wright, 1–18. London: Athlone Press.

Bayliss-Smith, Tim, Richard Bedford, Harold Brookfield, and Marc Latham. 1988. *Islands, Islanders, and the World: The Colonial and Post-Colonial Experience of Eastern Fiji.* Cambridge: Cambridge University Press.

Becker, Anne E. 1995. *Body, Self, and Society: The View from Fiji.* Philadelphia: University of Pennsylvania Press.

———. 1998. "Postpartum Illness in Fiji: A Sociosomatic Perspective." *Psychosomatic Medicine* 60, no. 4: 431–438.

Bell, Leland V. 1991. *Mental and Social Disorder in Sub-Saharan Africa: The Case of Sierra Leone, 1787–1990.* Westport, CT: Greenwood Press.

Belshaw, Cyril S. 1964. *Under the Ivi Tree: Society and Economic Growth in Rural Fiji.* London: Routledge & Kegan Paul.

Bemme, Doerte, and Nicole A. D'Souza. 2014. "Global Mental Health and Its Discontents: An Inquiry into the Making of Global and Local Scale." *Transcultural Psychiatry* 51, no. 6: 850–874.

Bender, Keith. 2013. "Obituary: Dr Donald Oldmeadow (1913–2013)." *Australasian Psychiatry* 21, no. 6: 611.

Bennett, Judy. 2006. "Malaria, Medicine and Melanesians: Contested Hybrid Spaces in World War II." *Health and History* 8, no. 1: 27–55.

Berne, Eric. 1959a. "Difficulties of Comparative Psychiatry: The Fiji Islands." *American Journal of Psychiatry* 116, no. 2: 104–109.

———. 1959b. "Psychiatric Epidemiology of the Fiji Islands." In *Progress in Psychotherapy,* vol. 4, edited by Frieda Fromm-Reichmann and Jacob Levy Moreno, 310–313. Oxford: Grune & Stratton.

———. 1960. "The Cultural Problem: Psychopathology in Tahiti." *American Journal of Psychiatry* 116, no. 12: 1076–1081.

Berrios, German E. 1995. "Mood Disorders: Clinical Section." In *A History of Clinical Psychiatry: The Origin and History of Psychiatric Disorders,* edited by German Berrios and Roy Porter, 384–408. New York: New York University Press.

———. 1996. *The History of Mental Symptoms: Descriptive Psychopathology since the Nineteenth Century.* Cambridge: Cambridge University Press.

Berrios, German E., and Roy Porter. 1995. Introduction to *A History of Clinical Psychiatry: The Origin and History of Psychiatric Disorders,* edited by German Berrios and Roy Porter, xvii–xix. New York: New York University Press.

Berrios, German E., Rogelio Luque, and José M. Villagrán. 2003. "Schizophrenia: A Conceptual History." *International Journal of Psychology and Psychological Therapy* 3, no. 2: 111–140.

Beuschel, Gail C. 2001. "Shutting Africans Away: Lunacy, Race and Social Order in Colonial Kenya, 1910–1963." PhD diss., School of Oriental and African Studies, University of London.

Bhugra, Dinesh, and Roland Littlewood, eds. 2001. *Colonialism and Psychiatry.* New Delhi: Oxford University Press.

Biumaiono, Solomoni. 2005. "Hospital Looks at New Unit." *Fiji Times,* February 18.

Booth, Heather. 1999. "Gender, Power and Social Change: Youth Suicide among Fiji Indians and Western Samoans." *Journal of the Polynesian Society* 108, no. 1: 39–68.

Bourne, Harold. 1953. "The Insulin Myth." *Lancet* 262 (November 7): 964–968.

Braslow, Joel T. 1997. *Mental Ills and Bodily Cures: Psychiatric Treatment in the First Half of the Twentieth Century.* Berkeley: University of California Press.

Brewster, Adolf . 1922. *The Hill Tribes of Fiji.* London: Seeley, Service & Co.

Brisbane Courier. 1913. "A Remarkable Incident." June 9. Accessed February 3, 2015. http://nla.gov.au/nla.news-article19870416.

British Medical Journal. 1984. "Obituary: D F Macgregor, BM, BCH, BSC, MRCPSYCH, DPM." Vol. 288, no. 6417: 648–649.

Brookes, Barbara. 1992. "Women and Madness: A Case Study of the Seacliff Asylum, 1890–1920." In *Women in History 2,* edited by Barbara Brookes, Charlotte Macdonald, and Margaret Tennant, 129–147. Wellington: Bridget Williams Books.

———. 1994. "Men and Madness in New Zealand, 1890–1916." In *New Countries and Old Medicine: Proceedings of An International Conference on the History of Medicine and Health,* edited by Linda Bryder and Derek A. Dow, 196–203. Auckland: Auckland Medical Historical Society.

———. 1998. "Women and Mental Health: An Historical Introduction." In *Folding Back the Shadows: A Perspective on Women's Mental Health,* edited by Sarah E. Romans, 15–22. Dunedin, NZ: University of Otago Press.

Brookes, Barbara, and Jane Thomson, eds. 2001. *"Unfortunate Folk": Essays on Mental Health Treatment 1863–1992.* Dunedin, NZ: University of Otago Press.

Brunton, Warwick. 2001. "'A Choice of Difficulties': National Mental Health Policy in New Zealand, 1840–1947." PhD diss., University of Otago.

Buchanan, John G., B. K. Jha, J. R. Matthews, and A. D. Nixon. 1979. "The Prevalence and Nature of Anaemia among Apparently Normal Subjects in Fiji." *Pathology* 11, no. 3: 369–376.

Buck, Albert H. 1900. *A Reference Handbook of the Medical Sciences: Embracing the Entire Range of Scientific and Practical Medicine and Allied Sciences.* New York: William Wood.

Buckingham, Jane. 2011. "The Inclusivity of Exclusion: Isolation and Community among Leprosy-Affected People in the South Pacific." *Health and History* 13, no. 2: 65–83.

Buckingham, Jane, and Vicki Luker, eds. 2017. "Leprosy in the Pacific." *Journal of Pacific History* 52, no. 3: 265–426.

Burton-Bradley, Burton Gyrth. 1973. *LongLong: Transcultural Psychiatry in Papua New Guinea*. Port Moresby: Public Health Department.

———. 1975. *Stone Age Crisis: A Psychiatric Appraisal*. Nashville, TN: Vanderbilt University Press.

Burton-Bradley, Burton Gyrth, Duncan Fleming Macgregor, and Georges Zeldine. 1967. "Report of the Advisors on Mental Health." In *Mental Health in the South Pacific: Report of a Meeting of Experts Held at Suva (Fiji) from 19 to 22 May, and at Noumea (New Caledonia) from 23 to 27 May*, by South Pacific Commission, vii–ix. Technical Paper no. 154. Nouméa: South Pacific Commission.

Busfield, Joan. 1986. *Managing Madness: Changing Ideas and Practice*. London: Hutchinson.

———. 1988. "Mental Illness as Social Product or Social Construct: A Contradiction in Feminists' Arguments." *Sociology of Health and Illness* 10, no. 4: 521–542.

———. 1996. *Men, Women and Madness*. London: Macmillan.

Campbell, Catherine, and Rochelle Burgess. 2012. "The Role of Communities in Advancing the Goals of the Movement for Global Mental Health." *Transcultural Psychiatry* 49, no. 3–4: 379–395.

Campbell, J. G. C. 1928. "Report by J. G. C. Campbell, Bacteriologist, on Bacteriological Work for Year, 1927." In Fiji Government, *Medical Department: Annual Report for 1927*. CP 57/28. Suva: Government Printer.

Capell, Arthur. 1941. *The Fijian Dictionary*. Suva: Government Printer.

Cassar, Paul. 1995. "Notes on the History of Psychiatry in Malta." *History of Psychiatry* 6, no. 24: 483–491.

Cavert, William. 2016. "At the Edge of an Empire: Plague, State, and Identity in New Caledonia 1899–1900." *Journal of Pacific History* 51, no. 1: 1–20.

Chand, Ganesh. 2017. "Whose Story Is It? Colonialism, Syria Ship Wreck, and Texting Race Relations in Fiji." *Fijian Studies: A Journal of Contemporary Fiji* 15, no. 1: 63–92.

Chand, Shalveen. 2014. "A First for Fiji's Court." *FT Online*, April 23. Accessed April 15, 2016. http://www.fijitimes.com/story.aspx?id=266375.

Chang, Odille A. 2011. "Mental Health Care in Fiji." *Asia-Pacific Psychiatry* 3, no. 1: 73–75.

Chang, Odille A., Myrielle M. Allen, and Balram Pandit. 2015. "Capacity Building for Pacific Island Countries: The Challenges and Benefits of Developing a Postgraduate Clinical Training Programme." *Australasian Psychiatry* 23, no. 6: 32–34.

Chapple, W. A. 1921. *Fiji: Its Problems and Resources*. Auckland: Whitcombe & Tombs.

Chesler, Phyllis. 1972. *Women and Madness*. Garden City, NY: Doubleday.

Chisholm, Donna. 2005. "Fiji Releases Insane Killer after Two Years." *Sunday Star-Times*, July 31.

———. 2008. "In the Name of God." *Sunday Star-Times*, March 16.

Churchward, C. Maxwell. 1940. *Rotuman Grammar and Dictionary*. New York: AMS Press.

Clark, Michael J. 1981. "The Rejection of Psychological Approaches to Mental Disorder in Late Nineteenth-Century British Psychiatry." In *Madhouses, Mad-Doctors, and*

Madmen: The Social History of Psychiatry in the Victorian Era, edited by Andrew Scull, 271–312. London: Athlone Press.

Clery, Tui. 2012. "The Art of Peace: Performative and Arts-Based Peace Practices in Contemporary Fiji." PhD thesis, University of Otago.

Clouston, Thomas Smith. 1911. *Unsoundness of Mind*. London: Methuen.

Cody, William J. T. 1974. "Psychiatry in Hawai'i: A Short History." *Hawai'i Medical Journal* 33, no. 6: 207–210.

Cohn, Bernard S. 1987. *An Anthropologist among the Historians*. Delhi: Oxford University Press.

Coleborne, Catharine. 1997. "'She Does Her Hair up Fantastically': The Production of Femininity in Patient Case Books of the Lunatic Asylum in 1860s Victoria." In *Forging Identities: Bodies, Gender and Feminist History*, edited by Jane Long, Jan Gothard, and Helen Brash, 47–68. Nedlands: University of Western Australia Press.

———. 2001. "Making 'Mad' Populations in Settler Colonies: The Work of Law and Medicine in the Creation of the Colonial Asylum." In *Law, History, Colonialism: The Reach of Empire*, edited by Diane Kirkby and Catharine Coleborne, 106–123. Manchester, UK: Manchester University Press.

———. 2007. *Reading "Madness": Gender and Difference in the Colonial Asylum in Victoria, Australia, 1848–1888*. Perth: API Network.

———. 2010. *Madness in the Family: Insanity and Institutions in the Australasian Colonial World, 1860–1914*. New York: Palgrave Macmillan.

———. 2014. "White Men and Weak Masculinity: Men in the Public Asylums in Victoria, Australia, and New Zealand, 1860s–1900s." *History of Psychiatry* 25, no. 4: 468–476.

———. 2015. *Insanity, Identity and Empire: Immigrants and Institutional Confinement in Australia and New Zealand, 1873–1910*. Manchester: Manchester University Press.

Coleborne, Catharine, and Dolly MacKinnon, eds. 2003. *"Madness" in Australia: Histories, Heritage and the Asylum*. St. Lucia: University of Queensland Press and API Network.

Comaroff, John, and Jean Comaroff. 1992. *Ethnography and the Historical Imagination*. Boulder, CO: Westview Press.

Crick, Malcolm. 1997. "Entangled Lives and Meanings: Colonisation and Its Cultural Legacy." In *Global Forces, Local Realities: Anthropological Perspectives on Change in the Third World*, edited by Bill Geddes and Malcolm Crick, 63–84. Geelong, AU: Deakin University Press.

Cumberland Argus and Fruitgrowers Advocate. 1913. "Left for Dead." September 13. Accessed February 3, 2015. http://nla.gov.au/nla.news-article85975934.

Cummins, C. J. 1979. *A History of Medical Administration in New South Wales 1788–1973*. Sydney: NSW Department of Health.

The Cyclopaedia of Fiji. 1984. Originally published 1907. Papakura, NZ: R. McMillan.

Cruz, Myrielle. 2004. *Consultancy Report on Mental Health Services in Fiji*. Suva: World Health Organization.

Davis, Gayle. 2008. *"The Cruel Madness of Love": Sex, Syphilis and Psychiatry in Scotland, 1880–1930*. Amsterdam: Rodopi.

———. 2012. "The Most Deadly Disease of Asylumdom: General Paralysis of the Insane and Scottish Psychiatry, c. 1840–1940." *Journal of the Royal College of Physicians Edinburgh* 42, no. 3: 266–273.

Dawson, Maree. 2012. " Halting the 'Sad Degenerationist Parade': Medical Concerns about Heredity and Racial Degeneracy in New Zealand Psychiatry, 1853–99." *Health and History* 14, no. 1: 38–55.

———. 2013. "National Fitness or Failure? Heredity, Vice and Racial Decline in New Zealand Psychiatry: A Case Study of the Auckland Mental Hospital, 1868–99." PhD thesis, University of Waikato.

de Bruce, Lucy. 2007. "Histories of Diversity: Kailoma Testimonies and 'Part-European' Tales from Colonial Fiji (1920–1970)." *Journal of Intercultural Studies* 28, no. 1: 113–127.

Deacon, Harriet. 1996. "Madness, Race and Moral Treatment: Robben Island Lunatic Asylum, Cape Colony, 1846–1890." *History of Psychiatry* 7, no. 26: 287–297.

———. 1999. "Racial Categories and Psychiatry in Africa: The Asylum on Robben Island in the Nineteenth Century." In *Race, Science and Medicine, 1700–1960,* edited by Waltraud Ernst and Bernard Harris, 101–123. London: Routledge.

Denholm, Carey, Phil McGowan, and Peter Tatham. 1996. "Emerging from the Shadows: Fijian Children and Youth with Disabilities." In *Beyond Basic Care: Special Education and Community Rehabilitation in Low Income Countries,* edited by Roy I. Brown, David Baine, and Aldred H. Neufeldt, 100–125. North York: Captus Press.

Denoon, Donald. 1989. *Public Health in Papua New Guinea: Medical Possibility and Social Constraint, 1884–1984.* Cambridge: Cambridge University Press.

Deo, Dhanjay. 2015. "Kaisau Has Not Expressed Remorse Verbally or in Writing for His Actions." Fijivillage.com, September 22. Accessed April 15, 2016. http://fijivillage.com/news/Kaisau-has-not-expressed-remorse-verbally-or-in-writing-for-his-actions-r29sk5.

Department of Immigration. 1879–1916. *General Register of Indian Immigrants, 1879–1916.* Microform. Fiji: Dept. of Immigration and Central Archives of Fiji and the Western Pacific High Commission.

Derrick, Ronald Albert. 1950. *A History of Fiji,* 2nd ed. Suva: Government Press.

Digby, Anne. 1996. "Contexts and Perspectives." In *From Idiocy to Mental Deficiency,* edited by David Wright and Anne Digby, 1–21. London: Routledge.

Dominion Post. 2005. "Civilising the Chicken Coop Wild Boy." June 14, TV5.

Douglas, Bronwen. 1998. "Dealing (with) Death in a Melanesian World: Indigenous Aetiologies of and the 'Sickness of the Christians.'" In *Across the Great Divide: Journeys in History and Anthropology,* 263-284. Amsterdam: Harwood.

Douglas, Mary. 1966. *Purity and Danger: An Analysis of Concepts of Pollution and Taboo.* London: Routledge & Kegan Paul.

Dow, Derek A. 2001. "'Pruned of Its Dangers': The Tohunga Suppression Act 1907." *Health and History* 3, no. 1: 41–64

Dowbiggin, Ian Robert. 1991. *Inheriting Madness: Professionalization and Psychiatric Knowledge in Nineteenth-Century France.* Berkeley: University of California Press.

Duncan, Nicole. 2000. "Death on Fiji Plantations, 1900–1909." In *Chalo Jahaji: On a Journey through Indenture in Fiji,* edited by Brij V. Lal, 291–323. Suva: Fiji Museum; Canberra: Division of Pacific and Asian History, Australian National University; Prashant Pacific Book.

Edington, Claire. 2013. "Going In and Getting Out of the Colonial Asylum: Families and Psychiatric Care in French Indochina." *Comparative Studies in Society and History* 55, no. 3: 725–755.

Edwards, Christopher, Andrea Hobkirk, LaBarron K. Hill, Rose Brown, Goldie Byrd, and Keith Whitfield. 2014. "Dementia." In *Cultural Sociology of Mental Illness: An A-to-Z Guide,* edited by Andrew Scull, vol. 1, 184–187. Thousand Oaks, CA: SAGE Reference.

Ernst, Waltraud. 1991a. "Colonial Psychiatry: The European Insane in British India, 1800–58." In *150 Years of British Psychiatry 1841–1991,* edited by German E. Berrios and Hugh Freeman, 152–162. London: Gaskell.

———. 1991b. "Racial, Social and Cultural Factors in the Development of a Colonial Institution: The Bombay Lunatic Asylum (1670–1858)." *Internationales Asienforum* 22, no. 3/4: 61–80.

———. 1996. "European Madness and Gender in Nineteenth-Century British India." *Social History of Medicine* 9, no. 3: 357–382.

———. 1997. "Idioms of Madness and Colonial Boundaries: The Case of the European and 'Native' Mentally Ill in Early Nineteenth-Century British India." *Comparative Studies in Society and History* 39, no. 1: 153–181.

———. 1998. "Asylum Provision and the East India Company in the Nineteenth Century." *Medical History* 42, no. 4: 476–502.

———. 1999a. "Colonial Policies, Racial Politics and the Development of Psychiatric Institutions in Early Nineteenth-Century British India." In *Race, Science and Medicine, 1700–1960,* edited by Waltraud Ernst and Bernard Harris, 80–101. London: Routledge.

———. 1999b. "Introduction: Historical and Contemporary Perspectives on Race, Science and Medicine." In *Race, Science and Medicine, 1700–1960,* edited by Waltraud Ernst and Bernard Harris, 1–29. London: Routledge.

———. 2007. "Beyond East and West: From the History of Colonial Medicine to a Social History of Medicine(s) in South Asia." *Social History of Medicine* 20, no. 3: 505–524.

———. 2013. *Colonialism and Transnational Psychiatry: The Development of an Indian Mental Hospital in British India, c. 1925–1940.* London: Anthem Press.

———, ed. 2016. *Work, Psychiatry and Society, c. 1750–2015.* Manchester: Manchester University Press.

Ernst, Waltraud, and Thomas Mueller, eds. 2010. *Transnational Psychiatries: Social and Cultural Histories of Psychiatry in Comparative Perspective, c. 1800–2000.* Newcastle-upon-Tyne, UK: Cambridge Scholars Publishing.

Eves, Richard. 1999. "Going Troppo: Images of White Savagery, Degeneration and Race in Turn-of-the-Century Colonial Fictions of the Pacific." *History and Anthropology* 11, no. 2: 351–385.

———. 2005. "Unsettling Settler Colonialism: Debates over Climate and Colonization in New Guinea, 1875–1914." *Ethnic and Racial Studies* 28, no. 2: 304–330.

Fabrega, H. 2009. *History of Mental Illness in India: A Cultural Psychiatric Retrospective.* Delhi: Motilal Banarsidass.

Fanon, Frantz. 1952. *Black Skin, White Masks.* Translated by Charles Lam Markmann. New York: Grove Press.

Feilding Star. 1884. "Fiji News." June 26.

Fernando, Suman. 2011. "A 'Global' Mental Health Program or Markets for Big Pharma." *Open Mind* 168 (September/October): 22.

———. 2014. *Mental Health Worldwide: Culture, Globalization and Development.* London: Palgrave Macmillan.

Ferraro, A. 1959. "Organic Conditions: Senile Psychosis." In *American Handbook of Psychiatry,* vol. 2, edited by Silvano Arieti, 1038–1045. New York: Basic Books.

Fiji Bureau of Statistics. 2012. "1.2A Census Population of Fiji by Ethnicity." Accessed March 30, 2016. http://www.statsfiji.gov.fj.

Fiji Government. 1884–1940. *Blue Book of Fiji.* Suva: Government Printer.

———. 1911a. *Annual Medical Report, 1910.* CP 40/11. Suva: Government Printer.

———. 1911b. *Report on the Census of the Population of Fiji, 1911.* CP 44/11. Suva: Government Printer.

———. 1912. *Annual Medical Report, 1911.* CP 28/12. Suva: Government Printer.

———. 1916. *Public Lunatic Asylum: Report for the Year 1916.* CP 54/16. Suva: Government Printer.

———. 1919. *Public Lunatic Asylum: Report for the Year 1918.* CP 21/19. Suva: Government Printer.

———. 1928. *Medical Department: Annual Report for 1927.* CP 57/28. Suva: Government Printer.

———. 1950. *Medical Department: Annual Report for 1949.* CP 24/50. Suva: Government Printer.

———. 1957. *Medical Department: Annual Report for 1956.* CP 36/57. Suva: Government Printer.

———. 1961. *Medical Department: Annual Report for 1960.* CP 32/61. Suva: Government Printer.

———. 1962. *Medical Department: Annual Report for 1961.* CP 39/62. Suva: Government Printer.

———. 1965. *Medical Department: Annual Report for 1964.* CP 12/65. Suva: Government Printer.

———. 1966. *Medical Department: Annual Report for 1965.* CP 30/66. Suva: Government Printer.

———. 1968. *Medical Department: Annual Report for 1966.* CP 12/68. Suva: Government Printer.

———. 1969. *Medical Department: Annual Report for 1968.* CP 39/6. Suva: Government Printer.

———. 1972. *Medical Department: Annual Report for 1970.* PP 17/72. Suva: Government Printer.

Fiji Times. 2005. "Beddoes Laments Killer's Release." August 29.
———. 2007. "The Sad Tale of Two Boys." July 7.
———. 2009. "St Giles Plans to Go Regional." October 24.
Finnane, Mark. 1985. "Asylums, Families and the State." *History Workshop Journal* 20, no. 1: 134–148.
———. 2003. "From Dangerous Lunatic to Human Rights?: The Law and Mental Illness in Australian History." In *"Madness" in Australia: Histories, Heritage and the Asylum*, edited by Catharine Coleborne and Dolly MacKinnon, 23–33. St. Lucia: University of Queensland Press and API Network.
Forsyth, Jenny. 2004. "Four Years Locked in a Poultry Coop, the Next 20 Tied to a Bed: The Boy who was Brought up as a Chicken." *The Guardian*, July 11. Accessed May 31, 2016. http://www.theguardian.com/world/2004/jul/11/fiji.jennyforsyth.
Foster, Kim, Kim Usher, Sainimere Gadai, and Rusieli Taukei. 2009. " 'There Is No Health without Mental Health': Implementing the First Mental Health Nursing Postgraduate Program in Fiji." *Contemporary Nurse* 32, nos. 1–2: 179–186.
Foucault, Michel. 1965. *Madness and Civilization*. Translated by Richard Howard. New York: Random House.
———. 1978. *The History of Sexuality, Volume 1: An Introduction*. Translated by Robert Hurley. New York: Random House.
Fowler, Glenn. 2000. "'A Want of Care': Death and Disease on Fiji Plantations, 1890–1900." In *Chalo Jahaji: On a Journey through Indenture in Fiji*, edited by Brij V. Lal, 272–290. Suva: Fiji Museum; Canberra: Division of Pacific and Asian History, Australian National University.
Frank, Leonard Roy, ed. 1978. *The History of Shock Treatment*. San Francisco: Leonard Roy Frank.
Fynes-Clinton, Matthew. 2007. "'Chicken Boy' Test Case for Humanity." *Courier-Mail*, March 20.
———. 2011. "A Ministry of One." *Courier-Mail*, March 26.
Garnham, Florence. 1918. *A Report on the Social and Moral Conditions of Indians in Fiji*. Sydney: F. E. Garnham.
Garrett, John. 1973. "Motivation, Values and Goals for Economic Development: The Case of Daku." In *Tourism in Fiji: Ray Parkinson Memorial Lectures*, 57–61. Suva: University of the South Pacific.
———. 1997. *Where Nets Were Cast: Christianity in Oceania since World War II*. Geneva: Institute of Pacific Studies, University of the South Pacific in association with World Council of Churches.
Garton, Stephen. 1988. *Medicine and Madness: A Social History of Insanity in New South Wales, 1880–1940*. Kensington: New South Wales University Press.
Gatty, Ronald. 2010. *Fijian-English Dictionary: With Notes on Fijian Culture and Natural History*. Suva: Southeast Asia Program, Cornell University.
Ghosh, Durba, and Dane Kennedy, eds. 2006. *Decentring Empire: Britain, India and the Transcolonial World*. Hyderabad: Orient Longman.
Gill, Kuldip. 2010. *Indian Women in Fiji: Their Health Choices*. Vancouver: Webzines of Vancouver.

Gillion, Ken L. 1962. *Fiji's Indian Migrants: A History to the End of Indenture in 1920.* Melbourne: Oxford University Press.
———. 1977. *The Fiji Indians: Challenge to European Dominance, 1920–1946.* Canberra: Australian National University Press.
Gilman, Sander L. 1985. *Difference and Pathology: Stereotypes of Sexuality, Race and Madness.* Ithaca, NY: Cornell University Press.
Gittins, Diana. 1998. *Madness in Its Place: Narratives of Severalls Hospital, 1913–1997.* London: Routledge.
Gluckman, Laurie Kalman. 1969. "Drau Ni Kau: The Ethnopsychiatry of Fiji in Historical and Clinical Perspective." *Australian and New Zealand Journal of Psychiatry* 3, no. 3: 152–158.
Goddard, Michael. 1988. "Psychiatry in Papua New Guinea: A Critique." PhD diss., University of Auckland.
———. 1992. "Bedlam in Paradise: A Critical History of Psychiatry in Papua New Guinea." *Journal of Pacific History* 27, no. 1: 55–72.
———. 1998. "What Makes Hari Run? The Social Construction of Madness in a Highland Papua New Guinea Society." *Critique of Anthropology* 18, no. 1: 61–81.
———. 2011. *Out of Place: Madness in the Highlands of Papua New Guinea.* New York: Berghahn Books.
Goldson, Anna. 2008. *An Island Calling.* 75 min. Auckland: Occasional Production.
Gounder, Kevin, and Luciana Brugnoli. 1998. "Mental Health Education." *Mental Health Nursing Newsletter,* February–March. St Giles Hospital file (STG) 2/3/9.
Grey River Argus. 1883. "Twelve Years' Penal Servitude." May 25.
Griffin, Chris, and Michael Monsell-Davis. 1986. *Fijians in Town.* Suva: Institute of Pacific Studies, University of the South Pacific.
Guthrie, Margaret W. 1979. *Misi Utu: Dr D. W. Hoodless and the Development of Medical Education in the South Pacific.* Suva: Institute of Pacific Studies, University of the South Pacific with the South Pacific Social Sciences Association.
Halliday, Emma Catherine. 2003. "Themes in Scottish Asylum Culture: The Hospitalisation of the Scottish Asylum 1880–1914." PhD thesis, University of Stirling.
Hare, Edward H. 1959. "The Origin and Spread of Dementia Paralytica." *British Journal of Psychiatry* 105, no. 440: 594–626.
———. 1998. *On the History of Lunacy: The 19th Century and After.* London: Gabbay.
Harper, Philip. 1916. "The Late Sequelae of Framboesia." *Lancet* 188 (4859): 678–679.
———. 1917. "Yaws as a Distinct Disease in Fiji." *Transactions of the Royal Society of Tropical Medicine and Hygiene* 10, no. 6: 114–116.
Harthorn, Barbara Herr. 2005. "Gender, Health Inequality, and Hidden Healers in Rural Fiji." *Fijian Studies: A Journal of Contemporary Fiji* 3, no. 2: 337–356.
Hattori, Anne Perez. 2004. *Colonial Dis-Ease: US Navy Health Policies and the Chamorros of Guam, 1898–1941.* Honolulu: University of Hawai'i Press.
Hawton, K. 2000. "Sex and Suicide: Gender Differences in Suicidal Behaviour." *British Journal of Psychiatry* 177, no. 6: 484–485.
Haynes, Ruth H. 1984. "Suicide in Fiji: A Preliminary Study." *British Journal of Psychiatry* 145, no. 4: 433–438.

——— 1987. "Suicide and Social Response in Fiji: A Historical Survey." *British Journal of Psychiatry* 151, no. 1: 21–26.

Hazlewood, David. 1872. *A Fijian and English and an English and Fijian Dictionary: With Examples of Common and Peculiar Modes of Expression and Uses of Words, also, Containing Brief Hints on Native Customs, Proverbs, the Native Names of Natural Productions, and Notices of the Islands of Fiji, and a Grammar of the Language, with Examples of Native Idioms,* edited by James Calvert. London: S. Low, Marston.

Healy, David. 2002. *The Creation of Psychopharmacology.* Cambridge, MA: Harvard University Press.

———. 2008. *Mania: A Short History of Bipolar Disorder.* Baltimore, MD: Johns Hopkins University Press.

Hellier, Charles. 1954. "The 1/- Drug that Halts Insanity." *Australasian Post,* February 25.

Henderson, George C. 1931. *Fiji and the Fijians 1835–1856.* Sydney: Angus and Robertson Ltd.

Hereniko, Vilsoni. 1995. *Woven Gods: Female Clowns and Power in Rotuma.* Honolulu: University of Hawai'i Press.

Holloway, Judith. 2001. "'Unfortunate Folk': A Study of the Social Context of Committal to Seacliff 1928–1937." In *"Unfortunate Folk": Essays on Mental Health Treatment 1863–1992,* edited by Barbara Brookes and Jane Thomson, 153–167. Dunedin, NZ: University of Otago Press.

Holt, Edgar K., Gladys Ward-Dunn, Bodhan Th. Nedilsky, and G. Donald Niswander. 1955. "Clinical Comparison of Raudixin and Rau-Sed in Chronic Mental Illness." *Diseases of the Nervous System* 16, no. 7: 222–223.

Hoodless, David Winn. 1947. *Central Medical School, Suva, Fiji.* Suva: Medical Department, Public Relations Office.

Howard, Alan. 1979. "The Power to Heal in Colonial Rotuma." *Journal of the Polynesian Society* 88, no. 3: 243–275.

Inglis, Kerri A. 2013. *Mai Lepera: Disease and Displacement in Nineteenth-Century Hawai'i.* Honolulu: University of Hawai'i Press.

———. 2014. "Disease and the 'Other': The Role of Medical Imperialism in Oceania." In *Native Diasporas: Indigenous Identities and Settler Colonialism in the Americas,* edited by Gregory D. Smithers and Brooke N. Newman, 385–410. Lincoln: University of Nebraska Press.

Jackson, Lynette A. 1997. "Narratives of 'Madness' and Power: A History of Ingutsheni Mental Hospital and Social Order in Colonial Zimbabwe, 1908–1959." PhD thesis, Columbia University.

———. 1999. "The Place of Psychiatry in Colonial and Early Postcolonial Zimbabwe." *International Journal of Mental Health* 28, no. 2: 38–71.

———. 2005. *Surfacing Up: Psychiatry and Social Order in Colonial Zimbabwe, 1908–1968.* Ithaca, NY: Cornell University Press.

Jackson, Will. 2013. *Madness and Marginality: The Lives of Kenya's White Insane.* Manchester: Manchester University Press.

Jaworski, Katrina. 2014. *The Gender of Suicide: Knowledge Production, Theory and Suicidology.* Farnham, UK: Ashgate.

Jayawardena, Chandra. 1975a. "Farm, Household and Family in Fiji Indian Rural Society: Part One." *Journal of Comparative Family Studies* 6, no. 1: 74–88.

———. 1975b. "Farm, Household and Family in Fiji Indian Rural Society: Part Two." *Journal of Comparative Family Studies* 6, no. 2: 209–221.

Jinna, Kantilal, and Francis Mangubhai, eds. 2008. *Gujaratis in Fiji Islands: Personal Glimpses.* Flynn: Gujarat Samaj of Fiji.

Jolly, Margaret. 1998. "Other Mothers: Maternal 'Insouciance' and the Depopulation Debate in Fiji and Vanuatu, 1890–1930." In *Maternities and Modernities: Colonial and Postcolonial Experiences in Asia and the Pacific,* edited by Kalpana Ram and Margaret Jolly, 177–212. Cambridge: Cambridge University Press.

Jones, Margaret. 2008. "The Most Cruel and Revolting Crimes: The Treatment of the Mentally Ill in Mid-Nineteenth-Century Jamaica." *Journal of Caribbean History* 42, no. 2: 290–309.

Joyce, Roger B. 1971. *Sir William MacGregor.* Melbourne: Oxford University Press.

Kakar, Sudhir. 1982. *Shamans, Mystics and Doctors: A Psychological Inquiry into India and Its Healing Traditions.* New Delhi: Oxford University Press.

Kale, Rajendra. 1997. "Bringing Epilepsy out of the Shadows." *British Medical Journal* 315, no. 7099: 2–3.

Kalinowsky, Lothar B. 1959. "Convulsive Shock Treatment." In *American Handbook of Psychiatry,* vol. 2, edited by Silvano Arieti, 1499–1520. New York: Basic Books.

Kaplan, Martha. 1989. "*Luve Ni Wai* as the British Saw It: Constructions of Custom and Disorder in Colonial Fiji." *Ethnohistory* 36, no. 4: 349–371.

———. 1990. "Meaning, Agency and Colonial History: Navosavakadua and the Tuka Movement in Fiji." *American Ethnologist* 17, no. 1: 3–22.

———. 1995. *Neither Cargo nor Cult: Ritual Politics and the Colonial Imagination in Fiji.* Durham, NC: Duke University Press.

Kaplan, Martha, and John Kelly. 1994. "Rethinking Resistance: Dialogics of 'Disaffection' in Colonial Fiji." *American Ethnologist* 21, no. 1: 123–151.

Karim, Issac. 1996. "A Brief History of St. Giles Hospital." Unpublished typescript, St Giles Hospital, Suva.

Karim, Isaac, and John Price. 1973. "Suicide in Fiji." *Fiji Medical Journal* 1, no. 3: 49–55.

Kasuga, Naoki. 1994. "Christ, the Devil, and Money: Witchcraft in Fijian Society." *Man and Culture in Oceania* 10, no. 1: 39–57.

Kate, Talebula. 2014. "Kaisau Insanity Case Back in Suva Court." *Fiji Sun Online,* April 23. Accessed March 11, 2019. http://fijisun.com.fj/2014/04/23/kaisau-insanity-case-back-in-suva-court.

———. 2015. "Mental Health Law Confusing." *Fiji Times,* September 23. Accessed March 12, 2019. https://www.fijitimes.com/mental-health-law-confusing.

Katz, Richard. 1999. *The Straight Path of the Spirit: Ancestral Wisdom and Healing Traditions in Fiji.* Rochester, VT: Park Street Press.

Keller, Richard C. 2001. "Madness and Colonization: Psychiatry in the British and French Empires 1800–1962." *Journal of Social History* 35, no. 2: 295–326.

———. 2007. *Colonial Madness: Psychiatry in French North Africa.* Chicago: University of Chicago Press.

Kelly, John Dunham. 1991. *A Politics of Virtue: Hinduism, Sexuality, and Countercolonial Discourse in Fiji.* Chicago: University of Chicago Press.

Kendler, Kenneth S. 1995. "Delusional Disorder: Clinical Section." In *A History of Clinical Psychiatry: The Origin and History of Psychiatric Disorders,* edited by German Berrios and Roy Porter, 360–383. New York: New York University Press.

Kimmich, Robert A. 1956. "100 Years of Hawaiian Psychiatry." *Hawaii Medical Journal* 15, no. 4: 345–347.

Kleinman, Arthur. 1988. *Rethinking Psychiatry: From Cultural Category to Personal Experience.* New York: Free Press.

Kleinman, Arthur, and Byron Good, eds. 1985. *Culture and Depression: Studies in the Anthropology and Cross-Cultural Psychiatry of Affect and Disorder.* Berkeley: University of California Press.

Knapman, Bruce. 1985. "The Rise and Fall of the White Sugar Planter in Fiji 1880–1925." *Pacific Studies* 9, no. 1: 53–82.

Knapman, Claudia. 1986. *White Women in Fiji, 1835–1930: The Ruin of Empire?* Sydney: Allen and Unwin.

Kritsotaki, Despo, Vicky Long, and Matthew Smith, eds. 2016. *Deinstitutionalisation and After: Post-War Psychiatry in the Western World.* Cham: Palgrave MacMillan.

Labrum, Bronwen. 1992. "Looking beyond the Asylum: Gender and the Process of Committal to Auckland, 1870–1919." *New Zealand Journal of History* 26, no. 2: 125–144.

———. 1994. "A Woman's World in a Male Universe: Treatment and Rehabilitation at the Auckland Lunatic Asylum, 1870–1910." In *New Countries and Old Medicine: Proceedings of an International Conference on the History of Medicine and Health,* edited by Linda Bryder and Derek A. Dow, 196–203. Auckland: Auckland Medical Historical Society.

———. 2005. "The Boundaries of Femininity: Madness and Gender in New Zealand, 1870–1910." In *Women, Madness and the Law: A Feminist Reader* edited by Wendy Chan, Dorothy E. Chunn, and Robert Menzies, 59–77. London: GlassHouse Press.

Laing, James M. 1889. "Hand Book for Surgeons Superintendent of the Coolie Emigration Service." British Colonial Office, March.

Laing, Ronald David. 1960. *The Divided Self: An Existential Study in Sanity and Madness.* London: Tavistock.

Lal, Brij V. 1983. *Girmitiyas: The Origins of the Fiji Indians.* Canberra: Journal of Pacific History.

———. 1985. "Veil of Dishonour: Sexual Jealousy and Suicide on Fiji Plantations." *Journal of Pacific History* 20, no. 3: 135–155.

———. 1986. "Murmurs of Dissent: Non-Resistance on Fiji Plantations." *Hawaiian Journal of History* 20: 188–214.

———. 1992. *Broken Waves: A History of the Fiji Islands in the Twentieth Century.* Honolulu: University of Hawai'i Press.

———. 1997. *A Vision for Change: A. D. Patel and the Politics of Fiji.* Canberra: Australian National University Press.

———. 1998. *Crossing the Kala Pani: A Documentary History of Indian Indenture in Fiji*. Canberra: Division of Pacific and Asian History, Australian National University; Suva: Fiji Museum.

———, ed. 2000. *Chalo Jahaji: On a Journey through Indenture in Fiji*. Suva: Fiji Museum; Canberra: Division of Pacific and Asian History, Australian National University.

Lambert, Sylvester Maxwell. 1929. "Yaws in the South Pacific." *American Journal of Tropical Medicine and Hygiene* s1-9, no. 6: 429–437.

———. 1946. *A Doctor in Paradise*. London: J. M. Dent.

Lateef, Shireen. 1990. "Rule by the *Danda*: Domestic Violence among Indo-Fijians." *Pacific Studies* 13, no. 3: 43–62.

Leckie, Jacqueline. 1997. *To Labour with the State: The Fiji Public Service Association*. Dunedin, NZ: University of Otago Press.

———. 2000. "Mapping and Managing Madness: Towards a History of Insanity in Fiji." Unpublished paper, Pacific History Association, Canberra.

———. 2002a. "The Complexities of Women's Agency in Fiji.' In *Gender Politics in the Asia-Pacific Region* edited by Brenda Yeoh, Peggy Teo, and Shirlena Huang, 156–180. London: Routledge.

———. 2002b. "Gendering Madness in Fiji." Unpublished paper, Association of Social Anthropologists of Oceania conference, Auckland.

———. 2003. "The Embodiment of Madness and Gender in Colonial Fiji." Unpublished paper, Association of Social Anthropologists of Oceania conference, Vancouver.

———. 2004a. "Modernity and the Management of Madness in Colonial Fiji." *Paideuma* 50, no. 1: 551–574.

———. 2004b. "The Qawa 'Epidemic.'" In *Bittersweet: The Indo-Fijian Experience*, edited by Brij V. Lal, 191–208. Canberra: Pandanus Books.

———. 2005a. "Discourses and Technologies of Mental Health in Post-War Fiji." In *The Defining Years, Pacific Islands, 1945–65*, edited by Brij V. Lal, 151–173. Canberra: Australian National University.

———. 2005b. "The Embodiment of Gender and Madness in Colonial Fiji." *Fijian Studies* 3, no. 2: 312–337.

———. 2007. "Unsettled Minds: Colonialism, Gender and Settling Madness in Fiji." In *Psychiatry and Empire*, edited by Sloan Mahone and Megan Vaughan, 99–123. Houndmills, UK: Palgrave Macmillan.

———. 2010. "Islands, Communities and Entangled Madness: Transferring Psychiatry to the Colonial Pacific, 1884–1964." In *Transnational Psychiatries: Social and Cultural Histories of Psychiatry in Comparative Perspective, c. 1800–2000*, edited by Waltraud Ernst and Thomas Mueller, 24–50. Newcastle-upon-Tyne, UK: Cambridge Scholars Publishing.

———. 2012. "'Lost Souls': Madness, Suicide and Migration in Colonial Fiji until 1920." In *Migration, Ethnicity, and Mental Health: International Perspectives, 1840–2010*, edited by Angela McCarthy and Catharine Coleborne, 123–140. New York: Routledge.

Leckie, Jacqueline, and Alumita Durutalo. 2015. "Kai Merika! Fijian Children of American Servicemen." In *Mothers' Darlings of the South Pacific: The Children of Indige-*

nous Women and US Servicemen, World War Two, edited by Judy Bennett and Angela Wanhalla, 283–310. Honolulu: University of Hawai'i Press.

Leckie, Jacqueline, and Frances Hughes. 2017. "Mental Health in the Smaller Pacific States." In *Mental Health in Asia and the Pacific: Historical and Comparative Perspectives,* edited by Harry Minas and Milton Lewis, 253–272. New York: Springer.

Leese, Peter. 2001. "Essay Review: Making Shell-shock." *British Journal of Psychology* 92, no. 2: 411–415.

Levine, Philippa. 2003. *Prostitution, Race and Politics: Policing Venereal Disease in the British Empire.* New York: Routledge.

Lewa, Sainimiu. 2002. "Madman Attacks Asylum Staff." *Fiji Times,* January 18.

Lewis, Aubrey. 1970. "Paranoia and Paranoid: A Historical Perspective." *Psychological Medicine* 1, no. 1: 2–12.

Lewis, Milton. 1988. *Managing Madness: Psychiatry and Society in Australia 1788–1980.* Canberra: Australian Government Publishing Service.

Lewis, Milton J., and Kerrie L. MacPherson, eds. 2008. *Public Health in Asia and the Pacific: Historical and Comparative Perspectives.* London: Routledge.

Lewis, Zoe. 2011. "Plight of 'Chicken Boy.'" *Knox Leader,* April 5.

Lidz, Theodore. 1946. "Psychiatric Casualties from Guadalcanal: A Study of Reactions to Extreme Stress." *Psychiatry* 9, no. 46: 193–213.

Lipphardt, Veronika, and Alexandra Widmer. 2016. Introduction to *Health and Difference: Rendering Human Variation in Colonial Engagements,* edited by Alexandra Widmer and Veronika Lipphardt, 1–19. New York: Berghahn Books.

LiPuma, Edward. 2000. *Encompassing Others: The Magic of Modernity in Melanesia.* Ann Arbor: University of Michigan Press.

Littlewood, Roland, and Simon Dein, eds. 2000a. *Cultural Psychiatry and Medical Anthropology: An Introduction and Reader.* London: Athlone Press.

———. 2000b. Introduction to *Cultural Psychiatry and Medical Anthropology: An Introduction and Reader,* edited by Roland Littlewood and Simon Dein, 1–34. London: Athlone Press.

Löckenhoff, Corinna E., Filip De Fruyt, Antonio Terraciano, Robert R. McCrae, Marleen De Bolle, Paul Costa, Martia Aguilar-Vafaie, et al. 2009. "Perceptions of Aging across 26 Cultures and Their Culture-Level Associates." *Psychology and Aging* 24, no. 4: 941–954.

López-Muñoz, Francisco, Ronaldo Ucha-Udabe, and Cecilio Alamo. 2005. "The History of Barbiturates a Century after Their Clinical Introduction." *Neuropsychiatric Disease and Treatment* 1, no. 4: 329–343.

Luker, Vicki. 2005. "A Tale of Two Mothers: Colonial Constructions of Indian and Fijian Maternity." *Fijian Studies* 3, no. 2: 357–374.

Lukere, Vicki. 2002. "Native Obstetric Nursing in Fiji." In *Birthing in the Pacific: Beyond Tradition and Modernity?* edited by Vicki Lukere and Margaret Jolly, 100–124. Honolulu: University of Hawai'i Press.

Lukere, Vicki, and Margaret Jolly, eds. 2002. *Birthing in the Pacific: Beyond Tradition and Modernity?* Honolulu: University of Hawai'i Press.

Lukere, Victoria. 1997. "Mothers of the Taukei: Fijian Women and 'the Decrease of the Race.'" PhD diss., Australian National University.

Lynch, G. W. A. 1917. "Yaws and Syphilis." *Transactions of the Royal Society of Tropical Medicine and Hygiene* 10, no. 6: 116–117.

Macgregor, Duncan F. 1967. "Notes of a Meeting between Three South Pacific Psychiatrists." In *Mental Health in the South Pacific: Report of a Meeting of Experts Held at Suva (Fiji) from 19 to 22 May, and at Noumea (New Caledonia) from 23 to 27 May,* by South Pacific Commission, 1–10. Technical paper no. 154. Nouméa: South Pacific Commission.

MacGregor, William. 1872. "Pathological Appendix." In *Medical Report of the Royal Lunatic Asylum of Aberdeen, for the Year Ending 31st December 1871,* 25–28. Aberdeen: Leslie and Russell.

MacKinnon, Dolly. 2003. "'Hearing Madness': The Soundscape of the Asylum." In *"Madness" in Australia: Histories, Heritage and the Asylum,* edited by Catharine Coleborne and Dolly MacKinnon, 73–82. St. Lucia: University of Queensland Press and API Network.

Macnaught, Timothy J. 1982. *The Fijian Colonial Experience: A Study of the Neotraditional Order under British Colonial Rule Prior to World War II.* Canberra: Australian National University.

Mageo, Jeannette Marie. 1998. *Theorizing Self in Samoa: Emotions, Genders, and Sexualities.* Ann Arbor: University of Michigan Press.

Mahone, Sloan, and Megan Vaughan, eds. 2007. *Psychiatry and Empire.* Houndmills, UK: Palgrave Macmillan.

Manson-Bahr, Philip Edmund Clinton. 1954. "Fijian Syphilis." *Transactions of the Royal Society of Tropical Medicine and Hygiene* 48, no. 3: 242–246.

Manson-Bahr, Philip Henry. 1928. "Yaws." *British Journal of Venereal Diseases* 4, no. 1: 44–54.

Marks, Shula. 1999. "'Every Facility that Modern Science and Enlightened Humanity Have Devised': Race and Progress in a Colonial Hospital, Valkenberg Mental Asylum, Cape Colony, 1894–1910." In *Insanity, Institutions and Society, 1800–1914: A Social History of Madness in Comparative Perspective,* edited by Joseph Melling and Bill Forsythe, 268–292. London: Routledge.

———. 2007. "The Microphysics of Power: Mental Nursing in South Africa in the First Half of the Twentieth Century." In *Psychiatry and Empire,* edited by Sloan Mahone and Megan Vaughan, 67–98. Houndmills, UK: Palgrave Macmillan.

Marland, Hilary. 1999. "'Destined to a Perfect Recovery': The Confinement of Puerperal Insanity in the Nineteenth Century." In *Insanity, Institutions and Society, 1800–1914: A Social History of Madness in Comparative Perspective,* edited by Joseph Melling and Bill Forsythe, 137–156. London: Routledge.

———. 2004. *Dangerous Motherhood: Insanity and Childbirth in Victorian England.* Basingstoke, UK: Palgrave Macmillan.

Marlborough Express. 1883. "Attempted Wife Murder in Fiji." February 28.

Marzan, Jean de. 1987. "Customs and Beliefs in Central Viti Levu: Papers from *Anthropos,* 1907–1913." Translated by Nicholas Thomas. *DomoDomo: Fiji Museum Journal* 5, no. 4: 28–62.

Masters, Catherine. 2008. "Scientists Want 'Chicken Boy' in Auckland to Pick His Brain." *New Zealand Herald*, September 6.

Mayer, Adrian C. 1973. *Peasants in the Pacific: A Study of Aspects of Fiji Indian Rural Society*, 2nd ed. London: Routledge & Kegan Paul.

McCarthy, Angela. 2015. *Migration, Ethnicity and Madness: New Zealand, 1860–1910*. Dunedin, NZ: Otago University Press.

McCarthy, Angela, and Catharine Coleborne. 2012a. "Introduction: Mental Health, Migration and Ethnicity." In *Migration, Ethnicity and Mental Health: International Perspectives, 1840–2010*, edited by Angela McCarthy and Catharine Coleborne, 1–14. New York: Routledge.

———, eds. 2012b. *Migration, Ethnicity and Mental Health: International Perspectives, 1840–2010*. New York: Routledge.

McClintock, Anne. 1995. *Imperial Leather: Race, Gender and Sexuality in the Colonial Contest*. New York: Routledge.

McCulloch, Jock. 1995. *Colonial Psychiatry and "The African Mind."* Cambridge: Cambridge University Press.

McDonagh, Patrick. 2008. *Idiocy: A Cultural History*. Liverpool: Liverpool University Press.

McLane, John Ryan. 2012. "Setting a Barricade against the East Wind: Western Polynesia and the 1918 Influenza Pandemic." PhD thesis, University of Otago.

Melling, Joseph. 1999. "Accommodating Madness: New Research in the Social History of Insanity and Institutions." In *Insanity, Institutions and Society, 1800–1914: A Social History of Madness in Comparative Perspective*, edited by Joseph Melling and Bill Forsythe, 1–30. London: Routledge.

Melling, Joseph, and Bill Forsythe, eds. 2006. *The Politics of Madness: The State, Insanity, and Society in England, 1845–1914*. London: Routledge.

Mercier, C. 1902. *A Text-Book of Insanity*. London: Swan, Sonnenschein.

Micale, Mark S. 1995. *Approaching Hysteria: Disease and Its Interpretations*. Princeton, NJ: Princeton University Press.

Miles, John. 1997. *Infectious Diseases: Colonising the Pacific?* Dunedin, NZ: University of Otago Press.

Mills, China. 2014. *Decolonizing Global Mental Health: The Psychiatrization of the Majority World*. London: Routledge.

Mills, James. 2000. *Madness, Cannabis and Colonialism: The Native Only Lunatic Asylums of British India 1857–1900*. Houndmills, UK: Macmillan.

———. 2001. "The History of Modern Psychiatry in India, 1858–1947." *History of Psychiatry* 12, no. 4: 431–458.

Minas, Harry, and Milton Lewis, eds. 2017. *Mental Health in Asia and the Pacific: Historical and Cultural Perspectives*. New York: Springer.

Mishra, Sudesh. 2012. "'Bending Closer to the Ground': Girmit as Minor History." *Australian Humanities Review* 52: n.p. Accessed March 11, 2019. http://australianhumanitiesreview.org/2012/05/01/bending-closer-to-the-ground-girmit-as-minor-history.

Montague, Aubrey. 1914. "Report by A. Montague, M.B. on the Use of Salvarsan at the Colonial Hospital, in 1913." In Fiji Government, *Annual Medical Report, 1913,* CP 44/14, 12. Suva: Government Printer.

———. 1930. "Native Medical Practitioners." *The Native Medical Practitioner* 1, no. 1: 2–4.

Morris, Pamela K., and Thambu Maniam. 2000. "Suicide in Fiji: A Review of the Literature." *Asia Pacific Journal of Public Health* 12, no. 1: 46–48.

Moss, Peter D., and Colin P. McEvedy. 1966. "An Epidemic of Overbreathing among Schoolgirls." *British Medical Journal* 2 (November): 1295–1300.

Mouchenik, Yoram. 2001–2002. "La psychiatrie colonial en Nouvelle-Calédonie." *Journal de la Société des Océanistes* 113: 109–119.

Mukherjee, Siddhartha. 2012. "Post-Prozac Nation." *New York Times*, April 19.

Munro, Doug. 1990. "The Origins of Labourers in the South Pacific: Commentary and Statistics." In *Labour in the South Pacific,* edited by Clive Moore, Jacqueline Leckie, and Doug Munro, xxxix–li. Townsville, AU: James Cook University of North Queensland.

———. 1993. "Patterns of Resistance and Accommodation." In *Plantation Workers: Resistance and Accommodation,* edited by Brij Lal, Doug Munro, and Edward Beechert, 1–43. Honolulu: University of Hawai'i Press.

Murphy, Henry B. M. 1978. *Mental Health Trends in the Pacific Islands: Report on a Tour of Pacific Territories, September 1977–March 1978.* Noumea, New Caledonia: South Pacific Commission.

Murphy, Henry B. M., and Ram Narayan. 1979. "Mental Hospitalisation in Fiji." *Fiji Medical Journal* 7, no. 1: 4–11.

Nabobo-Baba, Unaisi. 2006. *Knowing and Learning: An Indigenous Fijian Approach.* Suva: Institute of Pacific Studies, University of the South Pacific.

Nabukavou, Thelma Smith, Luke Butler Taveta, Joan Martin Teaiwa, and Teresia Teaiwa. 2013. "Reflecting back and Building on *Fright or Light*: Psychiatric Survivors and Contemporary Issues in Mental Health in Fiji." In *Pacific Identities and Well-Being: Cross-Cultural Perspectives,* edited by Margaret Nelson Agee, Tracey McIntosh, Philip Culbertson, and Cabrini 'Ofa Makasiale, 242–259. New York: Routledge.

Nabukavou, Thelma Smith, and Joan Teaiwa, eds. 2008. *Fright or Light: Surviving Mental Illness.* Suva: Leadership Fiji.

Naidu, Vijay. 1980. *The Violence of Indenture in Fiji.* Suva: World University Press in Association with the School of Social and Economic Development, University of the South Pacific.

Narayan, Dorine. 2008. "Ministry Links up with Society for Poor." *Fiji Times,* July 31.

Narayan, Ram. 1974. "Native Healing." Unpublished typescript, March 7. STG 2/3. St Giles Hospital.

———. 1975. "Report from St. Giles Hospital." *Fiji Medical Journal* 3, no. 12: 275–276, 280.

Narayan, Shishram. 2003. "Traditional Healers Accused of Abusing Mentally Ill." Interview with Dr. Shish Narayan. Radio Australia, February 6. Updated March 22, 2012.

National Health Promotion Council. 1998. *Fiji Health: Towards Healthy Fiji Islands, Final Report of the Mental Health Technical Working Party to the National Health Promotion Council.* Suva: National Health Promotion Council.

Nayacakalou, Rusiate Raibosa. 1963. "The Urban Fijians of Suva." In *Pacific Port Towns and Cities,* edited by Alexander Spoehr, 33–41. Honolulu: Bishop Museum.

———. 1975. *Leadership in Fiji.* Melbourne: Oxford University Press in Association with the University of the South Pacific.

Newman, Erica. 2018. "Colonial Intervention on Guardianship and 'Adoption' Practices in Fiji, 1874–1970." PhD thesis, University of Otago.

New Zealand Herald. 1907. "Suicide at Fiji." January 4.

———. 2008. "Flying above a Life with the Chickens." September 6.

Nicole, Robert. 2006. "Disturbing History: Aspects of Resistance in Early Colonial Fiji, 1874–1914." PhD thesis, University of Canterbury.

———. 2011. *Disturbing History: Resistance in Early Colonial Fiji.* Honolulu: University of Hawai'i Press.

Noricks, Jay. 1981. "The Meaning of Niutao fakavalevale (Crazy) Behaviour: A Polynesian Theory of Mental Disorder." *Pacific Studies* 5, no. 1: 19–33.

North Otago Times. 1883. "Benevolent Institution." June 5.

O'Connor, Maree. 2015. "Mobilizing Clouston in the Colonies? General Paralysis of the Insane at the Auckland Mental Hospital, 1868–99." *History of Psychiatry* 26, no. 1: 64–79.

Ohaeri, Jude U. 1997a. "Delirium and Dementia in the Older Person." *Fiji General Practitioner* 4, no. 4: 263–268.

———. 1997b. "The Drug Treatment of Schizophrenia." *Fiji General Practitioner* 4, no. 4: 277–279.

———. 1998. "Recent Classification and Drug Treatment of Depression." *Fiji General Practitioner* 5, no. 4: 397–402.

———. 1999a. "Directions for Mental Health Care Delivery in Fiji in the New Millennium." *Fiji General Practitioner* 6, no. 4: 529–531.

———. 1999b. "The General Practitioner as an Ally in Mental Health Care Delivery in Fiji." *Fiji General Practitioner* 6, no. 4: 532–533.

———, ed. 1999c. *Management of Mental Disorders and Promotion of Mental Health in Primary Care Settings in Fiji: Proceedings of National Workshops on Integrating Mental Health into the PHC in Fiji in 1999.* Suva: Quality Printers.

———. 1999d. "Psychotropic Drug Treatment of Psychotic and Other Severe Psychiatric Conditions in General Practice Settings." *Fiji General Practitioner* 6, no. 4: 536–538.

———. 1999e. "Technique of Appropriate Psychotherapy/Counselling in General Practice Settings: Brief Supportive Therapy." *Fiji General Practitioner* 6, no. 4: 534–535.

OneNews. 2013. "Schizophrenic Fiji Woman Locked in Shed for Years." YouTube video, 3:34. Accessed March 11, 2019. https://www.youtube.com/watch?v=YhrOMAkl6C4.

Pacific Review. 1970. "Are Mental Patients at Suva Subjected to Cruelty?" August 29.

Parke, Aubrey L. 1995. "The Qawa Incident in 1968 and Other Cases of 'Spirit Possession': Religious Syncretism in Fiji." *Journal of Pacific History* 30, no. 2: 210–226.

Parle, Julie. 2007. *States of Mind: Searching for Mental Health in Natal and Zululand, 1896–1918.* Scottsville, ZA: University of KwaZulu-Natal Press.

———. 2009. "'This Painful a Subject': Racial Politics and Suicide in Colonial Natal and Zululand." In *Histories of Suicide: International Perspectives on Self-destruction in the Modern World*, edited by John C. Weaver and David Wright, 156–177. Toronto: University of Toronto Press.

———. 2014. "Family Commitments, Economies of Emotions, and Negotiating Mental Illness in Late-Nineteenth to Mid-Twentieth-Century Natal, South Africa." *South African Historical Journal* 66, no. 1: 1–21.

Patel, Vikram. 2014. "Why Mental Health Matters to Global Health." *Transcultural Psychiatry* 51, no. 6: 777–789.

Patel, Vikram, Pamela Y. Collins, John Copeland, Ritsuko Kakuma, Sylvester Katontoka, Jagannath Lamichhane, Smita Naik, and Sarah Skeen. 2011. "The Movement for Global Mental Health." *British Journal of Psychiatry* 198, no. 2: 88–90.

Patel, Vikram, Crick Lund, Sean Hatherill, Sophie Plagerson, Joanne Corrigall, Michelle Funk, and Alan J. Flisher. 2010. "Mental Disorders: Equity and Social Determinants." In *Equity, Social Determinants and Public Health Programmes*, edited by Erik Blas and Anand Sivasankara Kurup, 115–134. Geneva: World Health Organization.

Peck, D. G. 1963. "Telecommunications in Fiji." *The Fiji Society: Transactions and Proceedings* 9, no. 2: 144–156.

Poltorak, Michael. 2007. "Nemesis, Speaking, and Tauhi Vaha'a: Interdisciplinarity and the Truth of 'Mental Illness' in Vava'u, Tonga." *The Contemporary Pacific* 19, no. 1: 1–35.

———. 2013. "From 'Evil Spirits' to 'Brain Disease': Shifting Agency, Humor and the Establishment of a Tongan Public Psychiatry." Paper presented at the conference of the American Anthropological Association's Society for Medical Anthropology, European Association of Social Anthropologists', Medical Anthropology Network, Universitat Rovira i Virgili, Tarragona, Spain, June 12–14.

Porter, Roy. 1987. *A Social History of Madness: Stories of the Insane*. London: Weidenfeld and Nicolson.

———. 1995. "Mood Disorders: Social Section." In *A History of Clinical Psychiatry: The Origin and History of Psychiatric Disorders*, edited by German Berrios and Roy Porter, 409–420. New York: New York University Press.

———. 2003. Introduction to *The Confinement of the Insane: International Perspectives, 1800–1965*, edited by Roy Porter and David Wright, 1–19. Cambridge: Cambridge University Press.

Porter, Roy, and David Wright, eds. 2003. *The Confinement of the Insane: International Perspectives, 1800–1965*. Cambridge: Cambridge University Press.

Price, John. 1979. "Review of Down's Syndrome in Fiji and Tonga: Some Medical Aspects." *Fiji Medical Journal* (February): 49–51.

Price, John, and Isaac Karim. 1975. "Suicide in Fiji: A Two-Year Survey." *Acta Psychiatrica Scandinavica* 52: 153–159.

———. 1976. "An Evaluation of Psychiatric After-Care in a Developing Country (Fiji)." *British Journal of Psychiatry* 129, no. 2: 155–157.

———. 1978. "Matiruku, a Fijian Madness: An Initial Assessment." *British Journal of Psychiatry* 133, no. 3: 228–230.

Price, Penny. 1996. "Developing Services in the South Pacific." In *Beyond Basic Care: Special Education and Community Rehabilitation in Low Income Countries,* edited by Roy I. Brown, David Baine, and Aldred H. Neufeldt, 63–99. North York: Captus Press.

Pridmore, Saxby. 1993. "Mental Health Service for Fiji." *Fiji Medical Journal* 19, no. 4: 9–12.

Quain, Buell. 1948. *Fijian Village.* Chicago: University of Chicago Press.

Quanchi, Max, and Alaima Talu. 1995. *Messy Entanglements: The Papers of the 10th Pacific History Association Conference, Tarawa, Kiribati.* Brisbane: Pacific History Association.

Randall, G. R. 1969. "Epidemic Hysteria." *Fiji School of Medicine Journal* 4, no. 12: 4–5.

Ravuvu, Asesala. 1983. *Vaka i Taukei: The Fijian Way of Life.* Suva: Institute of Pacific Studies, University of the South Pacific.

———. 1987. *The Fijian Ethos.* Suva: Institute of Pacific Studies, University of the South Pacific.

———. 1988. *Development or Dependence: The Pattern of Change in a Fijian Village.* Suva: Institute of Pacific Studies and Fiji Extension Centre, University of the South Pacific.

Ree, G. H. 1971. "Suicide in Macuata Province, Fiji." *The Practitioner* 207, no. 1241: 669–671.

Rensel, Jan, and Alan Howard. 1997. "The Place of Persons with Disabilities in Rotuman Society." *Pacific Studies* 20, no. 3: 19–50.

Roberts, Graham J. 2017. "The History of Mental Health in Papua New Guinea." In *Mental Health in Asia and the Pacific: Historical and Comparative Perspectives,* edited by Harry Minas and Milton Lewis, 223–235. New York: Springer.

Roberts, Graham J., Myrielle Cruz, and Elenoa S. Puamau. 2007. "A Proposed Future for the Care, Treatment and Rehabilitation of Mentally Ill People in Fiji." *Pacific Health Dialog* 14, no. 2: 107–110.

Roberts, Graham, Jacqueline Leckie, and Odille Chang. 2017. "The History of Mental Health in Fiji." In *Mental Health in Asia and the Pacific: Historical and Comparative Perspectives,* edited by Harry Minas and Milton Lewis, 237–251. New York: Springer.

Robertson, Robbie, and William Sutherland. 2001. *Government by the Gun: The Unfinished Business of Fiji's 2000 Coup.* Annandale, NSW: Pluto Press; London: Zed Books.

Robillard, Albert B. 1987. "Mental Health Services in Micronesia: A History." In *Contemporary Issues in Mental Health Research in the Pacific Islands,* edited by Albert B. Robillard and Anthony J. Marsella, 215–244. Honolulu: Social Science Research Institute, University of Hawai'i.

Roman, Gustavo C., and Lydia N. Roman. 1986. "Occurrence of Congenital, Cardiovascular, Visceral, Neurologic, and Neuro-Ophthalmologic Complications in Late Yaws: A Theme for Future Research." *Reviews of Infectious Diseases* 8, no. 5: 760–770.

Ross, S. G. 1950. "Pellagra in Fiji." *American Journal of Tropical Medical Hygiene* 30, no. 6: 921–928.

Roth, George Kingsley. 1935. "The Belief in Spells and a Suggested Treatment." *The Native Medical Practitioner* 2, no. 3: 262–264.

———. 1953. *Fijian Way of Life.* Melbourne: Oxford University Press.

Roth, Martin. 1955. "The Natural History of Mental Disorder in Old Age." *British Journal of Psychiatry* 101, no. 423: 281–301.

Rubinstein, Donald H. 1999. "Staking Ground: Medical Anthropology, Health, and Medical Services in Micronesia." In *American Anthropology in Micronesia: An Assessment,* edited by Robert C. Kiste and Mac Marshall, 327–359. Honolulu: University of Hawai'i Press.

Rubinstein, Donald H., and Geoffrey White. 1983. "Bibliography on Culture and Mental Health in the Pacific Islands." *Micronesia* 19, nos. 1–2: 183–245.

Russell, Denise. 1995. *Women, Madness and Medicine.* Cambridge: Polity Press.

Sadowsky, Jonathan. 1999. *Imperial Bedlam: Institutions of Madness in Colonial Southwest Nigeria.* Berkeley: University of California Press.

———. 2003. "The Social World and the Reality of Mental Illness: Lessons from Colonial Psychiatry." *Harvard Review of Psychiatry* 11, no. 4: 210–214.

Sahlins, Marshall. 1962. *Moala: Culture and Nature on a Fijian Island.* Ann Arbor: University of Michigan Press.

Sanadhya, Totaram. 1992. *My Twenty-One Years in the Fiji Islands and The Story of the Haunted Line.* Translated and edited by John Dunham Kelly and Uttra Kumari Singh. Suva: Fiji Museum.

———. 1998. "Hinduism under Indenture." In *Crossing the Kala Pani: A Documentary History of Indian Indenture in Fiji,* edited by Brij V. Lal, 103–120. Canberra: Division of Pacific and Asian History, Australian National University; Suva: Fiji Museum; Prashant Pacific Book.

Saunders, Kay. 1979. "'Troublesome Servants': The Strategies of Resistance Employed by Melanesian Indentured Labourers on Plantations in Colonial Queensland." *Journal of Pacific History* 14, no. 3: 168–183.

Sax, William. 2014. "Ritual Healing and Mental Health in India." *Transcultural Psychiatry* 51, no. 6: 829–849.

Scarr, Deryck. 1980. *Viceroy of the Pacific: The Majesty of Colour: A Life of Sir John Bates Thurston.* Canberra: Australian National University Development Studies Centre.

———. 1984. *Fiji: A Short History.* Laie, Hawai'i: Institute for Polynesian Studies, Brigham Young University; Sydney: George Allen & Unwin.

Scott, James C. 1985. *Weapons of the Weak: Everyday Forms of Peasant Resistance.* New Haven, CT: Yale University Press.

Scott, Owen. 2003. "Sex, Lies and Videotapes: The Long Road to Forgiveness." *Sunday Star Times,* August 24.

———. 2004. *Deep beyond the Reef: A True Story of Madness and Murder in the South Pacific.* Auckland: Penguin.

Scull, Andrew. 1989. *Social Order/Mental Disorder: Anglo-American Psychiatry in Historical Perspective.* Berkeley: University of California Press.

———. 1993. "Museums of Madness Revisited." *Social History of Medicine* 6, no. 1: 3–23.

———. 2006. *The Insanity of Place/The Place of Insanity: Essays on the History of Psychiatry.* London: Routledge.

———. 2015. *Madness in Civilization: A Cultural History of Insanity, from the Bible to Freud, from the Madhouse to Modern Medicine.* Princeton, NJ: Princeton University Press.

Scully, Matthew. 2002. "Man Accused of Double Murder Escapes." *Dominion,* January 12.

Sethi, Nichi, Elizabeth V. Robilotti, and Yariv Sadan. 2004. "Neurological Manifestations of Vitamin B-12 Deficiency." *Internet Journal of Nutrition and Wellness* 2, no. 1. http://ispub.com/IJNW/2/1/4476.

Shorter, Edward. 1997. *A History of Psychiatry: From the Era of the Asylum to the Age of Prozac.* New York: John Wiley & Sons.

Shorter, Edward, and David Healy. 2007. *Shock Therapy: A History of Electroconvulsive Treatment in Mental Illness.* New Brunswick, NJ: Rutgers University Press.

Showalter, Elaine. 1985. *The Female Malady: Women, Madness, and English Culture, 1830–1980.* New York: Pantheon Books.

Siegel, Jeff. 1985. "Origins of Pacific Islands Labourers in Fiji." *Journal of Pacific History* 20, no. 1: 42–54.

Singh, Sheetalpreet, Odille Chang, Michelle Funk, Laura Shields, Amelia Andrews, Frances Hughes, Kanna Sugiura, and Natalie Drew. 2013. *WHO Profile on Mental Health in Development (WHOproMIND): Fiji.* Geneva: World Health Organization. Accessed March 11, 2019. http://apps.who.int/iris/bitstream/10665/85325/1/9789241505659_eng.pdf.

Singh, Yadhu N. 1986. "Traditional Medicine in Fiji: Some Herbal Folk Cures Used by Fiji Indians." *Journal of Ethnopharmacology* 15, no. 1: 57–88.

Smith, Abel. 1996. "Community Psychiatric Nursing: The Fiji Experience." Presentation to Community Health Workshop, St Giles Hospital. April 15–19.

Smith, Leonard D. 2014. *Insanity, Race and Colonialism: Managing Mental Disorder in the Post-Emancipation British Caribbean, 1838–1914.* Houndmills, UK: Palgrave Macmillan.

Snow, Philip. 1997. *The Years of Hope: Cambridge, Colonial Administrator in the South Seas, and Cricket.* London: Radcliffe Press.

Spate, Oskar Hermann Khristian. 1959. "The Fijian People: Economic Problems and Prospects: A Report." Fiji Legislative Council Paper no. 13. Suva: Government Press.

Spencer, Dorothy. 1941. *Disease, Religion and Society in the Fiji Islands.* New York: J. J. Augustin.

Spiegel, John P. 1983. "Community Therapy in a Fiji Village." *Journal of Operational Psychiatry* 14, no. 1: 28–35.

Steele, Frances. 2011. *Oceania under Steam, Sea Transport and the Cultures of Colonialism, c. 1870–1914.* Manchester: Manchester University Press.

Stephenson, Elsie. 1997. *Fiji's Past on Picture Postcards.* Suva: Caines Jannif.

Stoler, Ann Laura. 1991. "Carnal Knowledge and Imperial Power: Gender, Race, and Morality in Colonial Asia." In *Gender at the Crossroads of Knowledge: Feminist Anthropology in the Postmodern Era,* edited by Micaela di Leonardi, 51–101. Berkeley: University of California Press.

———. 1995. *Race and the Education of Desire: Foucault's History of Sexuality and the Colonial Order of Things*. Durham, NC: Duke University Press.

———. 1997. "Making Empire Respectable: The Politics of Race and Sexual Morality in Twentieth-Century Colonial Cultures." In *Situated Lives: Gender and Culture in Everyday Life*, edited by Louise Lamphere, Helena Ragone, and Patricia Zavella, 374–399. New York: Routledge.

Stuart, Annie. 2006a. "Contradictions and Complexities in an Indigenous Medical Service." *Journal of Pacific History* 41, no. 2: 125–143.

———. 2006b. "We Are All Hybrid Here: The Rockefeller Foundation, Sylvester Lambert, and Health Work in the Colonial South Pacific." *Health and History* 8, no. 1: 56–79.

Summerfield, Derek. 2012. "Afterword: Against Global Mental Health." *Transcultural Psychiatry* 49, no. 3: 519–530.

———. 2013. "'Global Mental Health' is an Oxymoron and Medical Imperialism." *British Medical Journal* 346 (May): 346.

Suva Times. 1881. November 5, 2.

———. 1882. March 11, 2.

Suzuki, Akihito. 1999. "Framing Psychiatric Subjectivity: Doctor, Patient and Record-Keeping at Bethlem in the Nineteenth Century." In *Insanity, Institutions and Society, 1800–1914: A Social History of Madness in Comparative Perspective*, edited by Joseph Melling and Bill Forsythe, 115–136. London: Routledge.

———. 2006. *Madness at Home: The Psychiatrist, the Patient and the Family in England, 1820–1860*. Berkeley: University of California Press.

———. 2010. "Global Theory, Local Practice: Shock Therapies in Japanese Psychiatry, 1920–1945." In *Transnational Psychiatries: Social and Cultural Histories of Psychiatry in Comparative Perspective, c. 1800–2000*, edited by Waltraud Ernst and Thomas Mueller, 116–141. Newcastle-upon-Tyne, UK: Cambridge Scholars Publishing.

Swartz, Sally. 1995a. "The Black Insane in the Cape, 1891–1920." *Journal of Southern African Studies* 21, no. 3: 399–415.

———. 1995b. "Changing Diagnoses in Valkenberg Asylum, Cape Colony, 1891–1920: A Longitudinal View." *History of Psychiatry* 5: 431–451.

———. 1995c. "Colonizing the Insane: Causes of Insanity in the Cape, 1891–1920." *History of the Human Sciences* 8, no. 4: 39–57.

———. 1999. "Lost Lives: Gender, History and Mental Illness in the Cape, 1891–1910." *Feminism & Psychology* 9, no. 2: 152–158.

———. 2010. "The Regulation of British Colonial Lunatic Asylums and the Origins of Colonial Psychiatry, 1860–1864." *History of Psychology* 13, no. 2: 160–177.

———. 2015. *Homeless Wanderers: Movement and Mental Illness in the Cape Colony in the Late 19th Century*. Cape Town, ZA: UCT Press.

Sykes, Ingrid. 2016. "Disability, Leprosy, and Kanak Identity in Twentieth-Century New Caledonia." *Journal of Literary and Cultural Disability Studies* 10, no. 2: 173–189.

Szasz, Thomas. 1961. *The Myth of Mental Illness: Foundations of a Theory of Personal Conduct*. New York: Harper and Row.

Temkin, Owsei. 1971. *The Falling Sickness: A History of Epilepsy from the Greeks to the Beginnings of Modern Neurology*, 2nd ed. Baltimore, MD: Johns Hopkins University Press.

Tent, Jan. 2001. "A Profile of the Fiji English Lexis." *English World-Wide* 22, no. 2: 209–245.

Thomas, Nicholas. 1990. "Sanitation and Seeing: The Creation of State Power in Early Colonial Fiji." *Comparative Studies in Society and History* 32, no. 1: 149–170.

———. 1997. *In Oceania: Visions, Artifacts, Histories.* Durham, NC: Duke University Press.

Thompson, Laura. 1940. *Fijian Frontier.* San Francisco: American Council, Institute of Pacific Relations.

Thompson, Margaret. 1988. "The Wages of Sin: The Problem of Alcoholism and General Paralysis in Nineteenth-Century Edinburgh." In *The Anatomy of Madness: Essays in the History of Psychiatry*, vol. III: *The Asylum and Its Psychiatry,* edited by William F. Bynum, Roy Porter, and Michael Shepherd, 316–340. London: Routledge.

Thomson, Basil. 1908. *The Fijians: A Study of the Decay of Custom.* London: Heinemann.

Tomes, Nancy. 1990. "Historical Perspectives on Women and Mental Illness." In *Women, Health, and Medicine in America,* edited by Rima D. Apple, 143–171. New York: Garland.

———. 1994. "Feminist Histories of Psychiatry." In *Discovering the History of Psychiatry,* edited by Mark S. Micale and Roy Porter, 348–383. New York: Oxford University Press.

Tomlinson, Matt. 2013. "The Generation of the Now: Denominational Politics in Fijian Christianity." In *Christian Politics in Oceania,* edited by Matt Tomlinson and Debra McDougall, 78–102. New York: Berghahn Books.

Toren, Christina. 1990. *Making Sense of Hierarchy.* London: Athlone Press.

———. 1999. *Mind, Materiality and History: Explorations in Fijian Ethnography.* London: Routledge.

Tucker, George A. 1887. *Lunacy in Many Lands.* Sydney: Charles Potter, Government Printer.

Tuimaleali'ifano, Morgan A. 1990. *Samoans in Fiji: Migration, Identity and Communication.* Suva: Institute of Pacific Studies, Fiji, Tonga, and Western Samoa Extension Centres of the University of the South Pacific.

TV One (New Zealand). 2001a. "Double Lives." *60 Minutes*, November 18.

———. 2001b. "Saints or Sinners." *60 Minutes.* TV One (New Zealand), July.

———. 2005. *Expose: Saving a Wild Boy.* Reference no. TZP307510. New Zealand Archive of Film, Television and Sound (Ngā Taonga).

Ussher, Jane M. 2011. *The Madness of Women: Myth and Experience.* New York: Routledge.

Vakarewakobau, Brenda. 2004. "Relatives Bury 'Chained' Daughter." *Fiji Times,* January 13.

Vakaruru, Henry B. 1937. "An Undiagnosed Condition Which Does Not Yield to Medical Treatment but Yields to Fijian Medicine." *The Native Medical Practitioner* 2, no. 2: 360–363.

Vakatawa, Banuve. 1940. "What the Fijians Believe as the Cause of Disease." *The Native Medical Practitioner* 3, no. 2: 522–524.

Vallis, Mary, and Scott Stinson. 2004. "'Chicken Man' Learning to Love: Raised in Coop, Fijian 'Making up for Lost Time.'" *National Post* (Vancouver), July 15.

Vaughan, Megan. 1983. "Idioms of Madness: Zomba Lunatic Asylum, Nyasaland, in the Colonial Period." *Journal of Southern African Studies* 9, no. 2: 218–238.

———. 1991. *Curing Their Ills: Colonial Power and African Illness*. Cambridge: Polity Press.

Walmsley, Tom. 1991. "Psychiatry in Scotland." In *150 Years of British Psychiatry 1841–1991*, edited by German E. Berrios and Hugh Freeman, 294–305. London: Gaskell.

Weaver, John C. 2009. *A Sadly Troubled History: The Meanings of Suicide in the Modern Age*. Montréal: McGill-Queen's University Press.

Wells, Allen, and Gilbert M. Joseph. 1993. "Structure of Domination and Forms of Resistance on Yucatecan Estates during the late Pofiriato, ca. 1880–1915." In *Plantation Workers: Resistance and Accommodation*, edited by Brij Lal, Doug Munro, and Edward Beechert, 241–296. Honolulu: University of Hawai'i Press.

Westmore, Ann. 2003. "Reading Psychiatry's Archive: Academic Medicine and Psychiatric Medicine in Mid-Twentieth-Century Victoria." In *"Madness" in Australia: Histories, Heritage and the Asylum*, edited by Catharine Coleborne and Dolly MacKinnon, 207–216. St. Lucia: University of Queensland Press and API Network.

Whitley, Rob. 2015. "Global Mental Health: Concepts, Conflicts and Controversies." *Epidemiology and Psychiatric Sciences* 24, no. 4: 285–291.

Whyte, Peter. 1954. "Are Miracles Won by Nursing?" *Argus*, February 6.

Widmer, Alexandra. 2010. "Native Medical Practitioners, Temporality, and Nascent Biomedical Citizenship in the New Hebrides." *Political and Legal Anthropology Review* 33, supp. 1: 57–80.

Williams, Thomas. 1982. *Fiji and the Fijians, Vol. 1: The Islands and Their Inhabitants*. Edited by George Stringer Rowe with a new introduction by Fergus Clunie. Originally published 1858. Suva: Fiji Museum.

Wilson, D. M. 1921. "Report by Dr. D. M. Wilson, District Medical Officer, Ba." In Fiji Government, *Medical Department: Annual Report for 1920*, CP 43/21, 10. Suva: Government Printer.

Wilson, Glenn D. 1965. "'Europeanisation' and Admission to Mental Hospital in the Fiji Islands." *New Zealand Medical Journal* 64, no. 395: 364–367.

Wright, David. 1997. "Getting out of the Asylum: Understanding the Confinement of the Insane in the Nineteenth Century." *Social History of Medicine* 10, no. 1: 137–155.

———. 1998. "The Certification of Insanity in Nineteenth-Century England and Wales." *History of Psychiatry* 9, no. 35: 267–290.

———. 2004. "Delusions of Gender?: Lay Identification and Clinical Diagnosis of Insanity in Victorian England." In *Sex and Seclusion, Class and Custody: Perspectives on Gender and Class in the History of British and Irish Psychiatry*, edited by Jonathan Andrews and Anne Digby, 149–176. Amsterdam: Editions Rodopi.

Yap, Pow-Meng. 1974. *Comparative Psychiatry: A Theoretical Framework*. Toronto: Toronto University Press.

Yee-Chief, Theresa. 2000. "A Survey of Knowledge, Attitudes, Beliefs and Practices of Menopause in Fiji Women." MS thesis, Monash University.

Yeo, Stephen W., and Russell James Blong. 2010. "Fiji's Worst Natural Disaster: The 1931 Hurricane and Flood." *Disasters* 34, no. 3: 657–683.

Index

Page numbers in boldface type refer to figures, maps, and tables.

About the Author

Jacqueline Leckie's research and publications are on the history and anthropology of Asia Pacific, especially mental health, migration, gender, heritage, ethnicity, development and labor. Her books include *A University of the Pacific* (2018), *Indian Settlers: The Story of a New Zealand South Asian Community* (2007), *To Labour with the State* (1997), editing *Development in an Insecure and Gendered World* (2009), and co-editing *Migrant Cross-Cultural Encounters in Asia and the Pacific* (2016), *Asians and the New Multiculturalism in Aotearoa New Zealand* (2016), *Localizing Asia in Aotearoa* (2011), *Recentring Asia (2011),* and *Labour in the South Pacific* (1990). She has taught at the University of the South Pacific, Kenyatta University, and Otago University. In 2018, she was the JD Stout Research Fellow at the Stout Centre for New Zealand Studies, Victoria University of Wellington, where she is currently an adjunct research fellow. She is also a conjoint associate professor with the University of Newcastle in Australia.